S0-AYI-092

Nursing Theory

UTILIZATION & APPLICATION

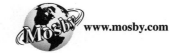
www.mosby.com

Nursing Theory

UTILIZATION & APPLICATION

Second Edition

Martha Raile Alligood, RN, PhD
Professor and Chair, MSN Program
College of Nursing, University of Tennessee,
Knoxville, Tennessee

Ann Marriner Tomey, RN, PhD, FAAN
Professor
Indiana State University School of Nursing
Leadership and Management Consultant
Terre Haute, Indiana

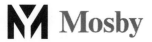 Mosby

A Harcourt Health Sciences Company

St. Louis   London   Philadelphia   Sydney   Toronto

NO LONGER THE PROPERTY

OF THE

UNIVERSITY OF R. I. LIBRARY

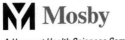

A Harcourt Health Sciences Company

Vice-President, Publishing Director: *Sally Schrefer*
Editor: *Yvonne Alexopoulos*
Developmental Editor: *Melissa K. Boyle*
Project Manager: *Deborah L. Vogel*
Designer: *Kathi Gosche*

SECOND EDITION
Copyright © 2002 by Mosby, Inc.

Previous edition copyrighted 1997

All rights reserved. No part of this publication may be reproduced or transmitted in any form or by any means, electronic or mechanical, including photocopy, recording, or any information storage and retrieval system, without permission in writing from the publisher.

Permission to photocopy or reproduce solely for internal or personal use is permitted for libraries or other users registered with the Copyright Clearance Center, provided the base fee of $4.00 per chapter plus $.10 per page is paid directly to the Copyright Clearance Center, 222 Rosewood Drive, Danvers, Massachusetts 01923. This consent does not extend to other kinds of copying, such as copying for general distribution, for advertising or promotional purposes, for creating new collected works, or for resale.

Mosby, Inc.
A Harcourt Health Sciences Company
11830 Westline Industrial Drive
St. Louis, Missouri 63146

Printed in the United States of America

Library of Congress Cataloging-in-Publication Data

Nursing theory : utilization and application / [edited by] Martha Raile Alligood, Ann Marriner-Tomey.—2nd ed.
    p. ; cm.
    Includes bibliographical references and index.
    ISBN 0-323-01194-2
    1. Nursing models.   2. Nursing—Philosophy.   I. Alligood, Martha Raile. II. Marriner-Tomey, Ann
    [DNLM: 1. Nursing Theory. 2. Models, Nursing. WY 86 N9758 2001]
RT84.5 .N94 2001
610.73—dc21
                                                                            2001031581

01 02 03 04 05 GW/FF 9 8 7 6 5 4 3 2 1

*C*ontributors

Martha Raile Alligood, RN, PhD
Professor and Chair, MSN Program
College of Nursing
University of Tennessee
Knoxville, Tennessee

Violeta A. Berbiglia, EdD, RN
Associate Professor/Clinical
School of Nursing
The University of Texas Health Science Center at San Antonio
San Antonio, Texas

Kimberly S. Bolton, RNC, MSN, WHCNP
Assistant Professor
Department of Nursing
Carson-Newman College
Jefferson City, Tennessee

Karen A. Brykczynski, RN, CS, FNP, DNSc
Associate Professor
University of Texas Medical Branch School of Nursing at Galveston
Galveston, Texas

Kaye Bultemeier, PhD, RNCS
Nurse Practitioner
Women's Health Associates
Oak Ridge, Tennessee

Margaret E. Erickson, RN, PhD
Holistic Healing Consultants
Austin, Texas

Jacqueline Fawcett, PhD, FAAN
Professor
College of Nursing
University of Massachusetts–Boston
Boston, Massachusetts

Maureen A. Frey, PhD, RN
Nurse Researcher
Children's Hospital of Michigan
Detroit, Michigan

Pamela J. Grace, PhD, RN, CS
Assistant Professor
Boston College School of Nursing
Chestnut Hill, Massachusetts

Bonnie Holaday, DNS, RN, FAAN
Dean, Graduate School and Associate Vice Provost for Research
Professor of Nursing
Clemson University
Clemson, South Carolina

Mary-Jean McGraw, RN, MSc[N], PhD[c]
Associate Professor
Laurentian University School of Nursing
Sudbury, Ontario, Canada, and
Consultant
Imaginings
Brooklin, Ontario, Canada

Mary M. (Molly) Meighan, RNC, PhD
Assistant Professor
Division of Nursing
Carson-Newman College
Jefferson City, Tennessee

Gail J, Mitchell, RN, PhD
Chief Nursing Officer
Sunnybrook & Women's College
Health Sciences Centre, and
Assistant Professor
Faculty of Nursing
University of Toronto
Toronto, Ontario, Canada

Marjorie G. Morgan, PhD, RN
Certified Nurse Midwife and Certified Transcultural Nurse
Department of Health and Environmental Control of South Carolina
Waccamaw District
Myrtle Beach, South Carolina

Diane M. Norris, PhD, RN
Assistant Professor
School of Nursing
Oakland University
Rochester, Michigan

Kenneth D. Phillips, PhD, RN
Assistant Professor
Department of Administrative and Clinical Nursing
College of Nursing
University of South Carolina
Columbia, South Carolina

Karen Moore Schaefer, RN, DNSc
Assistant Professor
Department of Nursing
Temple University College of Allied Health
Philadelphia, Pennsylvania

Norma Jean Schmieding, EdD, RN
Professor
College of Nursing
University of Rhode Island
Kingston, Rhode Island

Raphella Sohier, PhD, RN
Retired, Professor of Nursing
Bilzen, Belgium

Janet M. Witucki, PhD, RN
Nursing Faculty
College of Nursing
University of Tennessee–Knoxville
Knoxville, Tennessee

Angela F. Wood, PhD, RNC
Assistant Professor
Division of Nursing
Carson-Newman College
Jefferson City, Tennessee

Reviewers

Karolyn Kells, PhD, RN
Coordinator of Baccalaureate Outreach
Coordinator of Nursing Education Track
Department of Nursing
Fort Hays State University
Hays, Kansas

Rozzano C. Locsin, RN C, PhD
Associate Professor
College of Nursing
Florida Atlantic University
Boca Raton, Florida

Donna Scheideberg, CNM, PhD
Associate Professor, Nursing
Coordinator, Nurse-Midwifery
School of Nursing
University of Missouri—Columbia
Columbia, Missouri

Louise Selanders, RN, EdD
Associate Professor
College of Nursing
Michigan State University
East Lansing, Michigan

Mary Cipriano Silva, PhD, FAAN
Professor
George Mason University
Fairfax, Virginia

To our grandchildren:
Hunter Kent, Charlie Nicholas, and John Kent Alligood, Jr.

and

Kylie Anne and Taylor Marriner Bonomo
Allison and Laura Tomey

*P*reface

The first edition of this book was written to provide students and nurses with a text that demonstrated how theory guides nursing practice. This new, expanded second edition of *Nursing Theory: Utilization and Application* continues that purpose, building on the premises that the nature of knowledge needed for the practice of nursing is theoretical and that practice is central to nursing. On that basis, this current phase of utilization and application of theory is not only essential for our contributions to the health of society but also to the ongoing knowledge building process of a practice discipline such as nursing.

Like the first edition, this new edition of the text is designed for teaching nurses and students of nursing how philosophies, models, and theories of nursing guide the critical thinking process of professional nursing practice. The text is designed for courses in which nursing theory and theory-based practice are first introduced to students. In addition, the text will be especially useful to those committed to teaching theory-based nursing practice in baccalaureate nursing programs, in-service education programs for nursing staff development, and graduate-level nursing courses on the theoretical foundations of nursing and advanced practice nursing.

Nursing Theory: Utilization and Application builds on the premise of the need for nursing as a discipline to recognize the importance of theory utilization for nursing practice. Students using the text need a basic understanding of nursing philosophies, models, and theories; therefore, the reader is referred to *Nursing Theorists and Their Work,* fifth edition, by

Marriner Tomey and Alligood (2002)*, which introduces the reader to the nursing philosophies, models, and theories included in this text. For example, one might recommend that students review a chapter in *Nursing Theorists and Their Work* for the critical analysis of a philosophy, model, or theory as background for the corresponding chapter on its use in practice in *Nursing Theory: Utilization and Application*.

The content of the book is presented in three parts. Part One contextualizes the theme of the text, which is the use of theory to guide nursing practice. Chapter 1 sketches the historical background of a century of professional development toward the present phase of the theory era. The quest for nursing knowledge is viewed as a driving force that has shaped the nursing profession. Chapter 2 reviews areas in which theory-based nursing practice has been reported in the nursing literature. Three tables that illustrate the wide use of theory-based practice in various areas in which nursing is practiced are presented. Chapter 2 has been expanded in this new edition with a review of the nursing models using Kuhn's criteria (1970)[†] for "normal science."

Chapter 3 presents philosophies, models and theories as critical thinking structures from a "structure of knowledge" perspective; reviews the philosophies, models, and theories that point out the utility of middle-range theory for application in professional nursing practice; and provides guidelines for the student's use in the process of selecting a nursing model or theory for practice. Chapter 4, an exciting and unique new chapter added to this part, addresses the ethical obligations inherent in nursing's theoretical works and the moral imperatives of theory-based nursing practice.

Part Two, the heart of the text, has been greatly expanded in this new second edition, with nine new chapters, for a total of 16 (Chapters 5-20). These chapters demonstrate the utilization and application of philosophies, models, and theories as critical thinking structures with clinical cases in nursing practice. The chapters are written by clinical experts who apply the various philosophies, models, and theories in the nursing care of Debbie and in another case selected from their own practices. Each of these chapters features a table that aligns the content focus of the model with the process of critical thinking when using the model in practice. Critical thinking exercises are presented in each chapter to assist students with utilization and application of philosophies, models and theories to their own nursing practice.

---

*Marriner Tomey, A. & Alligood, M. R. (2002). *Nursing theorists and their work* (5th ed.). St. Louis: Mosby.
[†]Kuhn, T. S. (1970). *The structure of scientific revolutions* (2nd ed.). Chicago: University of Chicago Press.

Part Three of the text features Chapters 21 and 22, which call for the expansion of theory-based nursing practice. Chapter 21 mirrors Chapter 2 and identifies areas for expansion of the use of the models and their theories in areas of nursing practice in which theory-based practice has not been reported. In addition, middle-range theories for those areas of nursing practice based on the specifics of the nursing situations—such as nursing actions, client population, and area of practice—are proposed. Chapter 22 highlights the essential nature of theory-based nursing practice to the nursing profession and discipline. It also provides step-by-step guidelines for transforming one's practice by changing perspectives.

Organizational features of the text include the presentation of a contextual basis in Part One to introduce the premises of the text, including the ethical considerations of theory use. All of the applications in Part Two are organized with similar chapter length and content, including historical background; overview of the model; critical thinking in nursing practice with the model (presented in a table in each chapter); case history, followed by nursing care of Debbie; case history and nursing care of a second case; and critical thinking exercises. Part Three presents projections for future expansion of the areas of practice for theory-based nursing, and essential challenges for future theory-based nursing practice expansion argued on the basis of long-held philosophical values in nursing and the arduous task of changing one's perspective (growth). The process and strategies to accomplish such a change are presented.

SPECIAL FEATURES
- Ethical obligations and moral imperative inherent in theory-based nursing practice
- Cases that illustrate application of philosophies, models, and theories in nursing practice
- Use of the same case (Debbie) in the application chapters
- Critical thinking with each philosophy, model, or theory is illustrated with a table
- Critical thinking exercises at the end of each application chapter
- A glossary of terms from each chapter for student development

We believe this new, expanded second edition is a useful text for undergraduate programs because of the importance of theory use for professional nursing practice. Because theory is presented as a guide for reasoning and decision making, the critical thinking process of professional practice is clear for the student. Philosophies, nursing models, and theories are applied to clinical cases to illustrate their utilization and application in the practice of nursing. Nursing faculty who want to emphasize nursing approaches to nursing practice in their teaching will find this text clear and direct.

For core theory courses in master's programs, the text is useful in combination with a text such as *Nursing Theorists and Their Work*. Nursing faculty who want to move their students beyond a survey of the analyses of nursing theoretical works to the application of these works in nursing practice will find that this new second edition of the text provides a basis for theory-based practice, including nursing ethics, case examples that illustrate utilization and application of theory, and challenges and ideas for the future expansion of theory-based nursing practice.

ACKNOWLEDGMENTS

We would like to take this opportunity to thank the staff at Mosby for their work and support and the chapter authors for their expert clinical and theoretical knowledge, with a special thank you to Dr. Kenneth D. Phillips for developing the case history of Debbie for this text.

Martha Raile Alligood
Ann Marriner Tomey

Contents

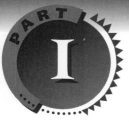

PART I

Conceptualization

The following conceptualizations provide the context for the premises of this text:

- Nursing's long search for a substantive body of knowledge has led to the development and discovery of nursing science to guide professional practice in the twenty-first century.
- There is evidence of "normal science" in the use of nursing's conceptual models.
- Theory utilization is documented in many areas of nursing practice.
- Nursing theoretical works in the form of philosophies, models, and theories specify approaches to practice for nursing outcomes.
- Critical thinking and decision making for professional nursing is directed by theoretical knowledge found in nursing philosophies, conceptual models, and nursing theories.
- Discussions of theory-based nursing practice include the ethical obligations of nursing practice and the moral imperatives of nursing's theoretical works.

CHAPTER 1

The Nature of Knowledge Needed for Nursing Practice

Martha Raile Alligood

"The systematic accumulation of knowledge is essential to progress in any profession . . . however, theory and practice must be constantly interactive. Theory without practice is empty and practice without theory is blind." (From Cross, P. [1981]. Adults as learners. *Washington, DC: Jossey-Bass. Copyright © 1981, Jossey-Bass. Reprinted by permission of Jossey-Bass Inc., a subsidiary of John Wiley & Sons, Inc.)*

This chapter highlights nursing's efforts toward the development of a body of knowledge to guide nursing practice in the last century. The significance of the achievements of professional nursing as we begin the twenty-first century are perhaps best understood from the perspective of the challenges within the nursing eras of the twentieth century. Therefore this chapter highlights nursing efforts toward the development of a body of substantive knowledge to guide nursing practice and to establish nursing as a profession. Within each era, there is an emphasis that contributed to the progress toward nursing becoming a profession with a substantive body of nursing knowledge on which to base nursing practice. We have come to understand that theory instructs the nurse in focus and content of that practice as well as guides nursing action. We also recognize that theory informs practice and that practice informs theory. Therefore we are coming to view the theory-research-practice relationship in new and different ways. Given our history and the challenges of today, utilization and application of nursing's theoretical works in the form of philosophies, nursing models, and theories of nursing are presented in this text as a means of helping you organize the process of critical thinking for professional nursing practice.

At the beginning of the twentieth century, nursing began its move from vocation toward profession (Alligood, 1994a; Alligood, 1994b; Johnson, 1974; Kalisch & Kalisch, 1995; Meleis, 1997; Rogers, 1961). Guided by the words of Nightingale and by the goal of professionalism, American nurses began to enter academia, first in individual courses and finally in collegiate nursing programs. The background of this movement toward professionalism is important in understanding the different emphases of the search for a body of knowledge over the decades.

These different emphases have been viewed as eras in nursing's march toward professionalism (Meleis, 1997). Despite the differences in each era, there is one criterion for the consideration of nursing as a profession that has been a constant force. This criterion specifies that nursing practice must be guided by a body of specialized knowledge (Bixler & Bixler, 1959). Today, our discussions are far beyond whether nursing is a profession, yet the criterion that calls for utilization of a specialized body of knowledge to guide nursing practice continues to be relevant to nursing as it embraces the challenges of an ever-changing society. The criterion that calls for nursing practice to be guided by specialized nursing knowledge clearly has been the most pertinent to the development of nursing as a profession.

A review of the efforts made to meet the criterion will help you understand the struggles of these eras and demonstrate how they lead us back to practice as nursing's central concern. Nursing's quest to answer the question of the nature of knowledge needed for the practice of nursing can be viewed as a driving force that has shaped our profession by guiding nurses and students of nursing in various directions that were often unclear and incompletely understood at the time.

ERAS OF NURSING KNOWLEDGE

Around the turn of the twentieth century, the idea that nurses needed knowledge to guide and improve nursing practice began to be noted. Signs of a new national consciousness for nursing can be traced back to the first national gathering of nurses at the World's Fair in Chicago in 1893 and to the publication of the first edition of the *American Journal of Nursing (AJN)*, the first national organ of communication for nurses, in October, 1900 (Kalisch & Kalisch, 1995). From these initial national efforts of nurses, the goal to move nursing to the professional level began to emerge.

At this early time, the focus was on practice and on teaching students to *do* nursing. These beginnings suggest, however, a move in the direction of recognizing the need for specialized knowledge to guide the practice of nursing. The journal *AJN* can be seen as an early symbol of nursing's movement toward becoming a profession and also as evidence that nurses needed to interact with each other about nursing practice as well as about training nurses and teaching nursing to others. With the boom of the industrial age, hospital training schools flourished in America, and the curriculum era of the 1920s and 1930s soon followed (Kalisch & Kalisch, 1995).

Curriculum Era

In the Curriculum Era, efforts to answer the question of the nature of the knowledge needed for nursing practice are evident from the emphasis on content and from movement toward the goal of standardization of curricula. The focus of this era is evident in state activities such as the 1933 curriculum survey of New York training schools (Kalisch & Kalisch, 1995). It was this emphasis on what nurses needed to know to practice nursing that led to the expansion of curricula beyond medical knowledge to include social sciences and nursing procedures. The fact that these classes were often called "fundamentals," which means "basic essentials," reflects an early valuing of nursing content specific to nursing action in this era. Nursing's initial embrace of science is also evident in the curricula of this early era.

It is interesting to note that nursing procedures were taught and practiced in a ward-like room called a "nursing arts" laboratory. In later decades, when nursing curricula emphasized science and research, these rooms were referred to as "skills labs." Reference to the art of nursing became unpopular and scarce in the nursing literature for a period of nursing's history. We are indebted to those scholars who maintained an emphasis on the art of nursing in this period as the emphasis on science gained popularity (Kalisch & Kalisch, 1995). The change in terminology noted earlier may also be related to the beginning of baccalaureate nursing programs in this era because with the move of nursing into schools of higher learning, there was an increased emphasis on science (Kalisch & Kalisch, 1995).

Once nursing began to be taught in colleges and universities, all of nursing was affected because nurses had to consider what that move meant with regard to them and the persistent question of the nature of the knowledge needed for nursing and the body of knowledge needed to guide nursing practice. The move of nursing into higher education was a major shift for the nursing profession; the effects of this transition are still being felt today as nurses continue to debate multiple levels of entry into nursing practice.

Nursing leaders at that time were beginning to advocate for nursing to be taught in a different educational environment and at a different level of education. The move of nursing into schools of higher learning brought with it a significant change in the search for a substantive body of knowledge and led to the research era.

Research Era

In the 1940s and 1950s, research became the driving force. Nurses were on the move to conduct research and to begin developing that specialized body of knowledge. The task was so great, however, that rather than being a means to an end, it often became an end in itself. Learning to carry out research led to an emphasis on statistics and research methods, which were new curriculum areas that needed to be mastered. Many believed that research alone was what was needed to generate the body of knowledge or science to form a basis for nursing practice.

This era emphasized scholarship and the need to disseminate research findings in scholarly publications. *Nursing Research,* the first nursing research journal, was established for this purpose in 1952. In addition, two programs funded by the federal government were instituted in 1955 to prepare nurses as researchers and teachers of research—the United States Public Health Service predoctoral research fellowships and the Nurse Scientist Training Program (Schlotfeldt, 1992).

These research beginnings influenced nursing, and as more and more nurse educators were introduced to research, a new emphasis on graduate education that included nursing research was emerging by the 1960s and 1970s. The research and graduate education eras seem to overlap, as other reviewers have noted (Meleis, 1997; Styles, 1982). The strong emphasis on nursing scholarship during both eras undoubtedly contributes to the close interrelationship of the two eras as well as the relationship of theory and research.

Graduate Education Era

During the graduate education era of the 1960s and 1970s, curricula for master's level preparation were proposed by regional groups and then standardized at national meetings of the National League for Nursing (NLN). By the end of the 1970s, most accredited nursing master's programs included courses in nursing research, clinical specialty practice, advanced physiology, and leadership. Many also included a course in nursing theory or nursing models in a core curriculum organized with a nursing philosophy and conceptual or organizing framework.

Although there were only three nursing doctoral programs at the beginning of this era, the continuing post–World War II shortage of nurses, which had generated the federally funded programs in the 1950s, meant that nurses with doctorates from a wide range of related disciplines were being prepared for research and teaching roles in nursing. Therefore although the American Nurses Association (ANA) had identified the need for nursing theory development in 1965, there was, at best, only a general consensus among nursing leaders as to what that consensus meant because of the variety of discipline perspectives held by nurses with doctorates.

During this era, a series of national conferences brought nurses together to exchange ideas and evaluate what had been learned in their doctoral programs in other fields that could address nursing's needs. The papers and discussions from these conferences were published in *Nursing Research* in 1968 and 1969, and they were republished in Nicoll's first edition (1986) under the unit heading "Three Landmark Symposia" (p. 91). The conferences, which centered on nursing science and theory development, were designed to facilitate the discussion of the application of knowledge from the various disciplines to nursing. The Nurse Scientist program is noteworthy in this history because it directly addressed the question of the nature of the body of nursing knowledge—that is, will nursing be other discipline–based or nursing-based? Dealing with this question was a turning point for nursing with regard to graduate education and understanding the nature of the body of knowledge needed for nursing practice.

Doctoral education began to flourish, and, by the end of the 1970s, there were 21 nursing doctoral programs and several more universities indicating the intent to develop programs. The driving force was undoubtedly the need to develop a specialized body of knowledge and the conclusion that it should be developed by nurses prepared in the discipline of nursing. Therefore it is not surprising that in this era we saw a distinction between nursing knowledge and borrowed knowledge in the nursing literature (Johnson, 1968). This awareness grew out of the understanding that theory from other disciplines was not specific to nursing and its nursing knowledge needs (Johnson, 1968; Rogers, 1970).

During this era, theorists began publishing their nursing frameworks. The works by Johnson (1980), King (1971), Levine (1967), Neuman (1972), Orem (1971), Rogers (1970), and Roy (1970) were evidence of the new emphasis on nursing theory.

Research continued to develop during this era of graduate education; however, many nurse scholars noted that the knowledge generated lacked form and direction. In fact, *Nursing Research* celebrated its twenty-fifth anniversary in 1977 (volume 26, number 3) with published reviews of the research progress. These reviews presented recommendations for development in five practice areas of nursing: medical-surgical, community, maternal-child, psychiatric, and gerontology. In general, the lack of conceptual or theoretical direction or connection in the research was identified as a weakness of the studies. It was also noted that the research focused on nurses or student nurses more often than on patients. The reviews were organized according to areas of medical practice, which reflected the lack of nursing theoretical structures.

From a comprehensive review of those first 25 years of published nursing research, Batey (1977) identified conceptualization as the greatest limitation of the projects. She emphasized the importance of the conceptual phase of research to provide a content basis as well as a connection with other studies to develop nursing science. It should be noted that reference to concepts and conceptualization was more common in that era and can now be considered a precursor to the theory era, which understands theory as a set of related concepts.

An indication of the shift of emphasis from research to theory at the national level began to be noted with the Nurse Educator conferences in Chicago (1977) and New York (1978). Although the first conference did not have a theory theme, Sister Callista Roy's workshop on how to use her conceptual framework as a guide for nursing practice was so popular that the second conference was planned with a nursing theory theme and brought nursing theorists together on the same stage for the first time. That second conference underscored a growing awareness that the nature of the knowledge needed for nursing practice was theoretical knowledge.

Other factors in the shift toward theory at this time were the publication of Carper's patterns of knowing for nursing (1978) and Fawcett's article on the relationship between theory and research (1978) in the first edition of a new nursing journal, *Advances in Nursing Science*. Carper (1978) described four types of nursing knowledge and clarified their contexts. Her work is significant in this history for distinguishing empirical from ethical, personal, and aesthetic knowledge. In the same issue, Fawcett (1978) clarified the relationship of theory and research in the development of science in her classic double-helix metaphor presentation. These events ushered in the theory era of the 1980s and 1990s.

Theory Era

The theory era began with a strong emphasis on development. Although in the previous two decades proponents of nursing theory and the nursing theorists had begun to publish their frameworks, it is noteworthy that they denied being theorists when they were introduced at the Nurse Educator Theory Conference in 1978. There was a strong sense among those attending the conference that they were theorists, and by the second day, the audience responded to their denials with laughter.

In only one decade—from 1980 to 1990—nursing theory development stimulated phenomenal growth, which has been noted to be the cornerstone of the development of the discipline of nursing (Meleis,

1983). The theory era, coupled with the research era, led to an understanding of the scientific process for the production of a scientific product (Whall, 1996). This era stimulated the growth of nursing scholarship in a way never before experienced in nursing history (Schlotfeldt, 1992). Proliferation of nursing literature and new nursing journals, national and international nursing conferences, and the opening of new nursing doctoral programs are evidence of the growth of this era.

Also during this decade, Fawcett (1984, 1989) significantly contributed to our understanding of the nature of nursing knowledge. She developed a metaparadigm explanation of the interconnectedness of the various nursing theoretical works and proposed a structure of nursing knowledge that began to clarify different levels of abstraction in nursing theoretical works according to Kuhn's philosophy of science (1970). Her work is particularly significant to this history because the structure she proposed led to an understanding of middle-range or practice theory for the theory utilization phase of the theory era. Although Fawcett's work focuses on analysis and evaluation of nursing models and theories, her structure demonstrates the decreasing level of abstraction in the direction of nursing practice. Most importantly, the structure shows how nursing theory is connected to or is derived from the models of nursing. This interconnection of nursing knowledge is vital to the development of nursing science.

It is important to note that the emphasis on the critique and analysis of theory was only one phase of the theory era that focused on the process of theory development. Although the process of theory development is essential for our progress, analysis and critique of the process or syntax and structure of theory will not tell about the use of the model or theory in practice. Therefore this text shifts the emphasis from theory development to theory utilization so that the value of theory for nursing practice can be known from its use in practice. Knowledge pertinent to further theory development and continued progress of nursing as a professional discipline will also be gained in this phase of the era (Whall, 1996).

This text recognizes the significance of the changing emphasis from theory development to theory utilization. From the perspective of theory utilization, the earlier eras take on a different light—that is, we come to understand that curriculum and education were very important but that they were not an end. Likewise, research, as important as it was to nursing's growth, was not an end, nor would research alone produce science but required an interrelationship with theory to do so (Fawcett, 1978). Neither is theory an end, although it might have seemed so during the past decade, considering the strong emphasis it received. Rather, theory and research together lead to science, which informs practice.

Education, research, and theory are all understood in this new alignment as tools of nursing practice. Only by clarifying the relationship of these important processes to nursing practice can nurses properly use them to advance the discipline. Theory utilization reestablishes practice as the central focus for the discipline of nursing. This text emphasizes nursing practice with a focus on knowledge utilization and clarifies theory and research as tools of practice (Alligood, 1994b; Allison, McLaughlin, & Walker, 1991; Field, 1987).

This position is in concert with the national agenda to move education from lower-order learning with a recall focus to higher-order learning with a reasoning focus. The Council of Baccalaureate and Higher Degree Programs (CBHDP) of the National League for Nursing (NLN) joined ranks with this initiative in the development of their criteria (1992) for accrediting member programs, as did the American Association of Colleges of Nursing (AACN) in the College Criteria for Nursing Education (CCNE) (1998). The National Council for Excellence in Critical Thinking Instruction defines critical thinking as "the intellectually disciplined process of actively and skillfully conceptualizing, applying, analyzing, synthesizing or evaluating information gathered from, or generated by, observation, experience, reflection, reasoning, or communication, as a guide to belief and action" (Paul & Nosich, 1991, p. 4). This text presents utilization of philosophies, nursing models, and theories of nursing as guides for the reasoning and decision-making process and information-processing skills for substantive critical thinking. These theoretical works become critical thinking structures that specify the focus and guide the clinical decision-making process of professional nursing practice.

To summarize these eras of nursing's search for a specialized body of nursing knowledge, progress has been evident most of this century. In the early era of the 1920s and 1930s, the emphasis was on curriculum and nursing education, and nursing experienced a phenomenal expansion of nursing programs with an emphasis on nursing principles and procedures and training for basic nursing. In the era of the 1940s and 1950s, nursing began the move into higher education; graduate programs were developed; and nursing research began to be conducted as nursing developed as a scientific discipline. In the 1960s and 1970s, the experiment of preparing nurse scientists in other disciplines ended, and the direction for the development of the discipline was clarified and led to an immediate expansion of nursing doctoral programs. The era of the 1980s and 1990s began with a theory development emphasis, which is shifting to theory utilization.

This brief history suggests how the emphasis of each era of nursing history led to a limited vision or partial view of the discipline's future. The point must be made that each of these eras was necessary for the growth and development of nursing, and continued progress toward theory-based practice is essential for the growth of nursing as a profession.

THE CENTRALITY OF NURSING PRACTICE

The premise that practice is central to nursing is vital. This text is an answer to the question "What is the nature of the knowledge needed for the practice of nursing?" This question has been a driving force for the nursing profession since its began. Nursing history suggests that it was in dealing with this question that the eras of growth have occurred. Although nursing practice has continued throughout these eras, efforts have often been divided. The focus on nursing practice will facilitate nursing unity for continued professional development and will pave the way for the recognition of professional nurses as key players in the healthcare delivery systems of the twenty-first century. It is a period in history for which we have waited a long time. More nurses are reimbursed primary providers of care in the United States today than ever before in history. This places the question of the nature of nursing practice at the forefront. If nurses define their practice in a manner similar to medicine, the very characteristics of practice that were valued and that contributed to this recognition as primary providers will no longer be present. It is a wonderful time of opportunity, but there are risks for the profession as a whole that cannot be overlooked (Fawcett, 1999).

For nurses to make their contribution, it is essential that they practice nursing in an organized manner. Nurses need to move beyond practice conventions based on physiological and psychosocial concerns to interventions using nursing works that are holistic and specific to nursing's concern (Sparacino, 1991). This move requires an approach to care that is consciously defined (Wardle & Mandle, 1989). The analytical process and complex reasoning for nursing judgments do not come automatically, as Wardle and Mandle (1989) found in their study of the frameworks nurses use in nursing practice. Rather, utilization of nursing's theoretical works requires knowledge and skill in practice. Finally—and most importantly—nursing must be practiced in a relationship with the patient rather than with the limited cross-sectional approach of the medical model (Alligood, 1994b).

Utilizing nursing's theoretical works in nursing practice provides frameworks for a nursing approach and guides the critical thinking process of reasoning and decision making for nurses to practice in an organized manner. The nursing literature continues to echo the urgent need for theory-based nursing practice (Algase & Whall, 1993; Fawcett, 1999; Tritsch, 1998; Whall, 1996). Mathwig (1975) said, even before the theory era began, that the first phase of translating theory into practice is the decision to do so. Similarly, use of a model in practice has been described as a habit to be formed (Broncatello, 1980), the practice of a true believer (Oliver, 1991), and the practice of one who has been properly persuaded (Levine, 1995).

The progression of nurses into theory utilization for theory-based practice is best explained by nursing's history. Change comes slowly and is greatly influenced by the preceding eras, but it does come. The application of theory in practice has been described as the acid test for theory, because the mark of its usefulness is its ability to guide practice (Martin, Forchuk, Santopinto, & Butcher, 1992). That understanding has led scholars to declare that it is essential that these models be tested and that testing be done in practice in a variety of settings (Huckabay, 1991; Whall, 1996). The theory utilization phase of the theory era is ushering in the next era of nursing history, which is an era of theory testing through the application of middle-range theory in nursing practice.

Evidence of theory utilization in the nursing literature is encouraging. Clarification of the levels of theory has increased references to middle-range theory (Fawcett, 1995). In 1997, the journal *Advances in Nursing Science* devoted an issue to middle-range theory. A recent review of middle-range theories in ten years of nursing literature (1988-1998) emphasized the theory-practice connection (Liehr & Smith, 1999). Liehr and Smith (1999) observed that the number of articles increased over the 10 years, with more appearing in the last five years than in the former five. It is also interesting to note that the 22 articles included in their study were from 10 different nursing journals—another sign of progress toward theory-based nursing practice.

In conclusion, nursing faces many challenges in this new century. Daiski (2000) discussed nursing's journey to professionalism in the era of managed care and concluded that "practice based in nursing theories will give nurses the necessary foundation to restructure healthcare where it counts: improving quality of care at the practice level" (p. 79). Similarly, Tritsch (1998) has observed that the transition into a capitated environment has heightened the need for theory-based practice to new levels. Rogers' premise (1970) of long ago is perhaps the most telling: "Nursing's potential for meaningful human service rests on the union of theory and practice for its fulfillment" (p. viii). This text is dedicated to the realization of that premise.

References

Algase, D. L. & Whall, A. F. (1993). Rosemary Ellis' views on the substantive structure of nursing. *Image, 25*(1), 69-72.

Alligood, M. R. (1994a). Evolution of nursing theory development. In A. Marriner-Tomey (Ed.), *Nursing theorists and their work* (3rd ed., pp. 58-69). St. Louis: Mosby.

Alligood, M. R. (1994b). Toward a unitary view of nursing practice. In M. Madrid & E. A. M.

Barrett (Eds.), *Rogers' scientific art of nursing practice* (pp. 223-237). New York: National League for Nursing.

Allison, S., McLaughlin, K., & Walker, D. (1991). Nursing theory: A tool to put nursing back into nursing administration. *Nursing Administration Quarterly, 15*(3), 72-78.

Batey, M. V. (1977). Conceptualization: Knowledge and logic guiding empirical research. *Nursing Research, 26*(5), 324-329.

Bixler, G. K. & Bixler, R. W. (1959). The professional status of nursing. *American Journal of Nursing, 59*(8), 1142-1147.

Broncatello, K. F. (1980). Auger in action: Application of the model. *Advances in Nursing Science, 3*(1), 13-23.

Carper, B. (1978). Fundamental patterns of knowing. *Advances in Nursing Science, 1*(1), 13-23.

College criteria for nursing education. (1998). Washington, DC: American Association of Colleges of Nursing.

Council of baccalaureate and higher degree accreditation criteria. (1992). New York: National League for Nursing.

Cross, P. (1981). *Adults as learners.* Washington, DC: Jossey-Bass.

Daiski, I. (2000). The road to professionalism in nursing: Case management or practice based in nursing theory? *Nursing Science Quarterly, 13*(1), 74-79.

Fawcett, J. (1978). The relationship between theory and research: A double helix. *Advances in Nursing Science, 1*(1), 49-62.

Fawcett, J. (1984). *Analysis and evaluation of conceptual models of nursing.* Philadelphia: F. A. Davis.

Fawcett, J. (1989). *Analysis and evaluation of conceptual models of nursing* (2nd ed.). Philadelphia: F. A. Davis.

Fawcett, J. (1995). *Analysis and evaluation of conceptual models of nursing* (3rd ed.). Philadelphia: F. A. Davis.

Fawcett, J. (1999). The state of nursing science: Hallmarks of the 20th and 21st centuries. *Nursing Science Quarterly, 12*(4), 311-315.

Field, P. A. (1987). The impact of nursing theory on the clinical decision-making process. *Journal of Advanced Nursing, 12,* 563-571.

Huckabay, L. M. (1991). The role of conceptual frameworks in nursing practice, administration, education, and research. *Nursing Administration Quarterly, 15*(3), 17-28.

Johnson, D. E. (1968). Theory in nursing: Borrowed and unique. *Nursing Research, 17*(3), 206-209.

Johnson, D. E. (1974). Development of theory: A requisite for nursing as a primary health profession. *Nursing Research, 23*(5), 372-377.

Johnson, D. E. (1980). The behavioral system model for nursing. In J. P. Riehl & C. Roy (Eds.), *Conceptual models for nursing practice* (2nd ed., pp. 207-216). Norwalk, CT: Appleton-Century-Crofts.

Kalisch, P. A. & Kalisch, B. J. (1995). *The advance of American nursing* (3rd ed.). Philadelphia: J. B. Lippincott.

King, I. (1971). *Toward a theory for nursing: General concepts of human behavior.* New York: John Wiley & Sons.

Kuhn, T. S. (1970). *The structure of scientific revolutions* (2nd ed.). Chicago: University of Chicago Press.

Levine, M. E. (1967). The four conservation principles of nursing. *Nursing Forum, 6,* 45-59.

Levine, M. E. (1995). The rhetoric of nursing theory. *Image, 27*(1), 11-14.

Liehr, P. & Smith, M. J. (1999). Middle range theory: Spinning research and practice to create knowledge for the new millennium. *Advances in Nursing Science, 21*(4), 81-91.

Martin, M., Forchuk, C., Santopinto, M., & Butcher, H. K. (1992). Alternative approaches to nursing practice: Application of Peplau, Rogers, and Parse. *Nursing Science Quarterly, 5*(2), 80-85.

Mathwig, G. (1975). Translation of nursing science theory to nursing education. In S. Ketefian (Ed.), *Translation of theory into nursing practice and education. Proceedings of the seventh annual clinical sessions,* Continuing Education in Nursing Division of Nursing, School of Education, Health, Nursing, and Arts Professions, New York University.

Meleis, A. (1983). The evolving nursing scholars. In P. Chinn (Ed.), *Advances in nursing theory development* (pp. 19-34). Rockville, MD: Aspen.

Meleis, A. I. (1997). *Theoretical nursing: Development and progress* (3rd ed.). Philadelphia: J. B. Lippincott.

National League for Nursing. (1992). *Criteria for evaluation of baccalaureate and higher degree programs in nursing* (7th ed.). New York: Author.

Neuman, B. (1972). A model for teaching total person approach to patient problems. *Nursing Research, 21*(3), 264-269.

Nicoll, L. H. (1986). *Perspectives on nursing theory.* Boston: Little, Brown.

Nurse Educator Conference, First Annual. (1977). *From student to effective professional.* Hyatt Regency, Chicago.

Nurse Educator Conference, Second Annual. (1978). *Nursing theory: Foundation for the future.* New York Hilton, New York City.

Oliver, N. R. (1991). True believers: A case for model-based nursing practice. *Nursing Administration Quarterly, 15*(3), 37-43.

Orem, D. E. (1971). *Nursing: Concepts of practice.* New York: McGraw-Hill.

Paul, R. W. & Nosich, G. M. (1991). *Proposal for the national assessment of higher-order thinking* (edited and revised version). Washington, DC: The United States Department of Education, Office of Educational Research and Improvement, National Center for Education Statistics.

Rogers, M. E. (1961). *Educational revolution in nursing.* New York: Macmillan.

Rogers, M. E. (1970). *An introduction to the theoretical basis of nursing.* Philadelphia: F. A. Davis.

Roy, C. (1970). Adaptation: A conceptual framework for nursing. *Nursing Outlook, 18*(3), 43-45.

Schlotfeldt, R. M. (1992). Why promote clinical nursing scholarship? *Clinical Nursing Research, 1*(1), 5-8.

Sparacino, P. (1991). The reciprocal relationship between practice and theory. *Clinical Nurse Specialist, 5*(3), 138.

Styles, M. M. (1982). *On nursing toward a new endowment.* St. Louis: Mosby.

Tritsch, J. M. (1998). Application of King's theory of goal attainment and the Carondelet St. Mary's case management model. *Nursing Science Quarterly, 11*(2), 69-73.

Wardle, M. G. & Mandle, C. L. (1989). Conceptual models used in clinical practice. *Western Journal of Nursing Research, 11*(1), 108-114.

Whall, A. L. (1996). Current debates and issues critical to the discipline of nursing. In J. J. Fitzpatrick & A. L. Whall (Eds.), *Conceptual models of nursing* (pp. 1-12). Norwalk, CT: Appleton & Lange.

Nursing Models: Normal Science for Nursing Practice

Angela F. Wood and Martha Raile Alligood

Nursing practice: "the acid test of nursing theory" (From M. Martin, C. Forchuk, M. Santopinto, & H. Butcher, Nursing Science Quarterly *5[2], p. 80-85, copyright © 1992 by Sage Publications, Inc. Reprinted by permission of Sage Publications, Inc.)*

"In the sciences, the formation of specialized journals, the foundation of specialist societies, and claim for a special place in the curriculum have usually been associated with a groups first reception of a single paradigm." (From Kuhn, T. S. [1970]. The structure of scientific revolutions *[2nd ed.]. Chicago: University of Chicago Press. © 1962, 1970 by The University of Chicago.)*

NURSING MODELS AND THEIR THEORIES IN NURSING PRACTICE

The use of nursing models and their theories in nursing practice is presented in this chapter, which documents various areas of application and utilization of the models as reported in the nursing literature. In line with the premise set forth in Chapter 1, the shift in emphasis from theory development to theory utilization restores a proper relationship between theory and practice for a professional discipline such as nursing. The importance of this shift is supported by Levine (1995), who noted in reference to Fawcett's clarification of models from theories, "It may be that the first prerequisite for effective use of theory in practice . . . rest[s] on just such a clarification" (p. 12). Nursing models and their theories have practical utility for nursing with details specific to practice in various areas.

Based on a review of the nursing literature, this chapter begins with examples of the areas in which nursing models and their theories guide nursing practice. Although all three tables present the use of the nursing models and their theories in nursing practice, these applications are described by their authors in various ways—(1) in terms of the medical conditions; (2) in terms of nursing based on human development, areas of practice, type of care, and type of health; and (3) in terms of nursing interventions or the nursing role. (See bibliography for references to applications of each model cited in Tables 2-1, 2-2, and 2-3.) Hilton (1997), who reviewed the theoretical perspectives of nursing in the literature, reports similar diversity. The chapter concludes with a review of the nursing models using the criteria for normal science set forth by Thomas Kuhn (1970) in *The Structure of Scientific Revolutions* and a discussion of whether the discipline of nursing has reached a period of normal science using the nursing models.

It became apparent from the literature review that nurses describe their practice in several ways. Some describe nursing practice in terms of the medical conditions. This view focuses on the patient or area of care, as noted in Table 2-1. Examples of this focus are the nursing of cardiovascular patients or of intensive care patients.

Several observations have been made about this focus (see Table 2-1). First, it represents the largest body of literature. Secondly, each of the models is represented within this focus. Although this large grouping is surprising in light of the efforts of the past 30 years to move nursing beyond the medical view to a nursing perspective, this focus reflects the practice area of the largest single group (68%) of practicing nurses, which, according to the American Nurses Association's Facts about Nursing (1988), continues to be acute or illness care in hospitals.

Table 2-2 presents model and theory use in publications in which nurses describe their practice in terms of a developmental or life-span focus, a particular group in society, a type of care, or a type of health. Examples of this focus are nursing of children, homeless, holistic care, and child health. Table 2-2 reflects the second largest group of articles. Like Table 2-1, Table 2-2 is represented by articles based on all seven of the nursing models. Although Table 2-2 is large, it represents a grouping of several perspectives nurses use to describe their practice: nursing groups according to a developmental category, areas of practice, types of care, and types of health or health promotion.

Table 2-3 presents model and theory use in publications with a focus on a nursing intervention or the nursing role. Examples of this focus are life review and counseling. This table is smaller than Tables 2-1 and 2-2 and also differs in that not all of the nursing models are represented in Table 2-3. Certain nurses practicing from the perspective of nursing

TABLE 2-1 Areas of Practice with Nursing Models Described in Terms of a Medical Conditions Focus							
Practice Areas	**Johnson**	**King**	**Levine**	**Neuman**	**Orem**	**Rogers**	**Roy**
Acute care						•	
Adolescent cancer							•
Adult diabetes		•			•		
AIDS management	•			•		•	•
Alzheimer's disease							•
Ambulatory care					•	•	
Anxiety		•			•		
Breast cancer							•
Burns			•				
Cancer			•		•	•	
Cancer pain management	•						
Cancer-related fatigue					•		
Cardiac disease		•			•		•
Cardiomyopathy							•
Chronic pain			•			•	
Cognitive impairment				•			
Congestive heart failure			•				
Critical care			•	•	•	•	•
Guillain-Barré syndrome					•		
Heart					•	•	
Hemodialysis	•				•		
Hypernatremia							•
Intensive care				•	•	•	•
Kawasaki disease							•
Leukemia							•
Long-term care			•		•		
Medical illness		•		•		•	
Menopause		•				•	
Neurofibromatosis		•					

Continued

TABLE 2-1 Areas of Practice with Nursing Models Described in Terms of a Medical Conditions Focus—cont'd

Practice Areas	Johnson	King	Levine	Neuman	Orem	Rogers	Roy
Oncology	•				•	•	
Orthopedics		•		•			
Osteoporosis							•
Ostomy care					•		
Pediatric						•	
Perioperative			•		•		•
Polio survivors						•	
Postanesthesia							•
Postpartum							•
Posttrauma							•
Preoperative adults			•				
Preoperative anxiety		•			•		
Pressure ulcers			•				
Renal disease		•		•	•		
Rheumatoid arthritis					•		
Schizophrenia							•
Substance abuse		•			•	•	
Terminal illness						•	•
Ventilator patient							•
Ventricular tachycardia	•						
Wound healing			•				

models seem to describe their practice in terms of a nursing intervention or nursing role. It is noted that the specificity of the language in Rogerian science has created several unique categories in this focus. This is not surprising, considering the following: (1) the development of a science calls for specific language; (2) a purpose of nursing science is to develop knowledge specific to the discipline perspective, so one would expect new intervention categories to be created rather than continuing to fit into other previously used categories; and (3) one would expect the categories to be descriptive of the uniqueness of the nurse's perspective.

The nursing categories in Tables 2-1, 2-2, and 2-3 can be considered in the context of Kuhn's discussion of normal science (1970). Paradigms (or nursing models) are not only frameworks to guide thinking about nursing but are also structures that guide research and practice. As such, their use by members of the profession produces knowledge that is a

TABLE 2-2 Areas of Practice with Nursing Models Based on Human Development, Type of Practice, Type of Care, or Type of Health Focus

Practice Areas	Johnson	King	Levine	Neuman	Orem	Rogers	Roy
Battered women					•		
Case management		•					
Cesarean father							•
Child health		•					
Child psychiatric				•			
Dying process						•	
Emergency		•	•	•			•
Gerontology		•		•	•	•	•
High-risk infants		•					
Holistic care			•				
Homeless			•				
Hospice			•		•		
Managed care		•		•			
Mental health	•			•	•	•	•
Neonates							•
Nursing administration		•		•	•	•	
Nursing adolescents	•	•			•		
Nursing adults		•	•	•	•	•	
Nursing children	•		•		•	•	•
Nursing community	•	•		•	•	•	•
Nursing elderly		•	•	•	•	•	•
Nursing families		•		•		•	
Nursing home residents						•	
Nursing infants			•		•		•
Nursing in space						•	
Nursing service						•	
Nursing women					•	•	
Occupational health					•		
Palliative care							•
Pregnancy					•		
Psychiatric nursing						•	
Public health				•			
Quality assurance	•						
Rehabilitation			•	•	•	•	•
Risk reduction				•			
Transcultural		•					

TABLE 2-3 Areas of Practice with Nursing Models with a Nursing Intervention or Role Focus

Practice Areas	Johnson	King	Levine	Neuman	Orem	Rogers	Roy
Breastfeeding				•			•
Community presence						•	
Counseling						•	
Family therapy		•		•			
Group therapy		•				•	•
Health patterning						•	
Humor						•	
Imagery						•	
Intentionality						•	
Knowing participation						•	
Laughter						•	
Leadership/scholarship				•			
Life-patterning difficulties						•	
Life review						•	
Movement						•	
Nutrition				•			
Parenting		•		•			
Storytelling						•	
Therapeutic touch						•	

guide to practice as well as further research and theory development. Normal science gives evidence of the growing maturity of a discipline as it moves beyond an emphasis on knowledge development to knowledge use. Model-based nursing practice literature reflects growth toward normal science.

In his book *The Structure of Scientific Revolutions,* Thomas Kuhn (1970) examines the nature of scientific discovery. He defines normal science as "research firmly based upon one or more past scientific achievements that some particular scientific community acknowledges for a time as supplying the foundation for its further practice" (Kuhn, 1970, p. 10). From this definition, Kuhn describes criteria that might be used for evaluation of a given paradigm (nursing model). These criteria include that the model would do the following: (1) be accepted by a community of scientists, (2) provide a basis for practice, and (3) be open-ended—that is, provide a guide for research that would broaden the scientific knowledge base of the discipline. Thus Kuhn's philosophy of science

(1970) is useful to examine the science of the discipline of nursing. Three possible interpretations will be presented.

EXAMINATION OF THE MODELS

Kuhn describes a paradigm that results in normal science as "an achievement sufficiently unprecedented to attract an enduring group of adherents away from competing modes of scientific activity" (Kuhn, 1970, p. 10) and as "leaving all sorts of problems for the redefined group of practitioners to resolve" (Kuhn, 1970, p. 10). In the attempt to develop nursing science, theory from numerous modes of scientific activity including medicine, social and physical science, education and even industrial management has been utilized (Wald & Leonard, 1964). However, it was not until the development of formal conceptual nursing models that nurses had "a systematic approach to nursing research, education, administration, and practice" (Fawcett, 1995) that ultimately resulted in normal science for the discipline of nursing. Each of the models will be reviewed with regard to Kuhn's definition and criteria of normal science.

Johnson

First presented in its entirety in the 1980 edition of *Conceptual Models for Nursing Practice* (Riehl & Roy, 1980), the Behavioral System Model, developed by Dorothy Johnson, has been a work in progress since 1959 (Fawcett, 1995). Begun as a basis for development of nursing core content, Johnson's work focuses on common human needs, care and comfort, and stress and tension reduction (Johnson, 1992). With its origins in Nightingale's work as well as in general system theory (Fawcett, 1995), Johnson's model has attracted a large following of nurse scientists who have linked her model with work from other disciplines to generate new theory (Fawcett, 1995). Use of the Behavioral System Model by educators, researchers, and practitioners all across the country (Fawcett, 1995; Meleis, 1997) indicates a significant number of nurses who are adherents to Johnson's Behavioral System Model. Although there is currently no organized group of nurses who support the use of the Johnson Behavioral System Model, Holaday reports that many nurses who use the model "stay in touch" (personal communication, January, 2000).

King

King (1964) first published work that would evolve into the General Systems Framework in 1964. Like many other theorists, King combined her own observations about nursing with knowledge from other disciplines and the theory from General System Theory to form a new conceptual framework for the discipline of nursing (King, 1990). With its focus on personal, interpersonal, and social systems, King's conceptual framework and the Theory of Goal Attainment that springs from it are widely used in nursing today (Frey & Sieloff, 1995). King's emphasis on the role of the client as well as the nurse in planning and implementation of healthcare is consistent with evolving philosophies of healthcare (Meleis, 1997). Adherents to this framework include nurse researchers and educators as well as staff nurses and administrators (Fawcett, 1995; Frey & Sieloff, 1995). The King International Nursing Group (KING) provides an organization for support and communication among nurses using King's General Systems Framework and Theory of Goal Attainment.

Levine

As is seen in Table 2-1, many nurse educators, researchers, and practitioners continue to rely on the medical model as their organizing framework. Levine perceived this as a problem for the development of nursing science and, in 1966, introduced a new paradigm to move nursing away from the medical model and provide nurses with a way to describe nursing care using the scientific method (Levine, 1966). Called the Conservation Model, Levine's work attempted to provide an organizing framework that could be used in a variety of nursing settings to facilitate nursing education (Levine, 1988). Focusing on adaptation as a way to maintain the integrity and wholeness of the person, Levine's work has attracted a large number of followers among nurse researchers, educators, administrators, and practitioners (Fawcett, 1995). Although use of Levine's work is evidenced in the nursing literature, currently there is no organization for Levine scholars (Schaefer, personal communication, January, 2000).

Neuman

Like many of the nursing models, the Neuman Systems Model had its beginnings in an educational setting, where it was developed and implemented to facilitate graduate education (McQuiston & Webb, 1995). Developed around the same time as several other nursing models, Neuman first published a description of her model in 1972 (Neuman & Young, 1972). Influenced by a variety of nurse scholars as well as knowledge from other disciplines, Neuman's model incorporates, among others, the concepts of adaptation and client wholism, with a strong emphasis on stress in the client environment.

The Neuman Systems Model continued its evolution and development for over 20 years. Nurse educators, researchers, administrators, and practitioners from around the world have made the Neuman Systems

Model one of the most recognized and used of the nursing paradigms. The Neuman archives are located at the library of Neuman College in Aston, Pennsylvania. Nurses who have attained a graduate degree may join the Neuman Systems Model Trustees Group, Inc.

Orem

A clinical nursing background in the medical-surgical nursing of adults and children, combined with readings in a variety of disciplines and her own personal reflection, contributed to Orem's development of the three-part theory of self-care (McQuiston & Webb, 1995). An early advocate of nursing conceptual models, Orem's work first began to take shape in the 1950s. From the beginning, Orem attempted to define the domain of nursing while providing a framework for nursing curricula development (Fawcett, 1995). Although a variety of nurse scholars and Orem herself have continued to refine her work, the basic conceptual elements have remained unchanged since 1970 (Orem, 1995).

Highly regarded for its usefulness in all aspects of nursing, Orem's Self-Care Model continues to be the organizing framework of many nurse researchers, educators, administrators, and providers of patient care (Fawcett, 1995). Nurses interested in the use of the Orem model have formed The International Orem Society for Nursing Science and Scholarship. This active organization sponsors publications and conferences on the Orem model, has formulated a list of schools of nursing that use the Orem model as an organizing framework, and is currently developing a list of institutions that use the model for care.

Rogers

Of all the nursing models discussed in this chapter, the work of Martha Rogers perhaps best fits Kuhn's description of a new paradigm as that which "forces scientists to investigate some part of nature in a detail and depth that would otherwise be unimaginable" (1970, p. 24). With its focus on unitary human beings as the central phenomenon of nursing (Fawcett, 1995), the Science of Unitary Human Beings (Rogers, 1970, 1992) introduced a set of concepts to nursing science to which other nursing models had not even hinted. Rejecting the idea of causality, Rogers' work moved beyond the reciprocal interaction worldview used by the other nursing models discussed in this chapter. Instead, Rogers' work with its pandimensional view of people and their world (Rogers, 1992) is consistent with the simultaneous action worldview (Fawcett, 1995).

Widely used by nurse researchers, educators, administrators, and clinical practitioners, The Science of Unitary Human Beings has established a worldwide following of nurses who have chosen a truly unique paradigm for their practice. The Society for Rogerian Scholars actively encourages the use of the Science of Unitary Human Beings through a program of publications and conferences that provide an avenue for work done in the model to be presented and discussed.

Roy

Beginning work on her model while she was a graduate student in the late 1960s, Sister Callista Roy drew the scientific basis for her adaptation model from both systems theory and adaptation-level theory (Roy & Andrews, 1999). Principles from these nonnursing disciplines were reconceptualized for implementation in nursing science (Meleis, 1997). In addition, threads from the work of other nurse scientists, particularly Johnson and Henderson (Meleis, 1997), contributed to what would become a new view of nursing. In a pattern seen in the development of many of the other scientific disciplines (Kuhn, 1970), Roy was able to weave the contributions from nonnursing disciplines as well as early nurse scientists into the fabric of her own original thoughts. This resulted in a new paradigm for nursing science, the Roy Adaptation Model.

Formally published in 1970 (Roy, 1970), the Roy Adaptation Model was implemented as the basis of the curriculum at Mount St. Mary's College, where the faculty has continued to work with Roy to develop and publish the elements of the model. The operationalizing of the theory in the curriculum at Mount St. Mary's College and the availability of literature and textbooks consistent with the model have resulted in its widespread adoption (Meleis, 1997).

DISCUSSION

The concept of normal science introduced by Kuhn describes the acceptance of a new paradigm for use by a discipline. According to Kuhn, normal science "means research firmly based upon one or more past scientific achievements, achievements that some particular scientific community acknowledges for a time as supplying the foundation for its further practice" (Kuhn, 1970, p. 10). The discipline of nursing moved toward normal science with widespread acceptance of the paradigm consisting of four concepts: person, health, environment, and nursing. However, these four concepts by themselves were not adequate for achievement of normal science. In a practice discipline such as nursing, the body of knowledge that is contained in the science of the discipline must be at a level of abstraction that is suitable for implementation.

The works of Johnson, King, Levine, Neuman, Orem, Rogers, and Roy, serving as frameworks for practice, education, and research, have provided this level of abstraction and, in doing so, have resulted in a body of normal science for the discipline of nursing. Kuhn points out that "paradigms gain their status because they are more successful than their competitors in solving a few problems that the group as practitioners has come to recognize as acute" (Kuhn, 1970, p. 23). Affirmation of the seven models and the theories that have developed as a result of them is evidenced repeatedly in the current nursing literature, as research studies are conducted, reported, and results implemented in client care.

Kuhn's definition of normal science thus could explain that the discipline of nursing has one body of normal science with seven branches—that is, the seven models. Although they are different in language, implementation, and research questions posed, each of the models is based on the four concept metaparadigm and so has many commonalities. Although the models certainly have their differences, they all have contributed to what we collectively call the body of nursing knowledge and, as such, can be considered nursing normal science.

A second possibility for interpretation of Kuhn's definition of normal science with regard to the discipline of nursing is to say that nursing has seven different bodies of normal science. Each of the seven nursing models has attracted a significant group of followers who utilize the models for practice, education, research, and development of nursing knowledge according to the specific views of nursing. This is evidenced by implementation of the models in healthcare institutions, schools of nursing, and textbooks. It is also evidenced by the fact that five of the seven models have professional organizations that have as their purpose to support and further the work in the models. In Kuhn's words, those "whose research is based on shared paradigms are committed to the same rules and standards for scientific practice. That commitment and the apparent consensus it produces are prerequisites for normal science" (Kuhn, 1970, p. 11). Thus according to the criteria described by Kuhn for normal science, it is possible to accept the view that at the present time, nursing does in fact have seven bodies of normal science.

The last viewpoint regarding the state of normal science within the discipline of nursing is that nursing has two bodies of normal science: one consisting of the knowledge produced from the work of Rogers (the Science of Unitary Human Beings) and the other consisting of knowledge developed from the works of Johnson, King, Levine, Neuman, Orem, and Roy. Evidence for this viewpoint springs from the underlying worldview of the models, Rogers' being based in the simultaneous action worldview, whereas the remaining six models are based in the reciprocal interaction worldview (Fawcett, 1995). A comparison of metaparadigm concept definitions from Rogers' model with the other models demonstrates the differences, such as the human/person viewed as an irreducible, indivisible whole rather than as parts of a whole. A comparison of the implementation in practice, education, and research yields a similar conclusion. Although each of the six reciprocal interaction models are able to make their unique contributions to the body of nursing knowledge, these contributions are similar in nature and thus can be viewed together as a body of normal science, separate from the knowledge developed from Rogers' model.

To summarize, a comparison of the body of nursing knowledge to the criteria that Kuhn sets forth for normal science indicates that the discipline of nursing has, through use of the seven nursing models examined above, reached the level of normal science. All of the models are accepted by groups of knowledge building nurse scientists. The models all can and do provide bases for the practice of the discipline of nursing. Finally, all the models are open-ended—that is, they provide a guide or framework for "further articulation and specification under new or more stringent conditions" (Kuhn, 1970, p. 23). Using three interpretations of the structure of the normal science in nursing to answer the basic question "has nursing achieved the level of normal science?", each interpretation has led to the conclusion that yes, nursing conceptual models have led to the achievement of normal science in the discipline of nursing.

References

American Nurses Association. (1988). *Facts about nursing.* Kansas City: Author.

Fawcett, J. (1995). *Analysis and evaluation of conceptual models of nursing* (3rd ed.). Philadelphia: F. A. Davis.

Frey, M. A. & Sieloff, C. L. (1995). *Advancing King's systems framework and theory of nursing.* Thousand Oaks, CA: Sage.

Hilton, P. A. (1997). Theoretical perspectives of nursing: A review of the literature. *Journal of Advanced Nursing, 26*(6), 1211-1220.

Holaday, B. Personal Communication. January, 2000.

Johnson, D. E. (1992). The origins of the behavioral system model. In F. Nightingale, *Notes on nursing: What it is and what it is not* (Commemorative edition, pp. 23-27). Philadelphia: J.B. Lippincott.

King, I. M. (1964). Nursing theory—problems and prospect. *Nursing Science, 2,* 394-403.

King, I. M. (1990). King's conceptual framework and theory of goal attainment. In M. E. Parker (Ed.), *Nursing theories in practice* (pp. 73-84). New York: National League for Nursing.

Kuhn, T. S. (1970). *The structure of scientific revolutions* (2nd ed.). Chicago: University of Chicago.

Levine, M. E. (1966). Trophicognosis: An alternative to nursing diagnosis. In *Exploring progress in medical-surgical nursing practice.* New York: American Nurses Association.

Levine, M. E. (1988). Making choices. In T. M. Shorr & A. Zimmerman, *Taking chances: Nurse leaders tell their stories* (pp. 215-228). St. Louis: Mosby.

Levine, M. E. (1995). The rhetoric of nursing theory. *Image, 27*(1), 11-14.

Martin, M., Forchuk, C., Santopinto, M., & Butcher, H. (1992). Alternate approaches to nursing practice: Application of Peplau, Rogers, and Parse. *Nursing Science Quarterly, 5*(2), 80-85.

McQuiston, C. & Webb, A. (1995). *Foundations of nursing theory.* Thousand Oaks, CA: Sage.

Meleis, A. I. (1997). *Theoretical nursing: Development & progress* (3rd ed.). New York: J. B. Lippincott.

Neuman, B. & Young, R. J. (1972). A model for teaching total person approach to patient problems. *Nursing Research, 21,* 264-269.

Orem, D. (1995). *Nursing: Concepts of practice* (5th ed.). St. Louis: Mosby.

Riehl, J. P. & Roy, C. (1980). *Conceptual models for nursing practice* (2nd ed.). New York: Appleton-Century-Crofts.

Rogers, M. E. (1970). *An introduction to the theoretical basis of nursing.* Philadelphia: F. A. Davis.

Rogers, M. E. (1992). Nursing science and the space age. *Nursing Science Quarterly, 5,* 27-34.

Roy, C. (1970). Adaptation: A conceptual framework for nursing. *Nursing Outlook, 18*(3), 43-45.

Roy, C. & Andrews, H. (1999). *The Roy Adaptation Model* (2nd ed.). Norwalk, CT: Appleton & Lange.

Schaefer, K. Personal Communication. January, 2000.

Wald, F. S. & Leonard, R. C. (1964). Towards development of nursing practice theory. *Nursing Research, 13*(4), 309-313.

Bibliography
Johnson

Broncatello, K. F. (1980). Auger in action: Application of the model. *Advances in Nursing Science, 2*(2), 13-24.

Derdiarian, A. K. (1990). Comprehensive assessment of AIDS patients using the behavioral systems model for nursing practice instrument. *Journal of Advanced Nursing, 15*(4), 436-446.

Derdiarian, A. K. (1990). Effects of using systematic assessment instruments on patient and nurse satisfaction with nursing care. *Oncology Nursing Forum, 17*(1), 95-101.

Derdiarian, A. K. (1991). Effects of using a nursing model—based assessment instrument on quality of nursing care. *Journal of Nursing Administration, 15*(3), 1-16.

Fruehwirth, S. E. S. (1989). An application of Johnson's behavioral model: A case study. *Journal of Community Health Nursing, 6*(2), 61-71.

Herbert, J. (1989). A model for Anna. *Nursing, 3*(42), 30-34.

Holaday, B. (1987). Patterns of interaction between mothers and their chronically ill infants. *Maternal-Child Nursing Journal, 16,* 29-45.

McCauley, K., Choromanski, J. D., Wallinger, C., & Liu, K. (1984). Current management of ventricular tachycardia: Symposium from the Hospital of the University of Pennsylvania. Learning to live with controlled ventricular tachycardia: Utilizing the Johnson model. *Heart and Lung, 13,* 633-638.

Niemela, K., Poster, E. C., & Moreau, D. (1992). The attending nurse: A new role for the advanced clinician in an adolescent inpatient unit. *Journal of Child and Adolescent Psychiatric and Mental Health Nursing, 5*(3), 5-12.

Rawls, A. C. (1980). Evaluation of the Johnson behavioral model in clinical practice. *Image, 12,* 13-16.

Spratlen, L. P. (1976). Introducing ethnic-cultural factors in models of nursing: Some mental health applications. *Journal of Nursing Education, 15*(2), 23-29.

Wilkie, D. J. (1990). Cancer pain management: State of the art nursing care. *Nursing Clinics of North America, 25*(2), 331-343.

King

Alligood, M. R. (1995). Theory of goal attainment: Application to adult orthopedic nursing. In M. A. Frey & C. Sieloff (Eds.), *Advancing King's systems framework and theory of nursing* (pp. 209-222). Thousand Oaks, CA: Sage.

Benedict, M. & Frey, M. (1995). Theory-based practice in the emergency department. In M. A. Frey & C. Sieloff (Eds.), *Advancing King's systems framework and theory of nursing* (pp. 317-324). Thousand Oaks, CA: Sage.

Davis, D. C. (1987). A conceptual framework for infertility. *Journal of Obstetric, Gynecologic, and Neonatal Nursing, 16*, 30-35.

DeHowitt, M. C. (1992). King's conceptual model and individual psychotherapy. *Perspectives in Psychiatric Care, 28*(4), 11-14.

Frey, M. A., Rooke, L., Sieloff, C., Messmer, P., & Kameoka, T. (1995). King's framework and theory in Japan, Sweden, and the United States. *Image, 27*(2), 127-130.

Fawcett, J. M., Vaillancourt, V. M., & Watson, C. A. (1995). Integration of King's framework into nursing practice. In M. A. Frey & C. Sieloff (Eds.), *Advancing King's systems framework and theory of nursing* (pp. 176-191). Thousand Oaks, CA: Sage.

Gonot, P. W. (1986). Family therapy as derived from King's conceptual model. In A. L. Whall (Ed.), *Family therapy theory for nursing: Four approaches* (pp. 33-48). Norwalk, CT: Appleton-Century-Crofts.

Hampton, D. C. (1994). King's theory of goal attainment as a framework for managed care implementation in a hospital setting. *Nursing Science Quarterly, 7*(4), 170-173.

Hanchett, E. S. (1990). Nursing models and community as client. *Nursing Science Quarterly, 3*, 67-72.

Hanna, K. M. (1995). Use of King's theory of goal attainment to promote adolescents' health behavior. In M. A. Frey & C. Sieloff (Eds.), *Advancing King's systems framework and theory of nursing* (pp. 239-250). Thousand Oaks, CA: Sage.

Heggie, M. & Gangar, E. (1992). A nursing model for menopause clinics. *Nursing Standard, 6*(21), 32-34.

Hughes, M. M. (1983). Nursing theories and emergency nursing. *Journal of Emergency Nursing, 9*, 95-97.

Husband, A. (1988). Application of King's theory of nursing to the care of the adult with diabetes. *Journal of Advanced Nursing, 13*(4), 484-488.

Husting, P. A. (1997). A transcultural critique of Imogene King's theory of goal attainment. *Journal of Multicultural Nursing and Health, 3*(3), 15-20.

Jolly, M. L. & Winker, C. K. (1995). Theory of goal attainment in the context of organizational structure. In M. A. Frey & C. Sieloff (Eds.), *Advancing King's systems framework and theory of nursing* (pp. 305-316). Thousand Oaks, CA: Sage.

Jonas, C. M. (1987). King's goal attainment theory: Use in gerontological nursing practice. *Perspectives, 11*(4), 9-12.

Kenny, T. (1990). Erosion of individuality in care of elderly people in hospital—An alternative approach. *Journal of Advanced Nursing, 15*, 571-576.

King, I. M. (1983). The family coping with a medical illness: Analysis and application of King's theory of goal attainment. In I. W. Clements & F. B. Roberts (Eds.), *Family health: A theoretical approach to nursing care* (pp. 383-385). New York: John Wiley & Sons.

King, I. M. (1983). The family with an elderly member: Analysis and application of King's theory of goal attainment. In I. W. Clements & F. B. Roberts (Eds.), *Family health: A theoretical approach to nursing care* (pp. 341-345). New York: John Wiley & Sons.

King, I. M. (1984). Effectiveness of nursing care: Use of a goal-oriented nursing record in end-stage renal disease. *American Association of Nephrology Nurses and Technicians Journal, 11*(2), 11-17, 60.

Kohler, P. (1988). Model of shared control. *Journal of Gerontological Nursing, 14*(7), 21-25.

Laben, J. K., Dodd, D., & Sneed, L. D. (1991). King's theory of goal attainment applied in group therapy for inpatient juvenile sexual offenders, minimum security state offenders, and community parolees using visual aids. *Issues in Mental Health Nursing, 12*(1), 51-64.

Laben, J. K., Sneed, L. D., & Seidel, S. L. (1995). Goal attainment in short-term group psychotherapy settings. In M. A. Frey & C. Sieloff (Eds.), *Advancing King's systems framework and theory of nursing* (pp. 261-277). Thousand Oaks, CA: Sage.

LaFontaine, P. (1989). Alleviating patient's apprehensions and anxieties. *Gastroenterology Nursing, 11,* 256-257.

McKinney, N. & Frank, D. I. (1998). Nursing assessment of adult females who are alcohol-dependent and victims of sexual abuse. *Clinical Excellence for Nursing Practitioners, 2*(3), 152-158.

Messmer, P. R. (1995). Implementation of theory-based nursing practice. In M. A. Frey & C. Sieloff (Eds.), *Advancing King's systems framework and theory of nursing* (pp. 294-304). Thousand Oaks, CA: Sage.

Messner, R. & Smoth, M. N. (1986). Neurofibromatosis: Relinquishing the masks: A quest for quality of life. *Journal of Advanced Nursing, 11,* 459-464.

Norris, D. M. & Hoyer, P. J. (1993). Dynamism in practice: Parenting within King's framework. *Nursing Science Quarterly, 1,* 145-146.

Sirles, A. T. & Selleck, C. S. (1989). Cardiac disease and the family: Impact, assessment, and implications. *Journal of Cardiovascular Nursing, 3*(2), 23-32.

Smith, M. C. (1988). King's theory in practice. *Nursing Science Quarterly, 1,* 145-146.

Steele, S. (1981). *Child health and the family: Nursing concepts and management.* New York: Masson Publishing USA.

Swindale, J. E. (1989). The nurse's role in giving preoperative information to reduce anxiety in patients admitted to hospital for elective minor surgery. *Journal of Advanced Nursing, 14,* 899-905.

Symanski, M. E. (1991). Use of nursing theories in the care of families with high-risk infants: Challenges for the future. *Journal of Perinatal and Neonatal Nursing, 4*(4), 71-77.

Temple, A. & Fawdry, K. (1992). King's theory of goal attainment: Resolving filial caregiver role strain. *Journal of Gerontological Nursing, 18*(3), 11-15.

Tritsch, J. M. (1998). Application of King's theory of goal attainment and the Carondelet St. Mary's case management model. *Nursing Science Quarterly, 11*(2), 69-73.

Woods, E. C. (1994). King's theory in practice with elders. *Nursing Science Quarterly, 7*(2), 65-69.

Levine

Bayley, E. W. (1991). Care of the burn patient. In K. M. Schaefer & J. A. B. Pond (Eds.), *Levine's conservation model: A framework for nursing practice* (pp. 91-99). Philadelphia: F. A. Davis.

Brunner, M. (1985). A conceptual approach to critical care using Levine's model. *Focus on Critical Care, 12*(2), 39-44.

Cooper, D. M. (1990). Optimizing wound healing: A practice within nursing's domain. *Nursing Clinics of North America, 25,* 165-180.

Cox, R. A. Sr. (1991). A tradition of caring: Use of Levine's model in long-term care. In K. M. Schaefer & J. A. B. Pond (Eds.), *Levine's conservation model: A framework for nursing practice* (pp. 179-197). Philadelphia: F. A. Davis.

Crawford-Gamble, P. E. (1986). An application of Levine's conceptual model. *Perioperative Nursing Quarterly, 2*(1), 64-70.

Dever, M. (1991). Care of children. In K. M. Schaefer & J. A. B. Pond (Eds.), *Levine's conservation model: A framework for nursing practice* (pp. 71-82). Philadelphia: F. A. Davis.

Fawcett, J., Archer, C. L., Becker, D., Brown, K. K., Gann, S., Wong, M. J., & Wurster, A. B. (1992). Guidelines for selecting a conceptual model of nursing: Focus on the individual patient. *Dimensions of Critical Care Nursing, 11,* 268-277.

Fawcett, J., Cariello, F. P., Davis, D. A., Farley, J., Simmaro, D. M., & Watts, R. J. (1987). Conceptual models of nursing: Application to critical care nursing practice. *Dimensions of Critical Care Nursing, 6,* 202-213.

Hanson, D., Langemo, D. K., Olson, B., Hunter, S., Sauvage, T. R., Burd, C., & Cathcart-Silberberg, T. (1991). The prevalence and incidence of pressure ulcers in the hospice setting: Analysis of two methodologies. *American Journal of Hospice and Palliative Care, 8*(5), 18-22.

Herbst, S. (1981). Impairments as a result of cancer. In N. Martin, N. Holt, & D. Hicks (Eds.), *Comprehensive rehabilitation nursing* (pp. 553-578). New York: McGraw-Hill.

Pasco, A. & Halupa, D. (1991). Chronic pain management. In K. M. Schaefer & J. A. B. Pond (Eds.), *Levine's conservation model: A framework for nursing practice* (pp. 101-117). Philadelphia: F. A. Davis.

Pond, J. A. B. (1991). Ambulatory care of the homeless. In K. M. Schaefer & J. A. B. Pond (Eds.), *Levine's conservation model: A framework for nursing practice* (pp. 167-178). Philadelphia: F. A. Davis.

Pond, J. A. B. & Taney, S. G. (1991). Emergency care in a large university emergency department. In K. M. Schaefer & J. A. B. Pond (Eds.), *Levine's conservation model: A framework for nursing practice* (pp. 151-166). Philadelphia: F. A. Davis.

Savage, T. A. & Culbert, C. (1989). Early intervention: The unique role of nursing. *Journal of Pediatric Nursing, 4,* 339-345.

Schaefer, K. M. (1991). Care of the patient with congestive heart failure. In K. M. Schaefer & J. A. B. Pond (Eds.), *Levine's conservation model: A framework for nursing practice* (pp. 119-131). Philadelphia: F. A. Davis.

Schaefer, K. M. & Pond, J. A. B. (1994). Levine's conservation model as a guide to nursing practice. *Nursing Science Quarterly, 7*(2), 53-54.

Webb, H. (1993). Holistic care following a palliative Hartmann's procedure. *British Journal of Nursing, 2,* 128-132.

Neuman

Anderson, E., McFarlane, J., & Helton, A. (1986). Community-as-client: A model for practice. *Nursing Outlook, 34,* 220-224.

Baerg, K. L. (1991). Using Neuman's model to analyze a clinical situation. *Rehabilitation Nursing, 16,* 38-39.

Beckingham, A. C. & Baumann, A. (1990). The aging family in crisis: Assessment and decision-making models. *Journal of Advanced Nursing, 15,* 782-787.

Beddome, G. (1995). Community-as-client assessment. In B. Neuman (Ed.), *The Neuman systems model* (3rd ed., pp. 567-579). Norwalk, CT: Appleton & Lange.

Beitler, B., Tkachuck, B., & Aamodt, D. (1980). The Neuman model applied to mental health, community health, and medical-surgical nursing. In J. P. Riehl & C. Roy (Eds.), *Conceptual models for nursing practice* (2nd ed., pp. 170-178). New York: Appleton-Century-Crofts.

Bergstrom, D. (1992). Hypermetabolism in multisystem organ failure: A Neuman systems perspective. *Critical Care Nursing Quarterly, 15*(3), 63-70.

Biley, F. C. (1989). Stress in high dependency units. *Intensive Care Nursing, 5,* 134-141.

Breckenridge, D. M. (1995). Nephrology practice and directions for nursing research. In B. Neuman (Ed.), *The Neuman systems model* (3rd ed., pp. 499-507). Norwalk, CT: Appleton & Lange.

Brown, M. W. (1988). Neuman's systems model in risk factor reduction. *Cardiovascular Nursing, 24*(6), 43.

Buchanan, B. F. (1987). Human-environment interaction: A modification of the Neuman systems model for aggregates, families, and the community. *Public Health Nursing, 4,* 52-64.

Bueno, M. M., & Sengin, K. K. (1995). The Neuman systems model for critical care nursing. In B. Neuman (Ed.), *The Neuman systems model* (3rd ed., pp. 275-291). Norwalk, CT: Appleton & Lange.

Chiverton, P. & Flannery, J. C. (1995). Cognitive impairment. In B. Neuman (Ed.), *The Neuman systems model* (3rd ed., pp. 249-261). Norwalk, CT: Appleton & Lange.

Cunningham, S. G. (1983). The Neuman systems model applied to a rehabilitation setting. *Rehabilitation Nursing, 8*(4), 20-22.

Delunas, L. R. (1990). Prevention of elder abuse: Betty Neuman health care systems approach. *Clinical Nurse Specialist, 4,* 54-58.

Evely, L. (1994). A model for successful breastfeeding. *Modern Midwife, 4*(12), 25-27.

Fawcett, J., Archer, C. L., Becker, D., Brown, K. K., Gann, S., Wong, J. J., & Wurster, A. B. (1992). Guidelines for selecting a conceptual model of nursing: Focus on the individual patient. *Dimensions of Critical Care Nursing, 11,* 268-277.

Fawcett, J., Cariello, F. P., Davis, D. A., Farley, J., Simmaro, D. M., & Watts, R. J. (1987). Conceptual models of nursing: Application to critical care nursing practice. *Dimensions of Critical Care Nursing, 6,* 202-213.

Foote, A. W., Piazza, D., & Schultz, M. (1990). The Neuman systems model: Application to a patient with a cervical spinal cord injury. *Journal of Neuroscience Nursing, 22,* 302-306.

Fulbrook, P. R. (1991). The application of the Neuman systems model to intensive care. *Intensive Care Nursing, 7,* 28-39.

Galloway, D. A. (1993). Coping with a mentally and physically impaired infant: A self-analysis. *Rehabilitation Nursing, 18,* 34-36.

Gavan, C. A. S., Hastings-Tolsma, M. T., & Troyan, P. J. (1988). Explication of Neuman's model: A holistic systems approach to nutrition for health promotion in the life process. *Holistic Nursing Practice, 3*(1), 26-38.

Herrick, C. A. & Goodykoontz, L. (1989). Neuman's systems model for nursing practice as a conceptual framework for a family assessment. *Journal of Child and Adolescent Psychiatric and Mental Health Nursing, 2,* 61-67.

Herrick, C. A., Goodykoontz, L., Herrick, R. H., & Hackett, B. (1991). Planning a continuum of care in child psychiatric nursing: A collaborative effort. *Journal of Child and Adolescent Psychiatric and Mental Health Nursing, 4,* 41-48.

Hiltz, D. (1990). The Neuman systems model: An analysis of a clinical situation. *Rehabilitation Nursing, 15,* 330-332.

Hoeman, S. P. & Winters, D. M. (1990). Theory-based case management: High cervical spinal cord injury. *Home Healthcare Nurse, 8,* 25-33.

Kelly, J. S. & Sanders, N. F. (1995). A systems approach to the health of nursing and health care organizations. In B. Neuman (Ed.), *The Neuman systems model* (3rd ed., pp. 347-364). Norwalk, CT: Appleton & Lange.

Kido, L. M. (1991). Sleep deprivation and intensive care unit psychosis. *Emphasis: Nursing, 4*(1), 23-33.

Knight, J. B. (1990). The Betty Neuman systems model applied to practice: A client with multiple sclerosis. *Journal of Advanced Nursing, 15,* 447-455.

Lindell, M. & Olsson, H. (1991). Can combined oral contraceptives be made more effective by means of a nursing care model? *Journal of Advanced Nursing, 16,* 475-479.

Mill, J. E. (1997). The Neuman systems model: Application in a Canadian HIV setting. *British Journal of Nursing, 6*(3), 163-166.

Millard, J. (1992). Health visiting an elderly couple. *British Journal of Nursing, 1,* 769-773.

Miner, J. (1995). Incorporating the Betty Neuman systems model into HIV clinical practice. *AIDS Patient Care, 9*(1), 37-39.

Moore, S. L. & Munro, M. F. (1990). The Neuman systems model applied to mental health nursing of older adults. *Journal of Advanced Nursing, 15,* 293-299.

Neuman, B., Newman, D., & Holder, P. (2000). Leadership-Scholarship integration: Using the Neuman systems model for 21st century nursing practice. *Nursing Science Quarterly, 13*(1), 60-63.

Piazza, D., Foote, A., Wright, P., & Holcombe, J. (1992). Neuman systems model used as a guide for the nursing care of an 8-year-old child with leukemia. *Journal of Pediatric Oncology Nursing, 9*(1), 17-24.

Pierce, A. G. & Gulmer, T. T. (1995). Application of the Neuman systems model to gerontological nursing. In B. Neuman (Ed.), *The Neuman systems model* (3rd ed., pp. 293-308). Norwalk, CT: Appleton & Lange.

Pierce, J. D. & Hutton, E. (1992). Applying the new concepts of the Neuman systems model. *Nursing Forum, 27,* 15-18.

Redheffer, G. (1985). Application of Betty Neuman's health care systems model to emergency nursing practice: Case review. *Point of View, 22*(2), 4-6.

Reed, K. S. (1993). Adapting the Neuman systems model for family nursing. *Nursing Science Quarterly, 6,* 93-97.

Ross, M. & Bourbonnais, F. (1985). The Betty Neuman systems model in nursing practice: A case study approach. *Journal of Advanced Nursing, 10,* 199-207.

Ross, M. & Helmer, H. (1988). A comparative analysis of Neuman's model using the individual and family as the units of care. *Public Health Nursing, 5,* 30-36.

Russell, J., Hileman, J. W., & Grant, J. S. (1995). Assessing and meeting the needs of home caregivers using the Neuman systems model. In B. Neuman (Ed.), *The Neuman systems model* (3rd ed., pp. 331-341). Norwalk, CT: Appleton & Lange.

Shaw, M. C. (1991). A theoretical base for orthopaedic nursing practice: *The Neuman systems model. Canadian Orthopaedic Nurses Association Journal, 13*(2), 19-21.

Smith, M. C. (1989). Neuman's model in practice. *Nursing Science Quarterly, 1,* 116-117.

Sohier, R. (1995). Nursing care for the people of a small planet: Culture and the Neuman systems model. In B. Neuman (Ed.), *The Neuman systems model* (3rd ed., pp. 101-117). Norwalk, CT: Appleton & Lange.

Stuart, G. & Wright, L. K. (1995). Applying the Neuman Systems Model to psychiatric nursing practice. In B. Neuman (Ed.), *The Neuman systems model* (3rd ed., pp. 263-273). Norwalk, CT: Appleton & Lange.

Sullivan, J. (1986). Using Neuman's model in the acute phase of spinal cord injury. *Focus on Critical Care, 13*(5), 34-41.

Trepanier, M. J., Dunn, S. I., & Sprague, A. E. (1995). Application of the Neuman systems model to perinatal nursing. In B. Neuman (Ed.), *The Neuman systems model* (3rd ed., pp. 309-320). Norwalk, CT: Appleton & Lange.

Utz, S. W. (1980). Applying the Neuman model to nursing practice with hypertensive clients. *Cardiovascular Nursing, 16,* 29-34.

Wallingford, P. (1989). The neurologically impaired and dying child: Applying the Neuman systems model. *Issues in Comprehensive Pediatric Nursing, 12,* 139-157.

Ware, L. A. & Shannahan, M. D. (1995). Using Neuman for a stable parent support group in neonatal intensive care. In B. Neuman (Ed.), *The Neuman systems model* (3rd ed., pp. 321-330). Norwalk, CT: Appleton & Lange.

Weinberger, S. L. (1991). Analysis of a clinical situation using the Neuman system model. *Rehabilitation Nursing, 16,* 278, 280-281.

Orem

Anderson, S. B. (1992). Guillain-Barré syndrome: Giving the patient control. *Journal of Neuroscience Nursing, 24,* 158-162.

Atkins, F. D. (1992). An uncertain future: Children of mentally ill parents. *Journal of Psychosocial Nursing and Mental Health Services, 30*(8), 13-16.

Beckmann, C. A. (1987). Maternal-child health in Brazil. *Journal of Obstetric, Gynecologic, and Neonatal Nursing, 16,* 238-241.

Berbiglia, V. A. (1991). A case study: Perspectives on a self-care deficit nursing theory—based curriculum. *Journal of Advanced Nursing, 16,* 1158-1163.

Blaylock, B. (1991). Enhancing self-care of the elderly client: Practical teaching tips for ostomy care. *Journal of Enterostomal Therapy Nursing, 18,* 118-121.

Buckwalter, K. C. & Kerfoot, K. M. (1982). Teaching patients self-care: A critical aspect of psychiatric discharge planning. *Journal of Psychiatric Nursing and Mental Health Services, 20*(5), 15-20.

Campbell, J. C. & Weber, N. (2000). An empirical test of a self-care model of women's responses to battering. *Nursing Science Quarterly, 13*(1), 45-53.

Campuzano, M. (1982). Self-care following coronary artery bypass surgery. *Focus on Critical Care, 9*(2), 55-56.

Cantanese, M. L. (1987). Vaginal birth after cesarean: Recommendations, risks, realities, and the client's right to know. *Holistic Nursing Practice, 2*(1), 35-43.

Caradus, A. (1991). Nursing theory and operating suite nursing practice. *ACORN Journal, 4*(2), 29-30, 32.

Clark, M. D. (1986). Application of Orem's theory of self-care: A case study. *Journal of Community Health Nursing, 3*(3), 127-135.

Comptom, P. (1989). Drug abuse: A self-care deficit. *Journal of Psychosocial Nursing and Mental Health Services, 27*(3), 22-26.

Connelly, C. E. (1987). Self-care and the chronically ill patient. *Nursing Clinics of North America, 22,* 621-629.

Cretain, G. K. (1989). Motivational factors in breast self-examination: Implications for nurses. *Cancer Nursing, 12,* 250-256.

Davidhizar, R. & Cosgray, R. (1990). The use of Orem's model in psychiatric rehabilitation assessment. *Rehabilitation Nursing, 15*(1), 39-41.

Dear, M. R. & Keen, M. F. (1982). Promotion of self-care in the employee with rheumatoid arthritis. *Occupational Health Nursing, 30*(1), 32-34.

Dropkin, M. J. (1981). Development of a self-care teaching program for postoperative head and neck patients. *Cancer Nursing, 4,* 103-106.

Duffy, J., Miller, M. P., & Parlocha, P. (1993). Psychiatric home care: A framework for assessment and intervention. *Home Healthcare Nurse, 11*(2), 22-28.

Dunn, B. (1990). Alcohol dependency: Health promotion and Orem's model. *Nursing Standard, 4*(40), 34.

Eichelberger, K. M., Kaufman, D. N., Rundahl, M. E., & Schwartz, N. E. (1980). Self-care nursing plan: Helping children to help themselves. *Pediatric Nursing, 6*(3), 9-13.

Eliopoulos, C. (1984). A self-care model for gerontological nursing. *Geriatric Nursing, 4,* 366-369.

Facteau, L. M. (1980). Self-care concepts and the care of the hospitalized child. *Nursing Clinics of North America, 15,* 145-155.

Fawcett, J., Archer, C. L., Becker, D., Brown, K. K., Gann, S., Wong, J. J., & Wurster, A. B. (1992). Guidelines for selecting a conceptual model of nursing: Focus on the individual patient. *Dimensions of Critical Care Nursing, 11,* 268-277.

Fawcett, J., Cariello, F. P., Davis, D. A., Farley, J., Simmaro, D. M., & Watts, R. J. (1987). Conceptual models of nursing: Application to critical care nursing practice. *Dimensions of Critical Care Nursing, 6*(4), 202-213.

Fields, L. M. (1987). A clinical application of the Orem nursing model in labor and delivery. *Emphasis: Nursing, 2,* 102-108.

Fitzgerald, S. (1980). Utilizing Orem's self-care model in designing an education program for the diabetic. *Topics in Clinical Nursing, 2*(2), 57-65.

Flanagan, M. (1991). Self-care for a leg ulcer. *Nursing Times, 87*(23), 67-68, 70, 72.

Foote, A., Holcombe, J., Piazza, D., & Wright, P. (1993). Orem's theory used as a guide for the nursing care of an eight-year-old child with leukemia. *Journal of Pediatric Oncology Nursing, 10*(1), 26-32.

Fridgen, R. & Nelson, S. (1992). Teaching tool for renal transplant recipients using Orem's self-care model. *CANNT, 2*(3), 18-26.

Geyer, E. (1990). Self-care issues for the elderly. *Dimensions in Oncology Nursing, 4*(2), 33-35.

Haas, D. L. (1990). Application of Orem's self-care deficit theory to the pediatric chronically ill population. *Issues in Comprehensive Pediatric Nursing, 13,* 253-264.

Hanchett, E. S. (1990). Nursing models and community as client. *Nursing Science Quarterly, 3,* 67-72.

Harris, J. K. (1980). Self-care is possible after cesarean delivery. *Nursing Clinics of North America, 15,* 191-204.

Hart, M. A. & Foster, S. N. (1998). Self-care agency in two groups of pregnant women. *Nursing Science Quarterly, 11*(4), 167-171.

Hurst, J. D. & Stullenbarger, B. (1986). Implementation of a self-care approach in a pediatric interdisciplinary phenylketonuria (PKU) clinic. *Journal of Pediatric Nursing, l,* 159-163.

Jacobs, C. J. (1990). Orem's self-care model: Is it relevant to patients in intensive care? *Intensive Care Nursing, 6,* 100-103.

Kam, B. W. & Werner, P. W. (1990). Self-care theory: Application to perioperative nursing. *Association of Operating Room Nurses Journal, 51,* 1365-1370.

Keohane, N. S. & Lacey, L. A. (1991). Preparing the woman with gestational diabetes for self-care: Use of a structured teaching plan for nursing staff. *Journal of Obstetric, Gynecologic, and Neonatal Nursing, 20,* 189-193.

Komulainen, P. (1991). Occupational health nursing based on self-care theory. *American Association of Occupational Health Nursing Journal, 39,* 333-335.

Kyle, B. A. S. & Pitzer, S. A. (1990). A self-care approach to today's challenges. *Nursing Management, 21*(3), 37-39.

Lacey, D. (1993). Using Orem's model in psychiatric nursing. *Nursing Standard, 7*(29), 28-30.

Mack, C. H. (1992). Assessment of the autologous bone marrow transplant patient according to Orem's self-care model. *Cancer Nursing, 15,* 429-436.

Meriney, D. K. (1990). Application of Orem's conceptual framework to patients with hypercalcemia related to breast cancer. *Cancer Nursing, 13,* 316-323.

Morse, W. & Werner, J. S. (1988). Individualization of patient care using Orem's theory. *Cancer Nursing, 11,* 195-202.

Moscovitz, A. (1984). Orem's theory as applied to psychiatric nursing. *Perspectives in Psychiatric Care, 22*(1), 36-38.

Mullin, V. I. (1980). Implementing the self-care concept in the acute care setting. *Nursing Clinics of North America, 15,* 177-190.

Murphy, P. P. (1981). A hospice model and self-care theory. *Oncology Nursing Forum, 8*(2), 19-21.

Norris, M. K. G. (1991). Applying Orem's theory to the long-term care of adolescent transplant recipients. *American Nephrology Nurses' Association Journal, 18,* 45-47, 53.

O'Donovan, S. (1990). Nursing models: More of Orem. *Nursing the Elderly, 2*(3), 22-23.

O'Donovan, S. (1990). Nursing models: More of Orem. *Nursing the Elderly, 2*(4), 20-22.

Padula, C. A. (1992). Self-care and the elderly: Review and implications. *Public Health Nursing, 9,* 22-28.

Park, P. B. (1989). Health care for the homeless: A self-care approach. *Clinical Nurse Specialist, 3,* 171-175.

Perras, S. & Zappacosta, A. (1982). The application of Orem's theory in promoting self-care in a peritoneal dialysis facility. *American Association of Nephrology Nurses and Technicians Journal, 9*(3), 37-39.

Raven, M. (1988-1989). Application of Orem's self-care model to nursing practice in developmental disability. *Australian Journal of Advanced Nursing, 6*(2), 16-23.

Ream, E. & Richardson, A. (1999). Continuing education. From theory to practice: Designing interventions to reduce fatigue in patients with cancer. *Oncology Nursing Forum, 26*(8), 1295-1305.

Rew, L. (1990). Childhood sexual abuse: Toward a self-care framework for nursing intervention and research. *Archives of Psychiatric Nursing, 4,* 147-153.

Richardson, A. (1991). Theories of self-care: Their relevance to chemotherapy-induced nausea and vomiting. *Journal of Advanced Nursing, 16,* 671-676.

Smith, M. C. (1977). Self-care: A conceptual framework for rehabilitation nursing. *Rehabilitation Nursing, 2*(2), 8-10.

Smith, M. C. (1989). An application of Orem's theory in nursing practice. *Nursing Science Quarterly, 2*(4), 159-161.

Swindale, J. E. (1989). The nurse's role in giving preoperative information to reduce anxiety in patients admitted to hospital for elective minor surgery. *Journal of Advanced Nursing, 14,* 899-905.

Taylor, S. G. (1988). Nursing theory and nursing process: Orem's theory in practice. *Nursing Science Quarterly, 1,* 111-119.

Taylor, S. G. (1989). An interpretation of family with Orem's general theory of nursing. *Nursing Science Quarterly, 1,* 131-137.

Taylor, S. G. (1990). Practical applications of Orem's self-care deficit nursing theory. In M. E. Parker (Ed.), *Nursing theories in practice* (pp. 61-70). New York: National League for Nursing.

Taylor, S. G. & McLaughlin, K. (1991). Orem's general theory of nursing and community nursing. *Nursing Science Quarterly, 4,* 153-160.

Titus, S. & Porter, P. (1989). Orem's theory applied to pediatric residential treatment, *Pediatric Nursing, 15,* 465-468, 556.

Tolentino, M. B. (1990). The use of Orem's self-care model in the neonatal intensive care unit. *Journal of Obstetric, Gynecologic, and Neonatal Nursing, 19,* 496-500.

Vasquez, M. A. (1992). From theory to practice: Orem's self-care nursing model and ambulatory care. *Journal of Post Anesthesia Nursing, 7,* 251-255.

Walborn, K. A. (1980). A nursing model for the hospice: Primary and self-care nursing. *Nursing Clinics of North America, 15,* 205-217.

Walsh, M. & Judd, M. (1989). Long term immobility and self-care: The Orem nursing approach. *Nursing Standard, 3*(41), 34-36.

Zach, P. (1982). Self-care agency in diabetic ocular sequelae. *Journal of Ophthalmic Nursing Techniques, 1*(2), 21-31.

Rogers

Alligood, M. R. (1989). Rogers' theory and nursing administration: A perspective on health and environment. In B. Henry, C. Arndt, M. DiVincenti, & A. Marriner-Tomey (Eds.), *Dimensions of nursing administration: Theory, research, education, and practice* (pp. 105-111). Boston: Blackwell Scientific.

Alligood, M. R. (1990). Nursing care of the elderly: Futuristic projections. In E. A. M. Barrett (Ed.), *Visions of Rogers' science-based nursing* (pp. 129-142). New York: National League for Nursing.

Alligood, M. R. (1994). Toward a unitary view of nursing practice. In M. Madrid & E. A. M. Barrett (Eds.), *Rogers' scientific art of nursing practice* (pp. 223-237). New York: National League for Nursing.

Anderson, M. D. & Smereck, G. A. D. (1994). Personalized nursing: A science-based model of the art of nursing. In M. Madrid & E. A. M. Barrett (Eds.), *Rogers' scientific art of nursing practice* (pp. 261-283). New York: National League for Nursing.

Barrett, E. A. M. (1988). Using Rogers' science of unitary human beings in nursing practice. *Nursing Science Quarterly, 1,* 50-51.

Barrett, E. A. M. (1990). Health patterning in clients in a private practice. In E. A. M. Barrett (Ed.), *Visions of Rogers' science-based nursing* (pp. 105-116). New York: National League for Nursing.

Barrett, E. A. M. (1990). Rogers' science-based nursing practice. In E. A. M. Barrett (Ed.), *Visions of Rogers' science-based nursing* (pp. 31-44). New York: National League for Nursing.

Barrett, E. A. M. (1992). Innovative imagery: A health patterning modality for nursing practice. *Journal of Holistic Nursing, 10,* 154-166.

Barrett, E. A. M. (1993). Virtual reality: A health patterning modality for nursing in space. Visions: *The Journal of Rogerian Nursing Science, 1,* 10-21.

Barrett, E. A. M. (1998). A Rogerian practice methodology for health patterning. *Nursing Science Quarterly, 11*(4), 136-138.

Black, G. & Haight, B. K. (1992). Integrality as a holistic framework for the life-review process. *Holistic Nursing Practice, 7*(1), 7-15.

Buczny, B., Speirs, J., & Howard, J. R. (1989). Nursing care of a terminally ill client. Applying Martha Rogers' conceptual framework. *Home Healthcare Nurse, 7*(4), 13-18.

Caroselli, C. (1994). Opportunities for knowing participation: A new design for the nursing service organization. In M. Madrid & E. A. M. Barrett (Eds.), *Rogers' scientific art of nursing practice* (pp. 243-259). New York: National League for Nursing.

Chapman, J. S., Mitchell, G. J., & Forchuk, C. (1994). A glimpse of nursing theory—based practice in Canada. *Nursing Science Quarterly, 7,* 104-112.

Christensen, P., Sowell, R., & Gueldner, S. H. (1993). Nursing in space: Theoretical foundations and potential practice applications within Rogerian science. *Visions: The Journal of Rogerian Nursing Science, 1,* 36-44.

Clarke, P. (1994). Nursing theory—based practice in the home and the community. *Advances in Nursing Science, 17*(2), 41-53.

Cowling III, W. R. (1990). A template for unitary pattern-based nursing practice. In E. A. M. Barrett (Ed.), *Visions of Rogers' science-based nursing* (pp. 45-66). New York: National League for Nursing.

Forker, J. E. & Billings, C. V. (1989). Nursing therapeutics in a group encounter. *Archives of Psychiatric Nursing, 3,* 108-112.

France, N. E. M. (1994). Unitary human football players. In M. Madrid & E. A. M. Barrett (Eds.), *Rogers' scientific art of nursing practice* (pp. 197-206). New York: National League for Nursing.

Green, C. A. (1998). Critically exploring the use of Rogers' nursing theory of unitary human beings as a framework to underpin therapeutic touch practice. *European Nursing, 3*(3), 158-169.

Griffin, J. (1994). Storytelling as a scientific art form. In M. Madrid & E. A. M. Barrett (Eds.), *Rogers' scientific art of nursing practice* (pp. 101-104). New York: National League for Nursing.

Gueldner, S. H. (1994). Pattern diversity and community presence in the human-environmental process: Implications for Rogerian-based practice with nursing home residents. In M. Madrid & E. A. M. Barrett (Eds.), *Rogers' scientific art of nursing practice* (pp. 131-140). New York: National League for Nursing.

Hanchett, E. S. (1990). Nursing models and community as client. *Nursing Science Quarterly, 3,* 67-72.

Heggie, J., Garon, M., Kodiath, M., & Kelly, A. (1994). Implementing the science of unitary human beings at the San Diego Veterans Affairs Medical Center. In M. Madrid & E. A. M. Barrett (Eds.), *Rogers' scientific art of nursing practice* (pp. 285-304). New York: National League for Nursing.

Heggie, J. R., Schoenmehl, P. A., Chang, M. K., & Crieco, C. (1989). Selection and implementation of Dr. Martha Rogers' nursing conceptual model in an acute care setting. *Clinical Nurse Specialist, 3,* 143-147.

Hill, L. & Oliver, N. (1993). Technique integration: Therapeutic touch and theory-based mental health nursing. *Journal of Psychosocial Nursing and Mental Health Services, 31*(2), 19-22.

Horvath, B. (1994). The science of unitary human beings as a foundation for nursing practice with persons experiencing life patterning difficulties: Transforming theory into motion. In M. Madrid & E. A. M. Barrett (Eds.), *Rogers' scientific art of nursing practice* (pp. 163-176). New York: National League for Nursing.

Johnson, R. L. (1986). Approaching family intervention through Rogers' conceptual model. In A. L. Whall (Ed.), *Family therapy theory for nursing: Four approaches* (pp. 11-32). Norwalk, CT: Appleton-Century-Crofts.

Joseph, L. (1990). Practical application of Rogers' theoretical framework for nursing. In M. E. Parker (Ed.), *Nursing theories in practice* (pp. 115-125). New York: National League for Nursing.

Jurgens, A., Meehan, T. C., & Wilson, H. L. (1987). Therapeutic touch as a nursing intervention. *Holistic Nursing Practice, 2*(1), 1-13.

Kodiath, M. F. (1991). A new view of the chronic pain client. *Holistic Nursing Practice, 6*(1), 41-46.

Madrid, M. (1990). The participating process of human field patterning in an acute-care environment. In E. A. M. Barrett (Ed.), *Visions of Rogers' science-based nursing* (pp. 93-104). New York: National League for Nursing.

Madrid, M. (1994). Participating in the process of dying. In M. Madrid & E. A. M. Barrett (Eds.), *Rogers' scientific art of nursing practice* (pp. 91-100). New York: National League for Nursing.

Magan, S. J., Gibbon, E. J., & Mrozek, R. (1990). Nursing theory applications: A practice model. *Issues in Mental Health Nursing, 11,* 297-312.

Malinski, V. M. (1986). Nursing practice within the science of unitary human beings. In V. M. Malinski (Ed.), *Explorations on Martha Rogers' science of unitary human beings* (pp. 25-32). Norwalk, CT: Appleton-Century-Crofts.

Malinski, V. M. (1994). Health patterning for individuals and families. In M. Madrid & E. A. M. Barrett (Eds.), *Rogers' scientific art of nursing practice* (pp. 105-117). New York: National League for Nursing.

Malinski, V. M. (1997). Rogerian health patterning: Evolving into the 21st century. *Nursing Science Quarterly, 10*(3), 115-116.

Matas, K. E. (1997). Human patterning and chronic pain. *Nursing Science Quarterly, 10*(2), 88-92.

Meehan, T. C. (1990). The science of unitary human beings and theory-based practice: Therapeutic touch. In E. A. M. Barrett (Ed.), *Visions of Rogers' science-based nursing* (pp. 67-82). New York: National League for Nursing.

Morwessel, N. J. (1994). Developing an effective pattern appraisal to guide nursing of children with heart variations and their families. In M. Madrid & E. A. M. Barrett (Eds.), *Rogers' scientific art of nursing practice* (pp. 147-161). New York: National League for Nursing.

Newshan, G. (1989). Therapeutic touch for symptom control in person with AIDS. *Holistic Nursing Practice, 3*(4), 45-51.

Novac, D. M. (1999). Perception of menopause and its application to Rogers' science of unitary human beings. *Visions: The Journal of Rogerian Nursing Science, 7*(1), 24-29.

Payne, M. B. (1989). The use of therapeutic touch with rehabilitation clients. *Rehabilitation Nursing, 14*(2), 69-72.

Sargent, S. (1994). Healing groups: Awareness of a group field. In M. Madrid & E. A. M. Barrett (Eds.), *Rogers' scientific art of nursing practice* (pp. 119-129). New York: National League for Nursing.

Smith, D. W. (1994). Viewing polio survivors through violet-tinted glasses. In M. Madrid & E. A. M. Barrett (Eds.), *Rogers' scientific art of nursing practice* (pp. 141-145). New York: National League for Nursing.

Thomas, S. D. (1990). Intentionality in the human-environment encounter in an ambulatory care environment. In E. A. M. Barrett (Ed.), *Visions of Rogers' science-based nursing* (pp. 117-128). New York: National League for Nursing.

Thompson, J. E. (1990). Finding the borderline's border: Can Martha Rogers help? *Perspectives in Psychiatric Care, 26*(4), 7-10.

Tudor, C. A., Keegan-Jones, L., & Bens, E. M. (1994). Implementing Rogers' science-based nursing practice in a pediatric nursing service setting. In M. Madrid & E. A. M. Barrett (Eds.), *Rogers' scientific art of nursing practice* (pp. 305-322). New York: National League for Nursing.

Tuyn, L. K. (1992). Solution-oriented therapy and Rogerian nursing science: An integrated approach. *Archives of Psychiatric Nursing, 6,* 83-89.

Tuyn, L. K. (1994). Rhythms of living: A Rogerian approach to counseling. In M. Madrid & E. A. M. Barrett (Eds.), *Rogers' scientific art of nursing practice* (pp. 207-221). New York: National League for Nursing.

Whall, A. (1981). Nursing theory and the assessment of families. *Journal of Psychiatric Nursing and Mental Health Services, 19*(1), 30-36.

Roy

Aaronson, L. & Seaman, L. P. (1989). Managing hypernatremia in fluid-deficient elderly. *Journal of Gerontological Nursing, 15*(7), 29-34.

Barnfather, J. S., Swain, M. A. P., & Erickson, H. C. (1989). Evaluation of two assessment techniques for adaptation to stress. *Nursing Science Quarterly, 2,* 172-182.

Bawden, M., Ralph, J., & Herrick, C. A. (1991). Enhancing the coping skills of mothers with developmentally delayed children. *Journal of Child and Adolescent Psychiatric Mental Health Nursing, 4,* 25-28.

Caradus, A. (1991). Nursing theory and operating suite nursing practice. *ACORN Journal, 4*(2), 29-30, 32.

DiMaria, R. A. (1989). Posttrauma responses: Potential for nursing. *Journal of Advanced Medical-Surgical Nursing, 2*(1), 41-48.

Doyle, R. & Rajacich, D. (1991). The Roy adaptation model: Health teaching about osteoporosis. *American Association of Occupational Health Nursing Journal, 39,* 508-512.

Ellis, J. A. (1991). Coping with adolescent cancer: It's a matter of adaptation. *Journal of Pediatric Oncology Nursing, 8,* 10-17.

Fawcett, J. (1981). Assessing and understanding the cesarean father. In C. F. Kehoe (Ed.), *The cesarean experience: Theoretical and clinical perspectives for nurses* (pp. 143-156). New York: Appleton-Century-Crofts.

Fawcett, J., Archer, C. L., Becker, D., Brown, K. K., Gann, S., Wong, M. J., & Wurster, A. B. (1992). Guidelines for selecting a conceptual model of nursing: Focus on the individual patient. *Dimensions of Critical Care Nursing, 11,* 268-277.

Galligan, A. C. (1979). Using Roy's concept of adaptation to care for young children. *American Journal of Maternal Child Nursing, 4,* 24-28.

Gerrish, C. (1989). From theory to practice. *Nursing Times, 85*(35), 42-45.

Giger, J. A., Bower, C. A., & Miller, S. W. (1987). Roy adaptation model: ICU application. *Dimensions of Critical Care Nursing, 6,* 215-224.

Hamner, J. B. (1989). Applying the Roy adaptation model to the CCU. *Critical Care Nurse, 9*(3), 51-61.

Hanchett, E. S. (1990). Nursing models and community as client. *Nursing Science Quarterly, 3,* 67-72.

Hughes, M. M. (1983). Nursing theories and emergency nursing. *Journal of Emergency Nursing, 9,* 95-97.

Innes, M. H. (1992). Management of an inadequately ventilated patient. *British Journal of Nursing, 1,* 780-784.

Jackson, D. A. (1990). Roy in the postanesthesia care unit. *Journal of Post Anesthesia Nursing, 5,* 143-148.

Janelli, L. (1980). Utilizing Roy's adaptation model from a gerontological perspective. *Journal of Gerontological Nursing, 6,* 140-150.

Kehoe, C. F. (1981). Identifying the nursing needs of the postpartum cesarean mother. In C. F. Kehoe (Ed.), *The cesarean experience: Theoretical and clinical perspectives for nurses* (pp. 143-156). New York: Appleton-Century-Crofts.

Kurek-Ovshinsky, C. (1991). Group psychotherapy in an acute inpatient setting: Techniques that nourish self-esteem. *Issues in Mental Health Nursing, 12,* 81-88.

Logan, M. (1986). Palliative care nursing: Applicability of the Roy model. *Journal of Palliative Care,* 1(2), 18-24.

Logan, M. (1988). Care of the terminally ill includes the family. *The Canadian Nurse, 84*(5), 30-33.

McIver, M. (1987). Putting theory into practice. *The Canadian Nurse, 83*(10), 36-38.

Miller, F. (1991). Using Roy's model in a special hospital. *Nursing Standard, 5*(27), 29-32.

Nash, D. J. (1987). Kawasaki disease: Application of the Roy adaptation model to determine interventions. *Journal of Pediatric Nursing, 2,* 308-315.

Nyquist, K. H. (1993). Advice concerning breastfeeding from mothers of infants admitted to a neonatal intensive care unit: The Roy adaptation model as a conceptual structure. *Journal of Advanced Nursing, 18*(1), 54-63.

Piazza, D. & Foote, A. (1990). Roy's adaptation model: A guide for rehabilitation nursing practice. *Rehabilitation Nursing, 15,* 254-259.

Piazza, D., Foote, A., Holcombe, J., Harris, M. G., & Wright, P. (1992). The use of Roy's adaptation model applied to a patient with breast cancer. *European Journal of Cancer Care, 1*(4), 17-22.

Schmidt, C. S. (1981). Withdrawal behavior of schizophrenics: Application of Roy's model. *Journal of Psychosocial Nursing and Mental Health Services, 19*(11), 26-33.

Sirignano, R. G. (1987). Peripartum cardiomyopathy: An application of the Roy adaptation model. *Journal of Cardiovascular Nursing, 2,* 24-32.

Smith, M. C. (1988). Roy's adaptation model in practice. *Nursing Science Quarterly, 1,* 97-98.

Thornbury, J. M. & King, L. D. (1992). The Roy adaptation model and care of persons with Alzheimer's disease. *Nursing Science Quarterly, 5,* 129-133.

Vavaro, F. F. (1991). Women with coronary heart disease: An application of Roy's adaptation model. *Cardiovascular Nursing, 27*(6), 31-35.

Weiss, M. E., Hastings, W. J., Holly, D. C., & Craig, D. I. (1994). Using Roy's adaptation model in practice: Nurses' perspectives. *Nursing Science Quarterly, 7,* 80-86.

Wright, P. S., Holcombe, J., Foote, A., & Piazza, D. (1993). The Roy adaptation model used as a guide for the nursing care of an 8-year-old child with leukemia. *Journal of Pediatric Oncology Nursing, 10,* 68-74.

Philosophies, Models, and Theories: Critical Thinking Structures

Martha Raile Alligood

"It is not simply knowing a lot of things; it is a way of knowing things." (Levine, 1988)

Application of nursing theory in practice depends on nurses having knowledge of the theoretical works as well as an understanding of how philosophies, models, and theories relate to each other. Fawcett (1993, 1995) has clarified nursing theory as less abstract than nursing models, but what does that mean for the practicing nurse? This chapter answers that question by describing the relationships of each of the seven nursing models included in this text with their theories as well as three philosophies of nursing and six theories of nursing. Based on the patterns of knowing in nursing (Carper, 1978), these works and their theories represent the empirical pattern or the science of nursing. Therefore they serve as organizing frameworks for substantive approaches to nursing. They do this by providing critical thinking structures to guide your reasoning in professional nursing practice. The linkage of nursing theoretical works (philosophies, models, and theories) with critical thinking is established based on the definition and process of critical thinking according to Paul and Nosich (1991). The chapter concludes with points to be considered in selecting a nursing theoretical work to guide your practice. The importance of a good fit between the nurse and the particular theoretical work is discussed. If you wish to review the philosophies, nursing models, and theories included in this text in more detail, see Units II, III, and IV of *Nursing Theorists and Their Work*

(Marriner Tomey & Alligood, 2002) for analyses and critiques of each philosophy, model, and theory. You are also encouraged to review the writings of the theorists themselves in the primary references of these works.

THE RELATIONSHIP OF PHILOSOPHIES, MODELS, AND THEORIES

The philosophies, models, and theories of a discipline are theoretical structures that address the central concepts of that discipline. The science of nursing is recognized as a fundamental pattern of knowing for nurses (Carper, 1978). Fawcett (1993, 1995) has proposed a structure for that science according to Kuhn's philosophy of science and scientific development (1970). This structure also provides a context to understand the interrelationship of the elements of the science (Fawcett, 1989, 1993, 1995, 2000).

Table 3-1 presents the knowledge structure with examples to illustrate the levels of nursing knowledge. The metaparadigm is the most abstract set of central concepts (i.e., person, environment, health, and nursing), and these concepts are defined by each conceptual model according to the philosophy of that model.

TABLE 3-1 Knowledge Structure Levels with Examples	
Structure Level	**Example**
Metaparadigm	Person, environment, health, nursing
Philosophy	Nightingale
Conceptual models	King's systems framework
Grand theory	King's theory of goal attainment
Theory	Goal attainment in hospital settings
Middle-range theory	Goal attainment in adolescent diabetic patients in the community

Modified from Fawcett, J. (1995). *Analysis and evaluation of conceptual models of nursing* (3rd ed.). Philadelphia: F. A. Davis; and Fawcett, J. (1993). *Analysis and evaluation of nursing theories.* Philadelphia: F. A. Davis.

Philosophies set forth the general meaning of nursing and nursing phenomena through reasoning and logical presentation of ideas (Alligood, 2000). Although Nightingale (1946) did not present her philosophy on the relationship of patients and their surroundings as a theory, such philosophies contain implicit theory that guides nursing practice. Conceptual models (also called paradigms or frameworks) such as King's systems framework are the next less abstract set of concepts in the structure. Grand theory (e.g., King's Theory of Goal Attainment) is next as the level of abstraction descends. Theory can be considered grand when it is nearly as abstract as the model itself and when the usefulness of the model depends on the soundness of that theory. Grand theory is very useful in research and practice because specific theories that contain the details of practice can be derived from it. Theory is the next less abstract level; it is more specific than grand theory but not as specific as middle-range theory (e.g., goal attainment in specific settings). Finally, as mentioned earlier, middle-range theory is the least abstract set of concepts and most specific to the details of nursing practice (e.g., goal attainment in adolescent, type II diabetic patients in the community). Therefore the theory terminology in the nursing literature is best understood according to the different levels of abstraction of sets of concepts (Alligood & Choi, 1998; Fawcett, 1989, 1995; Reynolds, 1971). Theory may also be differentiated by the way it is named or labeled. A model tends to be named for the person who authors it, such as King's General Systems Framework. Grand theories tend to be named for the outcome they propose, such as the Theory of Goal Attainment, and theories tend to be named for the characteristics its content demarcates as an explanatory shell of the outcomes the they propose, such as a theory of departmental power (Sieloff, 1991,1995).

Philosophies are theoretical works that address one or more of the metaparadigm concepts (person, environment, health, and nursing) and are of a philosophical nature. Philosophies address questions such as the following (Alligood, 2000):
- What is nursing?
- What is the nature of human caring?
- What is the nature of nursing practice?
- What is practice expertise and how do nurses develop it?

Therefore philosophies are broad and propose general ideas about what nursing is, what nursing's concerns are, and how the profession of nursing addresses its moral obligation to society. Each philosophy provides a unique view of nursing practice.

Nursing models are the frameworks or paradigms of the science of nursing that address the person, environment, health, and nursing metaparadigm. Nursing theories that are derived from models are guiding structures for reasoning about the person as well as about the determinants of nursing action. What this means in terms of nursing practice is that the way you think about people and about nursing has a direct impact on how you approach people, what questions you ask, how the information that is learned is processed, and what nursing activities are included in nursing care. Therefore a model provides a perspective of the person for whom you are caring, specifies the approach to be taken in the delivery of care, and is a structure for critical thinking, reasoning, and decision making in practice.

Theories are also sets of concepts, but they are less broad and propose more specific outcomes. Theories may have been derived from a philosophy, nursing model, or other model or framework. Theories guide propositions or relationship statements that are consistent with theoretical works from which they are derived, but a theory (e.g., Theory of Accelerating Change, Theory of the Person as an Adaptive System, Theory of Goal Attainment, or Theory of Health as Expanding Consciousness) proposes an outcome that is more specific. When you approach people from the perspective of a certain nursing theory and ask questions, process information, and carry out activities in a certain way, a specific outcome is anticipated based on the application of that theory. Therefore the outcome is directly related to the theory you are using to guide the delivery of nursing care.

Middle-range theory is the least abstract in the structure of knowledge. Grand theories are especially useful for the development of middle-range theory. Rogers' Theory of Accelerating Change, Roy's Theory of the Person as an Adaptive System, and King's Theory of Goal Attainment are considered grand theories because of their broad, abstract levels and the close relationship of the theory to the models from which they are derived. When a theory is at the grand theory level, many applications of that theory can be made in practice at the middle-range level by specifying such factors as the age of the patient, the situation, the health condition, the location, or the action of the nurse. This process of specifying the details of the theory makes it less abstract and less broad; therefore it applies to specific types of patients and makes specific propositions about the outcome of care.

Each philosophy provides a unique view for nursing practice. Similarly, each model provides a unique, comprehensive view of nursing. Likewise, the theories derived from the model have propositions that are specific to the theory and are also consistent with the view of the model. Middle-range theory, which is the least abstract level, may be derived from the philosophy, model, grand theory, or theory level. The relationship of these nursing theoretical works is best illustrated by reviewing the examples of each of them included in this text.

Philosophies

Philosophies set forth the meaning of nursing and nursing phenomena through reasoning and logical presentation of ideas. They provide broad general views of nursing that clarify values in answer to broad disciplinary questions. Three nursing philosophies have been selected for discussion here because they represent differing philosophical views of nursing (Alligood, 2000). Examples of philosophies of nursing may be seen in the works of Nightingale (1946), Watson (1979), and Benner (1984).

Nightingale's Philosophy of Nursing. Nightingale provides an answer to the question *what is nursing?* in her often-cited work *Nursing: What it is and What it is Not* (1946). In that work, Nightingale describes nursing as distinct from the household servant, draws a contrast between nursing and medicine, and specifies nursing's concern for health rather than illness. Within this work are directives for her unique theoretical perspective, which focused on the relationship of patients and their surroundings under the categories of pure air, pure water, efficient drainage, cleanliness, and light. Other discussions include diet, cleanliness, noise, rest, and the nurse's responsibility for protection and management of the care of the patient. Nightingale's work is relevant to current nursing practice, as is reflected by the nursing literature. For example, Corbett (1998) used Nightingale's ideas to critique nursing education according to the British National Health Service. Whall, Shin, and Colling (1999) suggest that Nightingale's emphasis on environment in health promotion is evident in general nursing in the United States and propose a Nightingale basis for a middle-range theory of dementia care in Korea. Bolton describes her nursing practice using Nightingale as a guide and illustrates with case applications in Chapter 5.

Watson's Philosophy of Nursing. Watson's work (1979) provides a unique approach to nursing as first set forth in *Nursing: The Philosophy and Science of Caring.* In her work, which is recognized as a human science, she has called for a return to earlier values of nursing, which emphasize its caring aspects (Watson, 1988). In this philosophical work, she sets forth theoretical propositions for the human-to-human relationships of nursing and specifies ten carative factors to guide its application in nursing practice. Transpersonal caring is the proposed approach to achieve connectedness in which the nurse and the patient change together. Emphasis is on harmony for unity in body, mind, and soul, and illness is seen as disharmony as the nurse and the patient participate together in relationship. Watson's work has been used to support conceptualizations of general practice (Chambers, 1998), psychiatric-mental health nursing practice (Tilley, 1995), and recently to address the caring needs of patients with rheumatoid arthritis (Nyman & Lutzen, 1999). McGraw discusses Watson's work in nursing practice and illustrates with case applications in Chapter 6.

Benner's Philosophy of Nursing. Benner (1984) provides a philosophical view of nursing practice that is focused on how the knowledge of practice is acquired and how it develops over time. In this way her work might be viewed as personal knowing using Carper's patterns (1978). Her interpretive research led to a description of the progression of nurses from novice to expert and an awareness of the importance of caring in nursing. Benner's work has been used to guide the examination of nursing practice innovations and changes. For example, it was used to examine threats to individualized care posed by critical pathways (Walsh, 1997). Alcock (1996) used Benner's work to study advanced practice nursing from an administrative point of view. Similarly, Dunn (1997) used it to examine advanced practice nursing in the nursing literature. Recently, Benner, Hooper-Kyriakidis, and Stannard (1999) published a book titled *Clinical Wisdom and Interventions in Critical Care: A Thinking in Action Approach.* Brykczynski reviews Benner's work, illustrates with case presentations, and discusses the interpretive approach to nursing practice in Chapter 7.

Nursing Models

Nursing conceptual models (or frameworks) provide a comprehensive view and guide for nursing practice. They are broad conceptual structures, and each provides a holistic view or perspective of nursing. They are organizing frameworks that guide the decision making of critical thinking in the processes of nursing (Alligood, 1997; Fawcett, 1995). This section reviews seven nursing models specified by Fawcett (1995).

Johnson's Behavioral System Model. When practicing nursing with the behavioral system model, the nurse views the person as a system of behaviors (Johnson, 1980). The actions and responses of the person comprise a system of interacting subsystems. Therefore assessment of the subsystems leads to an understanding of the whole behavior of the patient. Seven subsystems are identified to understand the activities of the person (Box 3-1).

BOX 3-1	SUBSYSTEMS OF JOHNSON'S BEHAVIORAL SYSTEM MODEL

1. Attachment or affiliative
2. Dependency
3. Ingestive
4. Eliminative
5. Sexual
6. Aggressive
7. Achievement

Three theories from Johnson's Behavioral System Model are listed in Box 3-2. The Theory of the Person as a Behavioral System is an implied grand theory of the model that has not been formalized. Two middle-range theories have been derived from the model: the Theory of a Restorative Subsystem (Grubbs, 1974), proposed as an additional subsystem to the seven subsystem model developed by Johnson, and the Theory of Sustenal Imperatives developed by Holaday, Turner-Henson, and Swan (1997) and based on the work of Holaday (1974) and Grubbs (1974). Holaday illustrates the application of this model and theory in nursing practice in Chapter 8.

BOX 3-2 THEORIES DERIVED FROM JOHNSON'S BEHAVIORAL SYSTEM MODEL

Theory of the person as a behavioral system
Theory of restorative subsystem (Grubbs, 1974)
Theory of sustenal imperatives (Holaday, Turner-Henson, & Swan, 1997)

King's Systems Framework. Nurses practicing with King's systems framework think in terms of three interacting systems: a personal system, an interpersonal system, and a social system (King 1971, 1981, 1995a, 1995b). Nursing practice in this framework is interactive, with the nurse viewing the patient as a personal system with interpersonal and social systems. King identifies each of the systems with a group of concepts, that, when considered together, specify the process of that system. The concepts of the three systems are presented in Box 3-3.

BOX 3-3 SYSTEM CONCEPTS OF KING'S SYSTEMS FRAMEWORK

Personal System	Interpersonal System	Social System
Perception	Interaction	Power
Self	Communication	Authority
Growth and development	Transaction	Status
Body image	Stress	Decision making
Time and space	Role	Role
		Organization

King (1981) developed the Theory of Goal Attainment from her own systems framework. Her theory that perceptual congruence and trans-actions in the nurse-patient interaction lead to the nursing outcome of goal attainment has been used in different areas of nursing practice (Alligood, 1995; Hanna, 1995) and more recently has been applied in case management (Tritsch, 1998). Other theories (Box 3-4) have been derived from King's systems framework by Frey (1989), Sieloff (1991, 1995), Brooks and Thomas (1997), and Alligood and May (2000). Frey and Norris present case applications in Chapter 9.

> **BOX 3-4   THEORIES DERIVED FROM KING'S SYSTEMS FRAMEWORK**
>
> Theory of goal attainment (King, 1981)
> Theory of social support and health (Frey, 1989)
> Theory of departmental power (Sieloff, 1991, 1995)
> Theory of perceptual awareness (Brooks & Thomas, 1997)
> Theory of personal system empathy (Alligood & May, 2000)

Levine's Conservation Model. Nursing practice with the conservation model and principles focuses on conserving the patient's energy for health and healing (Levine 1967, 1991). The principles (Box 3-5) constitute conservation for the whole person when considered together.

> **BOX 3-5   LEVINE'S CONSERVATION PRINCIPLES**
>
> 1. Conservation of energy
> 2. Conservation of structural integrity
> 3. Conservation of personal integrity
> 4. Conservation of social integrity

Three theories have been derived from Levine's model (Box 3-6). The first is a grand theory of conservation, which is implicit from the model and principles but has not yet been fully explicated. Two middle-range theories have been proposed by Levine: the Theory of Redundancy, which explains the fail-safe systems of the human body, and the Theory of Therapeutic Intention. Of these two theories, the Theory of Thera-peutic Intention has been noted by Schaefer (1991) as very relevant to nursing practice because of its linkage to intervention. She has practiced with Levine's model, principles, and theories and has written about their use in research, education, and practice. She illustrates the utilization of Levine's model and conservation principles in nursing practice with case applications in Chapter 10.

BOX 3-6	THEORIES DERIVED FROM LEVINE'S MODEL

Theory of conservation
Theory of therapeutic intention
Theory of redundancy

Neuman's Systems Model. When practicing nursing with the Neuman's Systems Model (1972, 1982, 1989, 1995), the nurse thinks of the client in terms of a system of variables interacting with the environment while focusing on stressors as they relate to client health. The nurse views the client with a central core of five variables: physiological, psychological, sociocultural, developmental, and spiritual. The variables interact systematically with the lines of resistance, normal line of defense, and the flexible line of defense as the client system acts or responds in a wholistic manner with intrapersonal, interpersonal, and extrapersonal stressors.

Two theories (Box 3-7) have been derived from the model: the Theory of Optimal Client Stability and the Theory of Prevention as Intervention (Neuman, 1995). The Theory of Optimal Client Stability is very useful with multiple client changes. The Theory of Prevention as Intervention is inherent in the systematic model because interventions are focused on increasing awareness of stress and stress reduction for a prevention outcome. Both theories are useful in practice because nursing action is linked to a nursing outcome for the client. These broad theories have numerous applications when age, health status, and nature of stressors are specified. Sohier demonstrates the application of Neuman's Systems Model in Chapter 11.

BOX 3-7	THEORIES DERIVED FROM NEUMAN'S SYSTEMS MODEL

Theory of optimal client stability
Theory of prevention as intervention

Orem's Conceptual Model. Nursing practice according to Orem's conceptual model (Orem, 1971, 1980, 1985, 1991, 1995) is a deliberate action of the nurse who views patients in terms of their self-care capacity. The concepts of Orem's model of nursing are presented in Box 3-8.

BOX 3-8	CONCEPTS OF OREM'S MODEL	
Major Concepts		**Peripheral Concept**
Self-care		Basic conditioning factors
Self-care agency		
Therapeutic self-care demand		
Self-care deficit		
Nursing agency		
Nursing system		

Orem has specified the relationships of her concepts in a set of theories: self-care, self-care deficit, and nursing system (Box 3-9). These three theories articulate to form an overall theory Orem calls "Self-Care Deficit Theory" (Orem, 1995, p. 170). The three theories form a system of complementary theories to guide nursing action. The theories specify a system of self-care and therapeutic self-care demand in relation to self-care requisites (or patient variables) and nursing agency, which is the nurse variable. The conceptual model with the system of theories provides guidance specific to patient activity and nursing action whether the patient is capable of self-care or needs compensation of care. Berbiglia illustrates practice with Orem's theories in Chapter 12.

BOX 3-9	OREM'S THEORIES
Self-care deficit theory or general theory of nursing	
Theory of self-care deficit or dependent-care deficit	
Theory of self-care	
Theory of nursing systems	

Rogers' Science of Unitary Human Beings. When practice is based on the Science of Unitary Human Beings (Rogers, 1970, 1986, 1990, 1992), the systematic focus is the life process or pattern of the human being. The four concepts are openness, energy field, pattern, and pandimensionality. The three homeodynamic principles—helicy, resonancy, and integrality—describe the relationship of the main concepts.

Many theories have been derived from Rogers' Science of Unitary Human Beings. The conceptual system and its theories guide research, education, and practice. The first three theories listed in Box 3-10 were derived by Rogers. The Science of Unitary Human Beings has also been used by others to generate theory, as is noted in the box. In addition to testing the theories derived by the theorist (for example, Alligood [1991]), the researcher may also develop a theory from either the model or a grand theory already proposed (Alligood, 1991, 1997; Alligood & McGuire, 2000; Fawcett, 1993). Bultemeier's Theory of Perception of Dissonant Pattern (1993) is an example of a middle-range theory derived from Rogers' Theory of Accelerating Change and tested in women who reported experiencing premenstrual syndrome (PMS). In Chapter 13, Bultemeier illustrates the use of the Science of Unitary Human Beings in her nursing practice with women.

BOX 3-10 THEORIES DERIVED FROM ROGER'S SCIENCE OF UNITARY HUMAN BEINGS

Theory of accelerating change
Theory of paranormal phenomena
Theory of rhythmical correlates of change

Theory of health as expanding consciousness (Newman, 1994)
Theory of human becoming (Parse, 1992)
Theory of human field motion (Ference, 1986)
Theory of power (Barrett, 1989)
Theory of perceived dissonance (Bultemeier, 1993)
Theory of aging (Alligood, 1997)

Roy's Adaptation Model. When nursing practice is based on the adaptation model, the focus is on the person as an adaptive system (Roy 1980, 1984; Roy & Roberts, 1981; Roy & Andrews, 1991). Adaptation occurs through cognator and regulator control processes that lead to coping behavior in four modes: physiological, self-concept, role function, and interdependence.

Roy has developed a Theory of the Person as an Adaptive System, and each of the four modes is also presented as a theory (Box 3-11). In terms of their specificity to nursing practice, the Theory of the Person as an Adaptive System is a grand theory, and the theories of the four modes are middle-range theories specific to the modes of coping.

BOX 3-11   THEORIES DERIVED FROM ROY'S ADAPTATION MODEL

Theory of the person as an adaptive system
   Theory of the physiological mode
   Theory of the self-concept mode
   Theory of the interdependence mode
   Theory of the role function mode

Phillips (1994) tested a middle-range theory from Roy's Adaptation Model and her Theory of the Person as an Adaptive System. He formed a middle-range theory of adaptation of persons living with Acquired Immunodeficiency Syndrome (AIDS). His work is an example of how a middle-range theory derives from a grand theory and specifies an outcome (coping in the four modes) in a specific patient population (persons living with AIDS). In Chapter 14, Phillips illustrates the use of Roy's model and theories in nursing practice with two cases.

Nursing Theories

Nursing theories are another type of theoretical work in the structure of nursing knowledge. They are sets of related concepts that propose something that is testable, e.g., King's Theory of Goal Attainment. Theories are less abstract than models and are more prescriptive because they propose specific outcomes. Theories are usually named for the outcome they propose or for characteristics of their content, such as Newman's Theory of Health as Expanding Consciousness or Parse's Theory of Human Becoming (Alligood, 2000).

Orlando's Theory of Nursing Process. Orlando's early work (1961) was stated as a Theory of Effective Nursing Practice and later as a Theory of Nursing Process (Orlando, 1990). Her work is a specific theory about how nurses process observations and respond to patients based on inferences from the nurse-patient interaction. She differentiates automatic action from deliberate action and specifies the latter. Therefore her work is a practice theory specific to the process of interaction of the nurse and the patient. Recent references to Orlando's work include application in perioperative nursing (Rosenthal, 1996) and nursing administration (Schmieding, 1999). Schmieding discusses her practice with Orlando's framework and illustrates with case applications in Chapter 15.

Modeling and Role-Modeling Nursing Theory. Modeling and Role-Modeling (Erickson, Tomlin, & Swain, 1983) is a theory of nursing that is specific enough to guide nursing practice yet abstract enough for middle-range theories to be derived from it. This theory is derived from developmental, inherent needs and stressors and from adaptation theory. Nurses and patients are in relationship as nurses learn from patients about their worlds. As nurses and patients understand the situation more clearly, resources are identified and move patients toward the goal of self-care action to satisfy their needs. Applications to the nursing care of the elderly include a middle-range theory of hope (Curl, 1992) and measuring their self-care action (Hertz, 1991). M. Erickson discusses the use of this theory in her practice and illustrates with case applications in Chapter 16.

Mercer's Theory of Maternal Role Attainment. Mercer's theory (1986, 1995) is specific to maternity nursing and the attainment of the maternal role by new mothers and mothers-to-be. She attributes the base of her theory to Rubin (1984), a nurse who had been her professor and had worked in this area. Mercer's work is a systematic approach to the dynamics of the interrelationship among the parents and the infant. She has isolated stages and identified factors that impact the role to assist the nurse in determining where the mothers (or parents) are in their development as they progress toward maternal (or parental) role attainment. Her work is discussed and illustrated with case applications by Meighan in Chapter 17.

Leininger's Theory of Culture Care Diversity and Universality. Leininger's work (1991) is a theory specific to culture and transcultural nursing. The goal of transcultural nursing is to plan care based on culturally defined knowledge and use the plan to provide care that is culturally congruent. Her theory is broad; it addresses the cultural aspects of all of human life with particular attention to the practices of health and caring (Alligood, 2000). Leininger's theory not only recognizes the culture from which patients come but also the one encountered when they seek health services. Care is focused on culture care preservation, accomodations, or repatterning according to the patients' needs. Numerous expressions of caring, such as vigilance (Carr, 1998), the needs of nurses in perinatal death (Gardner, 1999), and those for the aphasic Navajo (Huttlinger & Tanner, 1994) have been identified. Morgan presents the application of Leininger's theory with case illustrations in Chapter 18.

Parse's Theory of Human Becoming. Parse's theory is derived from Rogers' Science of Unitary Human Beings and phenomenology and is designated as a human science. Her work is specific to the nurse-patient relationship and is focused on patients and their health. Parse clarifies nursing from medicine and contributes to the differentiation of the two disciplines. Nursing is posed as a profession in its own right that is focused on human becoming and health. She defines health as a cocreation with the universe for patients as they experience the being and becoming of life. Parse sets forth three descriptive principles: (1) proposing human meaning as a developing structure of valuing and imaging from which reality emerges through languaging, (2) proposing a patterned unity of person and universe in rhythm, and (3) proposing the cotranscendence as the human capacity to grow in process with the universe (Alligood, 2000; Parse, 1992). There are many practice applications of Parse's theory in the nursing literature cited in Chapter 19, in which Mitchell discusses Parse's theory, presents its use in nursing practice, and illustrates with case applications.

Newman's Theory of Health as Expanding Consciousness. Newman's work (1994) is a theory of health derived from Rogers' Science of Unitary Human Beings. Coming from Rogers' perspective, she proposes a life process pattern focus to understand health (and illness) in a new way (Alligood, 2000). Therefore her work specifies a redefinition of health based on its meaning of wholeness. The nurse interacts with patients and views them in terms of the pattern of their whole lives. This is learned in relation to time, space, and movement which are correlates of consciousness. When practicing with Newman's theory, the nurse emphasizes the relationship with patients and their perceptions of their health. The nurse participates with patients to facilitate their discovery of inner strength as consciousness of their patterns unfold. There are many applications of Newman's theory, such as in patients with breast cancer (Mock, 1998) and in family caregiving (Yamashita, 1998, 1999) in the nursing literature. Witucki discusses her use of Newman's theory in nursing practice with case applications in Chapter 20.

NURSING THEORETICAL WORKS AND CRITICAL THINKING

As the nursing profession development continues, it has become quite clear that critical thinking and professional nursing practice are inextricably linked. When nursing theory guides the critical thinking of the decision-making process, it brings the knowing and doing of the nurse together in a nursing framework. Therefore theory utilization is essential in this phase of the development of the nursing profession because theory provides the basis for the nurse's knowing as well as a structure to guide nursing action (Mitchell, 1992; Sparacino, 1991).

Kuhn (1970) has said that it is the study of the models or paradigms of a scientific discipline that primarily prepares students for practice as members of that professional community. The paradigm (model or framework) plays a vital role in practice because without a framework, all of the information that the professional encounters seems to be equally relevant. Therefore students studying to enter a professional discipline are introduced to the models or paradigms as an orientation to the approaches used in the practice of that discipline. Following an introduction and survey of the models, students are ready to choose the model or models they will use in their practice. It is in studying these models and practicing with them that students "learn their trade" (Kuhn, 1970, p. 43).

In the past, critical thinking has been included in nursing curricula, but it has moved to a position of prominence as a required criterion in the National League for Nursing criteria for Baccalaureate and Higher

Degree Programs accreditation (1992) and in the more recent CCNE standards of the American Association of Colleges of Nursing (1998). This emphasis on critical thinking is not limited to nursing. Critical thinking has become a prevalent topic and research focus recently in higher education. This is reflected in the formation of a National Council for Excellence in Critical Thinking Instruction. That council adopted the following definition of critical thinking as presented by Paul and Nosich (1991):

> Critical thinking is the intellectually disciplined process of actively and skillfully conceptualizing, applying, analyzing, synthesizing, or evaluating information gathered from, or generated by, observation, experience, reflection, reasoning, or communication, as a guide to belief and action (p. 4).

The fact that nursing is a profession that is carried out for a certain purpose, according to the laws governing nursing practice in each state, makes it a purposeful activity. Further, the fact that nursing is an activity that answers a social mandate to determine an outcome from intelligible reasoning permits nursing to meet the criterion required for critical or higher-order thinking.

"Elements of thought, macro-abilities, traits of mind or affective dimensions and intellectual standards" have been proposed as the domains of critical thinking (Paul & Nosich, 1991, pp. 2-3). Nursing theoretical works have been identified to guide the reasoning of critical thinking (Alligood, 1997; Field, 1987; Mayberry, 1991; Sorrentino, 1991). A comparison of the eight elements of thought in critical thinking and nursing thought with nursing models supports the premise as illustrated in Table 3-2.

TABLE 3-2 Comparison of Critical Thinking and Nursing Thought	
Elements of Thought in Critical Thinking	**Nursing Thought**
1. Purpose, goal, or end in view	Patient health
2. Question at issue or problem	Health at risk
3. Point of view/frame of reference	Whole persons
4. Empirical dimensions	Person, environment, health, and nursing
5. Conceptual dimensions	Derived from model
6. Assumptions	Derived from model
7. Implications	Derived from model
8. Inferences	Derived from model

In this theory utilization phase of the theory era, the continuous development of the discipline of nursing is becoming more evident. The process and content of nursing that have often been viewed separately are now folded together in a unique way in theory-guided critical thinking. We move beyond the nursing process emphasis as we have known it, with its linear focus on what the nurse does in relation to the physiology and social science views of the patient, to a view of the whole person and a nursing approach to practice.

All three of the processes—nursing process, research process, and theory development process—beg the question "process of whom or what?" But theory-guided practice based on a nursing framework provides answers the question as the framework specifies the content as well as the process of nursing practice and guides both the thought and the action together. Therefore when viewed in the context of nursing practice, these processes can be considered tools of practice.

Mayberry (1991) calls for a merging of models, theories, and nursing practice and says, "theories and models reveal the relationship of one part of nursing to another. They provide a systematic approach for thinking about nursing matters, for observing the nursing situation, and for interpreting what is seen in the practice setting" (p. 47). Levine (1995) has called for a demonstration of how theory illuminates care as it specifies a perspective of the person, nursing action, and an expected outcome. Utilization of theory in practice has been noted as its most important function (Stevens, 1984; in Sorrentino, 1991). Similarly, Kerlinger (1979) has said that "the most important influence on practice is theory" (p. 296). Therefore theory-guided critical thinking is foundational to nursing practice (Mitchell, 1992).

SELECTING A FRAMEWORK FOR NURSING PRACTICE

The information presented so far forms a basis for selecting a model or theory for practice. However, in addition to knowledge of philosophies, models, and theories and an understanding of how they relate and form critical thinking structures to guide nursing practice, there is one additional factor to consider in selecting a theory for nursing practice. There needs to be a "fit" between the values inherent in the framework and your personal values. Identification of your personal values and the values within the framework will help you identify the model best suited to your practice. It is important to select the model or theory thoughtfully because it will serve as a tool for the reasoning process of your professional practice.

You may find that writing a brief philosophy of nursing clarifies your beliefs and values. This exercise can be done using the headings of *person, environment, health,* and *nursing* or other concepts that come to mind when you think about nursing and why you entered nursing. The process of thinking through and writing a philosophy forces you to consider the beliefs and values you truly hold. Once your beliefs are clarified, a survey of the definitions of *person, environment, health,* and *nursing* in the nursing theoretical works will lead you to particular works to be considered. Reviewing the assumptions of the philosophy, model, or theory and comparing them with your philosophy identifies linkage between the theoretical work and your values and beliefs. This process may be undertaken by considering whether the concepts in the theoretical work focus on ideas similar to the values expressed in your philosophy about the patient, environment, health, and nursing.

This survey and evaluation of various frameworks leads to the next step, which is to explore the particular philosophy, model, or theory in depth. This process is a bit like "trying them on." You should consider the frameworks that you have identified by making trial applications in selected areas of nursing practice. As you compare two or three frameworks on client focus, nursing action, and proposed outcome, you will find that a more in-depth understanding of the framework emerges. That is, using the framework in nursing practice expands your understanding and therefore your use of it. Also, you will want to review the nursing literature written by authors who use the frameworks in their practice and research. Reviewing applications in various areas of nursing practice highlights the flexibility of the model as you see its utility in these areas. Finally, select a nursing theoretical framework and develop its use for your practice. After you have practiced with the philosophy, model, or theory over time, it becomes more natural, and you can tailor it to the special aspects of your art of nursing. These guidelines (Box 3-12) may be used to identify a framework for theory-based nursing practice. The first step toward theory-guided practice is the decision to do so (Mathwig, 1975). It takes commitment to develop a base of understanding for professional nursing (Marriner-Tomey, 1998).

BOX 3-12 GUIDELINES FOR SELECTING A FRAMEWORK FOR NURSING PRACTICE

1. Consider values and beliefs truly held in nursing.
2. Write a philosophy of beliefs on person, environment, health, and nursing.
3. Survey definitions of person, environment, health, and nursing in the nursing models.
4. Select two or three frameworks that link best with your values.
5. Review the assumptions of the frameworks you have selected.
6. Make applications of those frameworks in a selected area of nursing practice (try them out).
7. Compare the frameworks on client focus, nursing action, and client outcome.
8. Review the nursing literature written by persons who have used the frameworks in nursing practice and research.
9. Select a framework and develop its use in your practice.

References

Alcock, D.S. (1996). The clinical nurse specialist, clinical nurse specialist/nurse practitioner, and other titled nurse in Ontario. *Canadian Journal of Nursing Administration, 9*(1), 23-44.

Alligood, M. R. (1991). Testing Rogers' Theory of Accelerating Change: The relationships among creativity, actualization, and empathy in persons 18-92 years of age. *Western Journal of Nursing Research, 13*(1), 84-96.

Alligood, M. R. (1995). Theory of Goal Attainment: Application to adult orthopedic nursing. In M. Frey & C. Sieloff (Eds.), *Advancing King's systems framework and theory of nursing* (pp. 209-222). Thousand Oaks, CA: Sage.

Alligood, M. R. (1997). Models and theories: Critical thinking structures. In M. R. Alligood & A. Marriner-Tomey (Eds.). *Nursing theorists and their work* (4th ed., pp. 31-45). St. Louis: Mosby.

Alligood, M. R. & Choi, E. C. (1998). Evolution of nursing theory development. In A. Marriner-Tomey (Ed.), *Nursing theorists and their work* (3rd ed., pp. 55-66). St. Louis: Mosby.

Alligood, M. R. (2000). Nursing theory: The basis for professional nursing practice. In K. K. Chitty (Ed.), *Issues in professional nursing* (3rd. ed., pp. 246-274). Philadelphia: W. B. Saunders.

Alligood, M. R. & May, B. (2000). A nursing theory of empathy discovered in King's personal system. *Nursing Science Quarterly, 13*(3), 243-247.

Alligood, M. R. & McGuire, S. (2000). Perception of time, sleep patterns, and activity in senior citizens: A test of a Rogerian Theory of Aging. *Visions: The Journal of Rogerian Nursing Science, 8*(1), 6-14.

Barrett, E. A. M. (1989). A theory of power for nursing practice: Derivation from Rogers' paradigm. In J. P. Riehl-Sisca (Ed.), *Conceptual models for nursing practice* (3rd ed., pp. 207-217). Norwalk, CT: Appleton & Lange.

Benner, P. (1984). *From novice to expert: Excellence and power in clinical nursing practice.* Menlo Park, CA: Addison-Wesley.

Benner, P., Hooper-Kyriakidis, P., & Stannard, D. (1999). *Clinical wisdom and interventions in critical care: A thinking in action approach.* Philadelphia: W. B. Saunders.

Brooks, E. M. & Thomas, S. (1997). The perception and judgment of senior baccalaureate student nurses in clinical decision making. *Advances in Nursing Science, 19,* 50-69.

Bultemeier, K. I. (1993). Photographic inquiry of the phenomenon premenstrual syndrome within a Rogerian-derived theory of perceived dissonance. Unpublished doctoral dissertation, University of Tennessee—Knoxville; Knoxville, Tennessee.

Carper, B. (1978). Fundamental patterns of knowing. *Advances in Nursing Science, 1*(1), 13-23.

Carr, J. M. (1998). Vigilance as a caring expression and Leininger's theory of cultural care diversity and universality. *Nursing Science Quarterly, 11*(2), 74-78.

Chambers, M. A. (1998). Some issues in the assessment of clinical practice: A review of the literature. *Journal of Clinical Nursing, 7*(3), 201-208.

Corbett, K. (1998). The captive market in nursing education and the displacement of nursing knowledge. *Journal of Advanced Nursing, 28*(3), 524-531.

Curl, E. D. (1992). Hope in the elderly: Exploring the relationship between psychosocial developmental residual and hope. Doctoral dissertation, University of Texas—Austin; Austin, Texas. *Dissertation Abstracts International, 47,* 992B.

Dunn, L. (1997). A literature review of advanced clinical nursing practice in the United States of America. *Journal of Advanced Nursing, 25*(4), 814-819.

Erickson, H., Tomlin, E., & Swain, M. (1983). *Modeling and role-modeling: A theory and paradigm for nursing.* Englewood Cliffs, NJ: Prentice-Hall.

Fawcett, J. (1989). *Analysis and evaluation of conceptual models of nursing* (3rd ed.). Philadelphia: F. A. Davis.

Fawcett, J. (1993). *Analysis and evaluation of nursing theories.* Philadelphia: F. A. Davis.

Fawcett, J. (1995). *Analysis and evaluation of conceptual models of nursing* (3rd ed.). Philadelphia: F. A. Davis.

Fawcett, J. (2000). *Contemporary nursing knowledge: Conceptual models and theories.* Philadelphia: F. A. Davis.

Ference, H. (1986). The relationship of time experience, creativity traits, differentiation, and human field motion. In V. M. Malinski (Ed.), *Explorations on Martha Rogers' Science of Unitary Human Beings* (pp. 95-106). Norwalk, CT: Appleton-Century-Crofts.

Field, P. A. (1987). The impact of nursing theory on the clinical decision-making process. *Journal of Advanced Nursing, 12,* 563-571.

Frey, M. A. (1989). Social support and health: A theoretical formulation derived from King's conceptual framework. *Nursing Science Quarterly, 2,* 138-148.

Gardner, J. M. (1999). Perinatal death: Uncovering the needs of midwives and nurses and exploring helpful interventions in the United States, England, and Japan. *Journal of Transcultural Nursing, 10*(2), 120-130.

Grubbs, J. (1974). An interpretation of the Johnson Behavioral System Model. In J. P. Riehl & C. Roy (Eds.), *Conceptual models for nursing practice* (pp. 160-197). Norwalk, CT: Appleton-Century-Crofts.

Hanna, K. M. (1995). Use of King's Theory of Goal Attainment to promote adolescents' health behavior. In M. A. Frey & C. L. Sieloff (Eds.), *Advancing King's systems framework and theory of nursing* (pp. 239-250). Thousand Oaks, CA: Sage.

Hertz, J. (1991). The perceived enactment of autonomy scale: Measuring the potential for self-care action in the elderly. Doctoral dissertation, University of Texas—Austin; Austin, Texas. *Dissertation Abstracts International, 52,* 1953B.

Holaday, B. (1974). Achievement behavior in chronically ill children. *Nursing Research, 23,* 25-30.

Holaday, B., Turner-Henson, A., & Swan, J. (1997). Explaining activities of chronically ill children: An analysis using the Johnson Behavioral System Model. In P. Hinton-Walker & B. Neuman (Eds.), *Blueprint for use of nursing models.* New York: National League for Nursing.

Huttlinger, K. W. & Tanner, D. (1994). The peyote way: Implications for culture care theory. *Journal of Transcultural Nursing, 5*(2), 5-11.

Johnson, D. E. (1980). The Behavioral System Model for nursing. In J. P. Riehl & C. Roy (Eds.), *Conceptual models for nursing practice* (pp. 207-216). Norwalk, CT: Appleton-Century-Crofts.

Kerlinger, F. N. (1979). *Behavioral research: A conceptual approach.* New York: Holt Rinehart & Winston.

King, I. (1971). *Toward a theory for nursing: General concepts of human behavior.* New York: John Wiley & Sons.

King, I. (1981). *A theory for nursing: Systems, concepts, process.* New York: John Wiley & Sons.

King, I. (1995a). A systems framework for nursing. In M. Frey & C. Sieloff (Eds.), *Advancing King's Systems Framework and theory of nursing* (pp. 14-22). Thousand Oaks, CA: Sage.

King, I. (1995b). The Theory of Goal Attainment. In M. Frey & C. Sieloff (Eds.), *Advancing King's Systems Framework and theory of nursing* (pp. 23-32). Thousand Oaks, CA: Sage.

Kuhn, T. S. (1970). *The structure of scientific revolutions* (2nd ed.). Chicago: University of Chicago Press.

Leininger, M. (1991). *Culture care diversity and universality: A theory of nursing.* New York: National League for Nursing.

Levine, M. E. (1967). The four conservation principles of nursing. *Nursing Forum, 6,* 45-59.

Levine, M. (1988). *The nursing theorist: Portraits of excellence.* [video]. Oakland, CA: Studio III.

Levine, M. E. (1991). The conservation principles: A model for health. In K. M. Schaefer & J. A. B. Pond (Eds.), *Levine's Conservation Model: A framework for nursing practice* (pp. 1-11). Philadelphia: F. A. Davis.

Levine, M. E. (1995). The rhetoric of nursing theory. *Image, 27*(1), 11-14.

Marriner-Tomey, A. (1998). Preface. In A. Marriner-Tomey & M. R. Alligood (Eds.), *Nursing theorists and their work* (4th ed., pp. xi-xii). St. Louis: Mosby.

Marriner-Tomey, A. & Alligood, M. R. (1998). *Nursing theorists and their work* (4th ed.). St. Louis: Mosby.

Marriner Tomey, A. & Alligood, M. R. (on press). *Nursing theorists and their work* (5th ed.). St. Louis.

Mathwig, G. (1975). Translation of nursing science theory to nursing education. In S. Ketefian (Ed.), *Translation of theory into nursing practice and education: Proceedings of the Seventh Annual Clinical Sessions.* Continuing Education in Nursing Division of School of Education, Health, Nursing, and Arts Professions, New York University.

Mayberry, A. (1991). Merging nursing theories, models, and nursing practice: More than an administrative challenge. *Nursing Administration Quarterly, 15*(3), 44-53.

Mercer, R. T. (1986). *First-time motherhood: Experiences from teens to forties.* New York: Springer.

Mercer, R. T. (1995). *Becoming a mother.* New York: Springer.

Mitchell, G. (1992). Specifying the knowledge base of theory in practice. *Nursing Science Quarterly, 5*(1), 6-7.

Mock, S. D. (1998). Health-within-illness: Concept development through research and practice. *Journal of Advanced Nursing, 28*(2), 305-310.

National League for Nursing. (1992). *Criteria and guidelines for the evaluation of baccalaureate and higher degree programs in nursing* (7th ed.). New York: Author.

Neuman, B. &Young, R. (1972). A model for teaching total person approach to patient problems. *Nursing Research, 21,* 264-269.

Neuman, B. (1982). *The Neuman Systems Model.* Norwalk, CT: Appleton-Century-Crofts.

Neuman, B. (1989). *The Neuman Systems Model* (2nd ed.). Norwalk, CT: Appleton & Lange.

Neuman, B. (1995). *The Neuman Systems Model* (3rd ed.). Norwalk, CT: Appleton & Lange.

Newman, M. (1994). *Health as expanding consciousness.* (2nd ed.). New York: Nursing League for Nursing.

Nightingale, F. (1946). *Notes on nursing: What it is and what it is not.* Philadelphia: J. B. Lippincott.

Nyman, C. S. & Lutzen, K. (1999). Caring needs of patients with rheumatoid arthritis. *Nursing Science Quarterly, 12*(2), 164-169.

Orlando, I. (1961). *The dynamic nurse-patient relationship: Function, process, and principles.* New York: G. P. Putnam's Sons.

Orlando, I. (1990). *The dynamic nurse-patient relationship: Function, process, and principles.* New York: National League for Nursing.

Orem, D. E. (1971). *Nursing: Concepts of practice.* New York: McGraw-Hill.

Orem, D. E. (1980). *Nursing: Concepts of practice* (2nd ed.). New York: McGraw-Hill.

Orem, D. E. (1985). *Nursing: Concepts of practice* (3rd ed.). New York: McGraw-Hill.

Orem, D. E. (1991). *Nursing: Concepts of practice* (4th ed.). St. Louis: Mosby.

Orem, D. E. (1995). *Nursing: Concepts of practice* (5th ed.). St. Louis: Mosby.

Parse, R. (1992). Human becoming: Parse's theory of nursing. *Nursing Science Quarterly, 5,* 35-42.

Paul, R. W. & Nosich, G. M. (1991). *Proposal for the national assessment of higher-order thinking, revised version.* Washington, DC: The United States Department of Education Office of Educational Research and Improvement, National Center for Education Statistics.

Phillips, K. D. (1994). Testing biobehavioral adaptation in person living with AIDS using Roy's Theory of the Person as an Adaptive System. Unpublished doctoral dissertation, University of Tennessee—Knoxville; Knoxville, Tennessee.

Reynolds, P. (1971). *A primer in theory construction.* Indianapolis: Bobbs-Merril.

Rogers, M. E. (1970). *An introduction to the theoretical basis of nursing.* Philadelphia: F. A. Davis.

Rogers, M. E. (1986). Science of Unitary Human Beings. In V. M. Malinski (Ed.), *Explorations on Martha Rogers' Science of Unitary Human Beings* (pp. 3-8). Norwalk, CT: Appleton & Lange.

Rogers, M. E. (1990). Nursing: Science of unitary, irreducible, human beings: Update 1990. In E. A. M. Barrett (Ed.), *Visions of Rogers' science-based nursing* (pp. 5-11). New York: National League for Nursing.

Rogers, M. E. (1992). Nursing science and the space age. *Nursing Science Quarterly, 5,* 27-34.

Rosenthal, B. C. (1996). An interactionist's approach to perioperative nursing. *Association of Operating Room Nurses Journal, 64*(2), 254-260.

Roy, C. (1980). The Roy Adaptation Model. In J. P. Riehl & C. Roy (Eds.), *Conceptual models for nursing practice* (2nd ed., pp. 179-188). Norwalk, CT: Appleton-Century-Crofts.

Roy, C. (1984). *Introduction to nursing: An adaptation model* (2nd ed.). Englewood Cliffs, NJ: Prentice-Hall.

Roy, C. & Andrews, H. (1991). *The Roy Adaptation Model: The definitive statement.* Norwalk, CT: Appleton & Lange.

Roy, C. & Roberts, S. L. (1981). *Theory construction in nursing: An adaptation model.* Englewood Cliffs, NJ: Prentice-Hall.

Rubin, R. (1984). *Maternal identity and the maternal experience.* New York: Springer.

Schaefer, K. (1991). Levine's conservation principles and research. In K. M. Schaefer & J. A. B. Pond (Eds.), *Levine's Conservation Model: A framework for nursing practice* (pp. 45-59). Philadelphia: F. A. Davis.

Schmieding, N. J. (1999). Reflective inquiry framework for nurse adminstrators. *Journal of Advanced Nursing, 30*(3), 631-639.

Sieloff, C. (1991). *Imogene King: A conceptual framework for nursing.* Thousand Oaks, CA: Sage.

Sieloff, C. (1995). Development of a theory of departmental power. In M. Frey & C. Sieloff (Eds.), *Advancing King's Systems Framework and theory of nursing* (pp. 46-65). Thousand Oaks, CA: Sage.

Sorrentino, E. A. (1991). Making theories work for you. *Nursing Administration Quarterly, 15*(3), 54-59.

Sparacino, P. (1991). The reciprocal relationship between practice and theory. *Clinical Nurse Specialist, 5*(3), 138.

Tilley, S. (1995). Notes on narrative knowledge in psychiatric nursing. *Journal of Psychiatric and Mental Health Nursing, 2*(4), 217-226.

Tritsch, J. M. (1998). Application of King's Theory of Goal Attainment and the Carondelet St. Mary's case management model. *Nursing Science Quarterly, 11*(2), 69-73.

Walsh, M. (1997). Will critical pathways replace the nursing process? *Nursing Standard, 11*(52), 39-42.

Watson, J. (1979). *Nursing: The philosophy and science of caring.* Boston: Little, Brown.

Watson, J. (1988). *Nursing: Human science human care.* New York: National League for Nursing.

Whall, A. L., Shin, Y., & Colling, K. (1999). A Nightingale-based model for dementia care and its relevance for Korean nursing. *Nursing Science Quarterly, 12*(4), 319-323.

Yamashita, M. (1998). Newman's Theory of Health as Expanding Consciousness: Research on family caregiving in mental illness in Japan. *Nursing Science Quarterly, 11*(3), 110-115.

Yamashita, M. (1999). Newman's theory of health applied in family caregiving in Canada. *Nursing Science Quarterly, 12*(1), 73-79.

Philosophies, Models, and Theories: Moral Obligations

Pamela J. Grace

"The end or purpose of nursing is the well-being of other people . . . it is a moral end. That is, it involves the seeking of a good, and it involves relationships with other human beings. The science learned and the technical skills developed are designed and shaped by this moral end." (From Curtin, L. & Flaherty, M. J. [1982]. Nursing ethics: Theories and pragmatics. *Bowie, MD: Brady Communications, Prentice Hall. Reprinted by permission of Pearson Education, Inc. Upper Saddle River, NJ 07458.)*

This chapter discusses the moral obligations inherent in nursing's theoretical works. An underlying assumption of this section is that nursing is a moral undertaking. This assumption is defensible because of the nursing profession's promise to provide a vital service to society. It proposes that it can address certain needs associated with human functioning. Thus nursing can be said to further a good for individuals and for society. The idea that nursing is engaged in providing for a good makes nursing actions worthy of moral criticism. We can say that these actions are good or bad, praiseworthy or blameworthy, to the degree that they honestly focus on advancing nursing's purpose.

It follows, then, that theory-guided practice, beyond helping to determine what is, in general, also assists the individual nurse in deciding appropriate courses of action for ethical practice in a variety of diverse situations. Additionally, theory-guided practice is able to suggest further responses when a problem appears to be beyond the student's or the nurse's singular ability to resolve it (Kenney, 1999).

An examination of nursing viewed as a moral endeavor is appropriately addressed via the explications of nursing's theorists and scholars.

This is so because theorizing in nursing is aimed at two main ends: (1) to describe and explain nursing, and (2) to provide a structure or framework that facilitates practice, research, and practitioner education. Within each of the theoretical works can be found moral implications and imperatives for the student, practitioner, researcher, or educator.

The moral concerns of nursing as a practice profession are derived primarily from the works of these original thinkers, who realistically can be considered nursing's philosophers. Whereas general philosophy engages in the search for knowledge or wisdom about humans and the world in which they find themselves, nursing philosophy has a more particular focus. Nursing philosophies attempt to answer the question "What is nursing?" as well as a related significant question—"Why is nursing important to human beings?" It is the task of other parts of this book to look at practice directed by various philosophical and theoretical frameworks and the purpose of a companion text by Marriner Tomey and Alligood (2002) to delineate more clearly the formulations of nursing's theorists and the distinctions among them. This chapter draws on such literature in an effort to clarify the moral responsibilities and obligations that accompany philosophically founded practice.

GUIDED PRACTICE

It has been said of nurses who do not suppose themselves to be practicing according to theory that they are in fact using some sort of internalized guide. That is, the individual is using a personal philosophy or theory to direct practice. Such frameworks also have inherent moral components. The tenets or assumptions of a personal or nonnursing framework used for nursing practice require examination for congruency with nursing's purpose. Critics have rightly questioned the capacity of such personal frameworks to adequately accomplish nursing's purposes. It is unlikely that individual nurses have engaged in the sort of rigorous investigation and analysis undertaken by nursing theorists in formulating their views; therefore the capacity of such practice to be consistent is questionable. Thus the following discussion is available to nurses who are openly utilizing the ideas of a theorist to guide practice and to those who are not—or at least are not at present.

The bases for nursing practice have been explicated in one or more of the following forms: philosophies, conceptual models, and/or theories. For simplicity and from this point forward in the chapter, when it is necessary to refer simultaneously to the terms *philosophies, models,* and *theories,* they will be grouped under the term *theoretical works.* An elucidation of the distinctions and relationships among these terms were introduced in Chapter 3 and are also discussed in Fawcett's writings (1993, 1995). Critiques regarding the validity of these distinctions are also available (Chinn & Kramer, 1995; Meleis, 1991). It is, however, generally understood that where distinctions are made, the conceptual progression of the theoretical works is from more abstract to less abstract. Philosophies are more abstract than conceptual models, which in turn are more abstract than theories. It should also be understood that a particular theorist may have developed a conceptual model and a theory or theories from a foundational philosophy or from a synthesis of one or more philosophies.

THE MORAL ENDEAVOR

The use of philosophies, models, and theories as guides for nursing practice and the reverse influence of practice experiences on theory development are factors critical to the development of nursing's knowledge base and thus to the maturation and evolution of the discipline. However, the importance of the discipline's contribution to the health of individuals and to the overall health of society is what makes nursing itself not just a practical but also a moral endeavor, as has been noted. It is worth reiterating at this point that the activity of nursing should be considered a moral endeavor because health is a human good; it is something valued by individuals and society. This main objective of the profession—to further health or well-being—constitutes nursing's promise to society. It is publicly articulated in codes of practice such as the American Nurses Association's (ANA) *Code for Nurses* (1985), the International Council of Nurses' (ICN) *Code for Nurses* (1973), and a variety of codes that have been developed in and thus speak more specifically to the cultural norms of other countries. Codes of ethics, as noted elsewhere, might be conceived of as the tentative end results of an evolving profession's political process (Grace, 1998). This is because codes of ethics are formulated as a result of a given profession's intradisciplinary conversations over time; they publicly articulate the purpose and the manner in which its services will be furnished to society. Therefore the influence of both scholars and practitioners of nursing—and, more indirectly, society—is brought to bear upon the formulation of codes of ethics for a discipline.

Codes of ethics are subject to change over time and in response to societal needs (Grace & Gaylord, 1999a). For this reason they are somewhat reflective of what society expects of the profession in question. Viens (1989) presents a good historical account of the development of the ANA's code over the last century. Although the ANA code provides guidelines for U.S. nurses, its pertinence to global nursing is unclear. The ANA periodically updates its code and is in the process of reformulation presently. An opportunity was provided for nurses to provide input as these changes were being considered. Because nursing's involvement in global health issues is a current and important topic of debate in the literature and other fora, it will be interesting to see whether global nursing issues have been addressed (Grace & Gaylord, 1999b; Ketefian & Redman, 1997; Kleffel, 1996).

It therefore becomes important to note that the scope of the present task, which is to uncover the moral responsibilities associated with theory-based practices, is somewhat broad. The moral implications of practicing according to a given theorist's works involve all of the following: individual, group, community, societal, and perhaps—although more debatably—global considerations. Both the writings of nursing's theorists and the profession's codes of ethics prove useful in highlighting the moral responsibilities of practice.

Health as a Metaparadigm Concept

Nursing's metaparadigm also proves important to the present discussion because the metaparadigm concepts are those "that identify the phenomena of interest to the discipline" (Fawcett, 1993, p. 2). They set out or identify the scope of concern for the profession. References to four concepts—*health, person, environment,* and *nursing* (viewed as a verb or action rather than as the discipline)—are explicitly or implicitly present in the writings of almost all of nursing's philosophers and/or theorists. One of the metaparadigm concepts, health, is (although perhaps arguably) a designator for nursing's main purpose with regard to the population of concern. How health is viewed and addressed depends, of course, on the particular theorist's definition, which will stem from a philosophy regarding the nature of human beings and of the world in which they find themselves or of which they are parts. Because the metaparadigm concepts are at a very high level of abstraction (Fawcett, 1993), they themselves do not provide guidance to the practitioner. They do, however, as already noted, delineate the scope of nursing's foci of concern.

It is from the description or definition of health, along with those of environment, person, and nursing as given by the nursing scholars that direction is provided for the practitioner. The characteristics of the metaparadigm concepts may be explicit in the scholar's writings, or they may be implicit. Thus actions taken by a nurse to further health may also vary in accordance with the philosophy, model, or theory used to guide practice, depending on a nurse's personal philosophy or belief system. It becomes important, then, that not only the philosophical and theoretical implications but also the moral implications of practicing according to a certain perspective are understood by nurses. Understanding is required because nursing actions that stem from a certain viewpoint may be inadequate for this purpose for a variety of reasons, although they are directed at fostering health.

Moral Implications of Philosophically or Theoretically Guided Practice

A grasp of the implications of certain viewpoints gives nurses the capacity for adjusting practice in such a way as to most consistently address health for the individual, group, or society. If the ramifications of a given perspective seem dissonant with any of or any combination of (1) the context or situation, (2) the nurse's philosophy, or (3) the patient's philosophy or beliefs, then the nurse has two main responsibilities. First, it is necessary to check that the framework is indeed being utilized as it was intended. An inadequate grasp of both the framework and its implications for practice has the potential for poor or inconsistent practice. Second, it is important to investigate whether it is the case that another framework is a better fit for the setting, the patient's situation and/or beliefs about health, or the practitioner's beliefs. Logically, then, it follows that practicing according to a well established theoretical framework generally results in more consistent and better care than does practice without such guides, even in those cases in which there is some disagreement about the underlying philosophical assumptions. Finally, a nurse who does choose to avoid the use of any of the discipline's theoretical structures in favor of a personal one should be capable both of articulating what this is and of justifying its use. One way to do this is by demonstrating that it leads to consistent practice and that it is capable of furthering the profession's purpose. Thus the practices of such nurses are also subject to moral critique.

There are a variety of reasons why a nurse who purports to be grounding practice in a given philosophical and/or theoretical point of view might be faced with or, worse, is ignorant of resulting problems. The following section provides a brief discussion of possible issues for nurses and for those receiving (or not receiving, as the case may be) care. The major questions that present themselves are important for theorists, practitioners, educators, and researchers as well as for students of nursing. They concern, among other things, the moral responsibilities or, more strongly, *obligations* attendant upon theory-based practice. This list is not intended to be exhaustive but rather to clarify some of the moral problems associated with directed practice.

MAJOR QUESTIONS FOR THEORY-BASED PRACTICE

In Chapter 3, the idea of theoretical frameworks as critical thinking structures was introduced. There it was noted that the first obligation of any nurse in selecting a framework for practice is reflection. The nurse reflects on the congruence of a personal philosophy of nursing with the underlying philosophical assumptions of the theorist. Examples of how this is accomplished are presented in the following sections. The next consideration entails an exploration of the specific responsibilities and/or obligations of a nurse practicing according to a particular theoretical or philosophical perspective. For example, nurses must ask themselves the following questions:

- What are my responsibilities to be faithful to the original intent of the theorist?
- What is the fit between the context of my practice and the framework I wish to use?
- To what am I committed by using this perspective?
- What further obligations exist when I find myself unable to practice according to the spirit of my chosen framework?
- Are there further obligations explicit or implicit in the guiding framework or philosophy when obstacles to practice present themselves?

These questions have serious implications for nursing's purpose of addressing health in whatever manner it is conceptualized by the philosopher or theorist. Thus they all represent crucial moral considerations for a nursing student, practitioner, researcher, or educator because health itself is defined differently in the various works.

Philosophical Fit

In addition to the guide presented in Chapter 3, several other authors have proposed helpful criteria for selecting a model or theory to use as a practice guide (Christensen, 1996; Kim, 1994; McKenna, 1997; Meleis, 1997). However, a fundamental concern of nurses, as stated earlier, is to ensure that their personal philosophies about the nature of human beings are congruent with the underlying philosophy of the theory. This is necessary because a philosophy, as Salsberry (1994) points out, "relates nursing to a particular world view" (p. 13). It highlights values that provide direction for practice and therefore for the practitioner (Salsberry, 1994). The following example illustrates this point. If a nurse's beliefs about human nature are that human beings are "bio-psycho-social beings" (Roy, 1980, p. 180), but he or she tries to practice according to Rogers' framework, which views persons as irreducible wholes (Rogers, 1987), there is a value mismatch. Thus there will also be some incoherence in practice. Practice incoherence not only interferes with the logical reasoning of the nurse but also has implications for the furtherance of health for the practice population.

The questions one asks of Roy's patients are framed in terms of the person viewed as a complex whole who behaves adaptively to changing (internal or external) environments (Andrews & Roy, 1991). Therapeutic nursing actions and the effects of these upon the individual are thus aimed at assisting adaptation. A nurse whose philosophical beliefs are more consistent with Rogers' view of persons as irreducible wholes that cannot be understood in terms of their parts will experience dissonance in trying to practice according Roy's framework. There are several reasons for the dissonance, not the least of which is that, in Rogers' view, a nurse is also an irreducible whole who brings this whole or self to the mutual interaction (Rogers, 1987) that is the nurse-patient relationship.

To label this as a moral problem for a nurse might seem extreme. However, if the aim of nursing action is health, both the definition of health and the approach to furthering it are dependent upon a particular philosophy and/or models and theories developed from it. To engage in therapeutic action stemming from one viewpoint while subscribing personally to another is likely to prove problematic in furthering nursing's purpose. This discussion highlights the importance of nurses having an in-depth awareness of their guiding frameworks. They should be capable both of explicating it and of comparing it with other theoretical works.

Commitment of the Framework

The pertinent parts of a given theoretical work may not be well understood by the practitioner who is using it. In such cases, practice is subject to inconsistency, as was noted earlier. Although it is understood that some inconsistency in practice will always exist because practice is necessarily contextual and thus affects practitioners no less than patients, nurses can, nevertheless, be held accountable for inadequate understanding of the framework they are utilizing. Accountability is a hallmark of professionals. Society has expectations of professionals, but if professionals are unable to at least make progress toward meeting these, then the very idea of professions becomes questionable. Newton (1988) has asserted that the professional "comprehends both the person ultimately served and the knowledge essential to the service in his perception of his obligations" (p. 49). This proposition has societal implications for several reasons. The discipline is both present- and future-oriented. It has strategies for addressing immediate problems and is concerned with predicting future areas of need. The person in question might be a potential rather than an actual patient. That is, a person may not yet be susceptible to formal identification because he or she is serving as a placeholder for one who has future nursing needs.

The knowledge that Newton's professional possesses varies. This draws attention to the idea that not only do frameworks guide practice, but they also guide knowledge development and knowledge acquisition for practitioners. Thus the use of theoretical works has moral implications not just for practice itself but for the education of practitioners and for research. This idea is explored later.

Newton's conceptualizations concerning professional activity are reflected in tenets of the ANA's *Code for Nurses* (1985). Practice inadequacy that results from misinterpretation, misrepresentation, or uninformed adaptation of any elements of the theoretical works or inadequate grasp of the prescriptions of one's personal framework is implicitly proscribed by the ANA's code. Plank 4 notes that "the nurse assumes responsibility and accountability for individual nursing judgments and actions," and Plank 5 asserts, "The nurse maintains competence in nursing." Many of the frameworks contain inherent guidelines, although these may be subtle, regarding what constitutes competence in the particular perspective.

For example, Nightingale's ideas about nursing, which have been classified as a philosophy (Marriner-Tomey & Alligood, 1998), had unmistakably moral foundations. Nightingale's work stemmed from a desire to serve humankind. She encouraged nurses to attend to the environment of the patient, who could be sick or well. Manipulation of a patient's environment was necessary to "put the patient in the best condition for nature to act upon him" (Nightingale, 1946, p. 74). Observation, experience, and reflection were required to both learn the laws of health and to apply them in practice (Nightingale, 1946). Furthermore, Nightingale's philosophy, evident both in her life work and in her writings, placed expectations on nurses to tackle the social forces that got in the way of "putting the patient in the best condition for nature to act upon him" (Nightingale, 1946, p. 74).

A professional nurse practicing according to Nightingale's philosophy would be committed both to gathering and analyzing data about a given patient's environment and, more broadly, to assessing the environment for its potential for making patients of persons either as yet unaffected or only at risk for an illness. Thus a nurse whose only interest is in handling immediate situations yet professes to attend to the environment of patients with smoking-related illnesses is committed to attend to the wider situation (Reed & Zurakowski, 1996). For example, a pulmonary rehabilitation nurse who is not interested in the problem of tobacco distribution and advertising is morally culpable from Nightingale's perspective. We may reaffirm here that a firm grasp of the implications of a given framework is a moral responsibility or moral obligation of the nurse.

Nightingale-style education of nurses would also necessarily include strategies that enable one to attend to the immediate situation and also to any wider environmental problems implicated. Political activity might well be within a nurse's domain of practice activity. The idea that nursing education includes the development of skills necessary for immediate practice and for political activity on behalf of actual or possible patients constitutes a moral obligation of nursing educators with regard to teaching theory-based practice that is based on Nightingale's perspective. Researchers, no less than educators, are subject to moral critique based on the questions they ask, the information they seek to uncover, and the methods they use. Moral critique, as noted throughout this chapter, is based on the idea that nursing as a discipline makes promises to society and may be criticized to the extent that it does or does not make efforts to keep its promises.

Keeping to the Theorist's Intent

Nurses who are very conversant with the intent of a given model or theory and who find the philosophical underpinnings congruent with their own views may nevertheless wish to do the following: (1) derive a middle-range theory that is more specific to a certain aspect of care or particular population (as described in Chapter 3), (2) take the theory further, (3) test it via research questions, and (4) apply it in practice situations. Once again, self-reflection is required to discover whether beliefs about persons, health, and environment are indeed pertinent to the particular situation.

It is also important to reflect collaboratively with others who have expertise in both the area of concern and in the theory to be used. One source for theoretical questions is the theorist herself, when this is possible. Contemporaneously, there is a growing number of scholars, including doctoral students, who have extended the work of various theorists. Some examples of these can be found in the later chapters of this text, in which a variety of clinical experts provide descriptions of their applications of specific theoretical works in practice. Additionally, there are various communities of scholars that have been formed for the express purposes of studying and/or furthering the works of a particular theorist. This self-reflection and reflection on the proposed project is a moral responsibility for the reasons given previously and because theory development and testing provide important contributions toward knowledge development for the profession and ultimately for the benefit of the population of concern.

Fit Between the Framework and Practice Context

Fit is an important consideration for theory-based practice. Professional nursing practice makes demands on a nurse to use knowledge and reasoning both in the choice of a guiding framework and in practice that stems from a framework. Although it is true that most of the theories will provide for consistent patient care, the setting and the nurse's personal value system may suggest a particular framework as best suiting both requirements. In deciding which theoretical work is a good fit for an individual's personal practice, the clinician should clearly understand the inherent moral implications of practicing according to this particular theorist's conceptions and in this particular setting. The majority of nursing's philosophers derived their frameworks as a result of engagement with specific populations. For example, Newman's emphasis (1986) on grasping human patterns might be difficult (although not necessarily impossible) to accomplish in an ambulatory surgery center because of time constraints. It is thus a responsibility of nurses to examine a variety of theories with which they have philosophical congruence to discover those that are best able to further nursing's goals in the specific setting.

There may be occasions when a nurse is faced with working on a floor or in a setting where practice is structured by a particular framework with which he or she is either not familiar or does not like. In the former case, one should familiarize oneself with the theoretical work to comprehend both in what manner it structures care for these patients and what the moral imperatives of the framework are. Take, for example, a neurological unit that has adopted Orem's framework (1991) as a guide for practice. Nurses on this floor are committed to assisting patients to regain self-care agency, when this is possible. Assisting patients with a variety of neurological impairments to meet therapeutic self-care demands (Orem, 1991) often requires more time and patience of a nurse than does the giving of total care or doing everything for the patient. However, it is a moral imperative of the framework that we take the longer route when this is what will best serve a patient viewed through Orem's lens. Obstacles to facilitating self-care, such as inadequate staffing or lack of appropriate supportive equipment, present an Orem nurse with further obligations to address these shortcomings. Such shortcomings may require a nurse to serve on policy-making committees or to become politically aware and active.

Even if a nurse has an aversion to a given framework, it may still be, as argued earlier, that the resulting care will be better than unstructured care. Nevertheless, if a nurse believes another framework will better address the needs of a particular patient population, then that nurse has further options. For example, some institutions, settings, or floors have adopted a nursing framework in an effort to ensure consistency in practice. This may pose a challenge for the nurse who has a personal philosophy that is incommensurable with the prevailing perspective. What are the nurse's responsibilities in this regard? This is a difficult question. First, and before employment, the nurse should try to ascertain what the philosophy of the institution is and whether the values are congruent with his or her personal views regarding nursing care. It is understood, however, that there may be occasions when employment choices are limited. In such instances, a nurse is faced with a difficult balancing decision. Second, a nurse can investigate whether the framework is actually being used correctly. Theoretical works, as previously argued, generally have the capacity to structure good nursing care. Third, a nurse can present a reasoned case for a change of framework or for the freedom to choose from a variety of frameworks.

If, however, there are serious concerns about whether the model being used to direct unit care has suffered distortion in institutional hands and/or is being used to serve institutional rather than patient needs, then this abuse needs to be addressed. For example, a professional nurse recently reported being asked by her employing institution (where Benner's work is used) to provide an exemplar that demonstrates her practice expertise. When she replied that she wasn't sure she could do this, she was asked by a superior, "You can embellish a story, can't you?" The institution was apparently collecting these exemplars as part of accreditation documentation. In such cases, it is a moral responsibility of the nurse to address this inaccurate and thus unethical use of nursing theory.

This may require supervisory help, or it may require seeking guidance from a professional group or organization. It is, however, a moral responsibility of the nurse to take appropriate steps toward addressing those problems that constitute either injustice or distortion of purpose and that ultimately find expression in the quality of patient care and the facilitation of health.

Finally, there may be obligations to discover whether a patient's beliefs and goals are congruent with the approach to care suggested by the particular framework the nurse is using. For example, a patient may believe that one accepts one's fate and that effects have causes that are beyond our control. This is a deterministic view. A patient with such beliefs might find a philosophical framework geared to assisting individuals to discover meaning in illness problematic, whereas one that attempts to alleviate suffering, address stressors, or help adaptation might be more appropriate. Thus among other obligations, it is also important to discover a given patient's view of health.

Inherent Moral Implications of Theoretical Works: Some Examples

Examples of the moral implications of several theoretical works have already been given throughout this part of the book. Some further examples are offered here to assist in addressing the questions posed earlier in the chapter. A crucial aspect of theory-guided practice for the nursing student, practitioner, researcher, or educator to consider, as noted throughout this chapter, involves understanding the commitments of the particular framework.

The pivotal hypothesis of Parse's Theory of Human Becoming (1992) is that "humans participate with the universe in the cocreation of health" (p. 37). In Parse's view, persons are free-willed and capable of making meaning from life. Health is defined as "lived value priorities" that cannot be judged as "good, bad, more, or less" (Parse, 1987, p. 159). Health is an existential concept related to personal evolution as persons select or create meaning from their interactions with the world in which they find themselves. Nursing is concerned with the patient's (or group's) process by "illuminating meaning, synchronizing rhythms, and mobilizing transcendence" (Parse, 1987, p. 167). The nurse is interactive with the patient. This interaction facilitates the patient's grasp of meaning in the situation or phenomenon. It is the patient, in this perspective, who decides the value of a given experience. A nurse practicing from Parse's framework is committed to this approach. She or he must guard against practicing from personal value priorities when these are at odds with the patient's priorities. For example, it may be that a nurse's beliefs include the idea that it is a patient's duty to hang on to life as long as possible. Perhaps the clinician's belief is that life is sacred and that this means one should never give up. However, if the patient is in the process of discovering that he or she is ready to stop life-sustaining treatment, then the nurse must continue to facilitate the patient's development of meaning rather than his or her own.

To understand Parse's theory is to grasp this fact. Practice will be erratic if the nurse uses Parse's theory for only part of her relationship with the patient. The nurse is morally committed to following through because this is what will best serve the patient's health as Parse conceptualizes it. Parse notes that her theory requires "special education" (1987, p. 166). This education is to assist the clinician in suspending personal judgments about patient situations. Parse argues that "[i]t is essential to go with the person where the person is, rather than attempting to judge, change, or control the person" (1992, p. 40).

The nurse's obligations are perhaps less clear when obstacles to practice occur. Extrapolating from theory, one could surmise that nurses have obligations to politically address obstructive environments.

The responsibilities of a nurse practicing according to Orlando's Theory of the Deliberative Nursing Process can be contrasted with those of a Parse nurse. Orlando's background includes experience with psychiatric nursing and education (Fawcett, 1993). An important aspect of this theory involves interpersonal processes occurring between nurse and patient that, optimally, result in improvement in the patient's behavior. This improvement is accomplished as a result of "finding out (what are) and (thus) meeting the patient's immediate needs for help" (Orlando, 1990, p. viii). The nurse engages both his or her cognitive processes and personal and professional knowledge base to perceive, interpret, and react to patients' needs. These needs become discernable in the course of the nurse-patient interaction.

The implication is that the nurse rather than the patient recognizes and interprets, from the interaction, the need for help that exists and grasps what strategies are most likely to meet the need. If the need is not met, as is evidenced by unchanged or worsened patient behavior, then the process is repeated. Further efforts on the part of a nurse are made to correct misunderstanding or misinterpretation of the problem by validating these with the patient.

Thus the nurse individualizes care to a patient situation and needs. This is a moral responsibility attendant upon using Orlando's theory. The development of a trusting relationship is also important because trust is more likely to facilitate revelation of a patient's needs. A patient's unique needs may commit a nurse to enlisting other appropriate services when a particular need is beyond that nurse's capacity to address it. When the patient's needs cannot be met because of institutional constraints, the nurse is obliged to undertake further action.

This can be considered a political obligation that is inherent in this particular (as well as in many of the other) theoretical works. For example, perhaps it becomes clear that the patient needs to have her hospital stay to be extended another day to meet her psychological support needs, but pressure is being placed to send her home. Thus there are responsibilities that take a nurse out of the demands of the immediate nurse-patient relationship to meet a patient's actual needs.

It is not as clear what this theory commits the nurse to in terms of addressing the needs of those people who are unable, for a variety of reasons, to access the healthcare system and thus gain assistance from Orlando's theory. It is reasonable to assert that those nurses who choose to structure practice by Orlando's theory do have commitments to political or policy activities on behalf of those who could be assisted by a deliberative nursing process.

Theory-Based Practice: Nursing's Commitments

It can be noted, then, that subsequent to the work of self-reflection and theory selection, there are further moral commitments inherent in theoretical frameworks for the nursing student and practicing nurse. These commitments also extend to nursing educators and researchers. For example, as discussed both earlier and later in this text, responsibilities to address obstacles to structuring care according to a given framework are implicit in theoretical works. The moral commitment for nurse educators who are charged with teaching nursing philosophies, models, and theories is to elucidate by discussion and by other means the inherent moral responsibilities of theory usage. The responsibilities of educators (in their position as educators rather than as practitioners, which many also are) with regard to theoretical works are thus somewhat more general. They include highlighting not just the importance of theory use but also moral commitments inherent in particular theories. Additionally, educators are accountable for elucidating theory implications for policy formulation and for the profession's political efforts on behalf of patients.

Political Implications

In summary, a given framework will generally direct professionals when obstacles to providing service in the envisioned manner arise. For example, if there are insufficient nurses on a floor to provide even the minimal interventions implied by a particular framework, it becomes obvious that health issues cannot be addressed adequately and that further responsibilities exist. The practitioner should be able to articulate what further obligations accrue to the practitioner using a particular theoretical work when such barriers exist. Possible barriers include time constraints, conflicts of interest, access to care problems, economic concerns, and a host of other problems associated with profit-driven and other forms of healthcare delivery.

Healthcare provision in the United States and elsewhere is continually evolving—and not necessarily in a positive manner. That is, it is not evolving in a manner designed to actually facilitate health either as it is envisioned by nursing or by any other interested or susceptible parties. Because many of nursing's theoretical works were conceptualized in an earlier era, in which more time was available for hands-on nursing care, those using theory are increasingly faced with time constraints and other barriers to their ability to accomplish goals. This does not mean that theoretical frameworks are obsolete; rather, it implies that individuals and society are not getting their health needs met. Thus the important question for nursing to consider is "what are our individual and collective obligations when circumstances are such that nursing cannot be practiced in the manner envisioned by its theorists?" The answer to this question should be implicit in any conceptualization regarding the furtherance of health. It is pointless to urge actions facilitative of health for individuals (from any perspective of what this might look like) if conditions are such that what is postulated as necessary cannot possibly be accomplished. Thus theoretical works should be able to assist the profession in demonstrating the importance of nursing to the health of persons in society by illuminating the nature and location of problems.

Theories should help the nursing profession avoid the philosophical problem of 'ought implies can,' which recognizes the futility of obliging persons to actions they cannot possibly complete. Newton's view (1988) of professional obligation may be helpful here. She notes the following:

> The professional must respond . . . if practices in his field are inadequate at any stage of the rendering of the service: if the client the ultimate consumer is unhappy; if he is happy but unknowing, badly served by shabby products or service; or if he is happy and well served but the state of the art is not adequate to his real needs (p. 49).

Newton's conclusion, although not written specifically about health professions, is pertinent to theory-based nursing and highlights some of the obligations that are attendant upon providing a societally-based service. Her conclusions are borne out both in the ANA *Code for Nurses* (1985) and its *Social Policy Statement* (1995).

CONCLUSION

Professional nursing practice that is guided by any or all of the elements of philosophies, models, and/or theories carries with it a number of moral responsibilities and obligations. These responsibilities have moral force because the nursing discipline professes to be capable of furthering health for its population of concern. It is to this purpose and for this end that nursing endeavors to increase its knowledge base. The development of this knowledge base is dependent in part upon theory-based practice and research and in part upon theory informed by practice and research. Thus members of the profession are obliged to examine the bases for their practice and the potential of these bases for accomplishing nursing's—and thus society's—goals.

CRITICAL THINKING EXERCISES

1. What creative strategies could be used to deal with conflict between personal philosophy and the philosophical assumptions underlying a setting-imposed framework?
2. The ANA's *Social Policy Statement* (1995) has adopted Pender's assertion that "nurses help people to identify both short- and long-term health goals and act as advocates for people dealing with barriers encountered in obtaining health care" (p. 3). What moral implications does this statement hold for nurses who use theoretically guided practice, research, or teaching?
3. What are the implications of permitting a patient's philosophy to guide the choice of an appropriate model or theory for practice?
4. What are the moral implications of a clash between a nurse's personal philosophy and a patient's personal philosophy?
5. What avenues are open to a nurse attempting to address broader societal obstacles to providing theory-guided care?

References

American Nurses Association. (1985). *Code for nurses with interpretive statements.* Kansas City, MO: Author.

American Nurses Association. (1995). *Social policy statement.* Washington, DC: American Nurses Publishing.

Andrews, H. A. & Roy, C. (1991). Essentials of the Roy Adaptation Model. In C. Roy & H. A. Andrews (Eds.), *The Roy Adaptation Model: The definitive statement* (pp. 3-25). Norwalk, CT: Appleton & Lange.

Chinn, P. L. & Kramer, M. K. (1995). *Theory and nursing: A systematic approach* (4th ed.). St. Louis: Mosby.

Christensen, P. J. (1996). *Nursing process: Application of conceptual models* (4th ed.). St. Louis: Mosby.

Curtin, L. & Flaherty, M. J. (1982). *Nursing ethics: Theories and pragmatics.* Bowie, MD: Brady Communications, Prentice Hall.

Fawcett, J. (1993). *Analysis and evaluation of nursing theories.* Philadelphia: F. A. Davis.

Fawcett, J. (1995). *Analysis and evaluation of conceptual models of nursing* (3rd ed.). Philadelphia: F. A. Davis.

Grace, P. J. (1998). A philosophical analysis of the concept "advocacy": Implications for provider-patient relationships. *UMI Dissertation Abstracts,* 9923287.

Grace, P. & Gaylord, N. (1999a). Transcendental health care ethics: Beyond the medical model. *Ethical Human Sciences and Services, 1*(3), 243-253.

Grace, P. J. & Gaylord, N. (1999b, June). *Philosophical inquiry in nursing: A moral endeavor.* Paper presented at the International Nursing Research Conference—Post Conference Workshop: Philosophical Inquiry in Nursing. Edmonton, Alberta, Canada.

International Council of Nurses. (1973). *Code for Nurses: Ethical concepts applied to nursing.* Geneva, Switzerland: Author.

Kenney, J. W. (1999). Theory-based advanced practice nursing. In J. W. Kenney (Ed.), *Philosophical and theoretical perspectives for advanced practice nursing* (2nd ed., pp. 324-343). Sudbury, MA: Jones and Bartlett.

Ketefian, S. & Redman, R. W. (1997). Nursing science in the global community. *Image, 29*(1), 11-15.

Kim, H. S. (1994). Practice theories in nursing and a science of nursing practice. *Scholarly Inquiry for Nursing Practice, 8*(2), 145-158.

Kleffel, D. (1996). Environmental paradigms: Moving toward an ecocentric perspective. *Advances in Nursing Science, 18*(4), 1-10.

Marriner-Tomey, A. & Alligood, M. R. (1998). *Nursing theorists and their work* (4th ed.). St. Louis: Mosby.

Marriner Tomey, A. & Alligood, M. R. (2002). (on press). *Nursing theorists and their work* (5th ed.). St. Louis: Mosby.

McKenna, H. (1997). Choosing a theory for practice. In H. McKenna (Ed.), *Nursing theories and models* (pp. 127-157). New York: Routledge.

Meleis, A. I. (1991). *Theoretical nursing: Development and progress* (2nd ed.). Philadelphia: Lippincott.

Meleis, A. I. (1997). *Theoretical nursing: Development and progress* (3rd ed.). Philadelphia: Lippincott.

Newman, M. A. (1986). *Health as expanding consciousness.* St. Louis: Mosby.

Newton, L. H. (1988). Law-giving for professional life: Reflections on the place of the professional code. In A. Flores (Ed.), *Professional ideals* (pp. 47-56). Belmont, CA: Wadsworth.

Nightingale, F. (1946). *Notes on nursing: What it is and what it is not.* Philadelphia: J. B. Lippincott.

Orem, D. E. (1991). *Nursing: Concepts of practice* (4th ed.). St. Louis: Mosby.

Orlando, I. J. (1961). *The dynamic nurse-patient relationship: Function, process and principles.* New York: J. P. Putnam & Sons.

Orlando, I. J. (1990). *The dynamic nurse-patient relationship.* New York: National League for Nursing. (Reprint of the 1961 text).

Parse, R. R. (1987). *Nursing science: Major paradigms, theories, and critiques.* Philadelphia: W. B. Saunders.

Parse, R. R. (1992). Human becoming: Parse's theory of nursing. *Nursing Science Quarterly, 5,* 35-42.

Reed, P. G. & Zurakowski, T. L. (1996). Nightingale: Foundations of nursing. In J. J. Fizpatrick & A. L. Whall (Eds.), *Conceptual models of nursing: Analysis and application* (3rd ed., pp. 27-54). Stamford, CT: Appleton & Lange.

Rogers, M. E. (1987). Rogers science of unitary human beings. In R. R. Parse (Ed.), *Nursing science: Major paradigms, theories and critiques* (pp. 139-147). Philadelphia: W. B. Saunders.

Roy, C. (1980). The adaptation model. In J. P. Riehl & C. Roy (Eds.), *Conceptual models for nursing* (2nd ed., pp. 179-188). New York: Appleton-Century-Crofts.

Salsberry, P. J. (1994). A philosophy of nursing: What is it? What is it not? In J. F. Kikuchi & H. Simmons (Eds.), *Developing a philosophy of nursing.* Thousand Oaks, CA: Sage.

Viens, D. (1989). A history of nursing's code of ethics. *Nursing Outlook, 37*(1), 45-49.

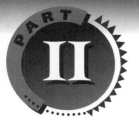

A pplication

The application of nursing theoretical works in nursing practice illustrates their utility. Each philosophy, model, and theory provides a unique perspective of the care, as is seen in the case of Debbie:

Philosophies

- Patients and their environmental surroundings when Nightingale is applied
- A transpersonal way of caring when Watson is applied
- A clinical hermeneutic of the nurse-patient narrative when Benner is applied

Models

- A system of behaviors when Johnson is applied
- A framework of interacting systems when King is applied
- A set of conservation principles when Levine is applied
- A system response to stressors when Neuman is applied
- A set of theories for self-care when Orem is applied
- A human/environmental field pattern when Rogers is applied
- A system of adaptive modes when Roy is applied

Theories

- The deliberate approach to patient needs when Orlando is applied
- The life ways of the patient when modeling and role-modeling is applied
- The nature of maternal role development when Mercer is applied
- The view of culture for total care when Leininger is applied
- The unique contribution of presence to human becoming when Parse is applied
- The nature of health as expanding consciousness when Newman is applied

Nightingale's Philosophy in Nursing Practice

Kim Bolton

"Nursing ought to signify the proper use of fresh air, light, warmth, cleanliness, quiet, and the proper selection and administration of diet—all at the least expense of vital power to the patient." (Nightingale, 1969)

HISTORY AND BACKGROUND

Nightingale was born in 1820 in Florence, Italy. Her parents were very wealthy and often traveled abroad. Nightingale was very beautiful and was expected to behave like every other Victorian lady, filling her time before marriage with music, reading, embroidery, and learning how to be the perfect hostess (Brown, 1988).

Nightingale had other ideas. She had felt different from those around her even at a young age and by the time she was 17 believed she was called into service by God (Woodham-Smith, 1951). She had great compassion and sympathy for people of all types, and as she grew older, she believed she had been called to help mankind. She desired to help the truly poor but suffered in silence for years because it was improper for someone of her upbringing to involve herself with actual physical work (Brown, 1988).

At the age of 24, Nightingale decided she needed to help the suffering masses and wished to work in a hospital. This was met with opposition from her family, and they fought about it for years before finally allowing her to go to Kaiserworth, Germany to learn nursing from the Institution of Deaconesses (Brown, 1988; Woodham-Smith, 1951). She studied there for 3 months and then returned to the service of her family. It was another 2 years before she was allowed to practice nursing (Brown, 1988; Woodham-Smith, 1951).

She developed what we have come to refer to as her nursing theory after her travel to Scutari to care for wounded soldiers during the Crimean War. Her writings, which included philosophy and directives, were developed from a need to define nursing and reform hospital environments rather than give nursing new knowledge. Nightingale worked endlessly during her lifetime to bring about all types of reform, in areas as diverse as the British military and the environment of England (Woodham-Smith, 1951; Brown, 1988). Because of her work in reforming nursing, she has come to be called *the founder of modern nursing* (Dennis & Prescott, 1985; Henry, Woods, & Nagelkerk, 1990). She started a school of nursing at St. Thomas Hospital in England and wrote many manuscripts about hospital reform and nursing care (Woodham-Smith, 1951; Brown, 1988). Nightingale believed that "nursing knowledge is distinct from medical knowledge" (1969, p. 3).

OVERVIEW OF NIGHTINGALE'S ENVIRONMENTAL PHILOSOPHY

Nightingale's philosophy is environmentally oriented. This is evidenced by her many writings and her book *Notes on Nursing: What It Is and What It Is Not* (Nightingale, 1969). She believed that the environment of the patient could be altered so as to allow nature to act on the patient (Nightingale, 1969; McKenna, 1997). Her work focuses mostly on the patient and the environment but also includes the nurse and health. For instance, it was the nurse's duty to alter the patient's environment so that nature could act on the patient and repair health. The components of Nightingale's philosophy, which is recognized as theory in this theory era, are the following:

- *Environment: Environment* can be defined as anything that can be manipulated to place a patient in the best possible condition for nature to act (Selanders, 1998). This theory has both physical and psychological components. The physical components of the environment refer to ventilation, warmth, light, nutrition, medicine, stimulation, room temperature, and activity (Lobo, 1995; Nightingale, 1969; Reed & Zurakowski, 1996; Selanders, 1998). The psychological components include avoiding chattering hopes and advices and providing variety (Lobo, 1995; Nightingale, 1969).
- *Person:* Although most of Nightingale's writings refer to the person as the one who is receiving care, she did believe that the person is a dynamic and complex being. Reed and Zurakowski (1996) state,

"Nightingale envisioned the person as comprising physical, intellectual, emotional, social, and spiritual components" (p. 33).

- *Health:* Nightingale (1954b) wrote, "Health is not only to be well, but to be able to use well every power we have" (p. 357). From this statement, we can infer that she believed in prevention and health promotion in addition to nursing patients from illness to health.
- *Nursing:* Nightingale believed nursing to be a spiritual calling. Nurses were to assist nature to repair the patient (Chinn & Jacobs, 1987; Nightingale, 1969; Reed & Zurakowski, 1996; Selanders, 1998). She defined different types of nursing as *nursing proper* (nursing the sick), *general nursing* (health promotion), and *midwifery nursing* (Reed & Zurakowski, 1996; Selanders, 1998). Nightingale saw nursing as the "science of environmental management" (Whall, 1996, p. 23). Nurses were to use common sense, observation, and ingenuity to allow nature to effectively repair the patient (deGraaf, Marriner-Tomey, Mossman, & Slebodnik, 1994).

Although the model seems linear, it has been observed that the nurse initiates mutuality of care and outcome between the nurse and the patient (Selanders, 1998). Nightingale assumed that the patient wanted to be healthy and would cooperate with and assist the nurse to allow nature to help the patient (deGraaf, Marriner-Tomey, Mossman, & Slebodnik, 1994). Using Nightingale's philosophy in practice today fits well with the use of the nursing process. The nurse assesses the patient situation, identifies a need, implements a plan of care, reevaluates the situation, and finally changes the plan to better serve the patient. This is done as often as necessary until the main goal of nursing (improved health state) is accomplished. At each phase of the process, documentation occurs to allow other caregivers to follow the plan of care (Selanders, 1998).

CRITICAL THINKING USING NIGHTINGALE'S THEORETICAL PHILOSOPHY

The term *critical thinking* was not in use in Nightingale's day; however, she expected nurses to use their powers of observation in caring for patients. In her book *Notes on Nursing: What It Is and What It Is Not* (1969) she developed a whole section on observation of the sick. She wanted her nurses "to be clear thinkers and independent in their judgments" (Reed & Zurakowski, 1996, p. 47). She advocated for nurses to have educational backgrounds and knowledge that was different from that of physicians (Nightingale, 1969; Reed & Zurakowski, 1996; Selanders, 1998). She believed in and rallied for nursing education to be a combination of clinical experience and classroom learning. Nightingale states, "Neither can [nursing] be taught by lectures or by books, though these are

TABLE 5-1   Critical Thinking with Nightingale's Theory

Nightingale's Canons (Nightingale, 1969; Selanders, 1998)	Nursing Process and Thought
Ventilation and warmth	Assess the client's body temperature, room temperature, and room for fresh air (or adequate ventilation) and foul odors. Develop a plan to keep the room airy and free of odor while maintaining the client's body temperature.
Light	Assess the room for adequate light. Sunlight works best. Develop and implement adequate light in the client's room without placing the client in direct light.
Cleanliness of rooms and walls	Assess the room for dampness, darkness, and dust or mildew. Keep the room free from dust, dirt, mildew, or dampness.
Health of houses	Assess the surrounding environment for pure air, pure water, drainage, cleanliness, and light. Examples include removing garbage or garments from the area, removing any standing water (or ensuring that water drains away from the area), and ensuring that air and water are clean and free from odor and that there is plenty of light.
Noise	Assess the noise level in the client's room and surrounding area. Attempt to keep noise level to a minimum, and refrain from whispering outside the door.
Bed and bedding	Assess the bed and bedding for dampness, wrinkles, and soiling, and check the bed for height. Keep the bed dry, wrinkle-free, and at the lowest height to ensure the client's comfort.
Personal cleanliness	Attempt to keep the client dry and clean at all times. Frequent assessment of the client's skin is needed to maintain adequate skin moisture.
Variety	Attempt to stimulate variety in the room and with the client. This is accomplished with cards, flowers, pictures, books, or puzzles. Encourage friends and relatives to engage the client in some sort of stimulating conversation.
Chattering hopes and advices	Avoid talking without reason or giving advice that is without fact. Continue to talk to the client as a person, and continue to stimulate the client's mind. Avoid personal talk.
Taking food	Assess the diet of the client. Take note of the amount of food and drink ingested by the client at every meal or snack.
What food	Continue with the assessment of the diet to include type of food and drink the client likes or dislikes. Attempt to ensure that the client always has some food or drink available that he or she enjoys.
Petty management	Petty management ensures continuity of care. Documentation of the plan of care and all evaluation will ensure others give the same care to the client in your absence.
Observation of the sick	Observe everything about your client. Record all observations. Observations should be factual and not merely opinions. Continue to observe the client's surrounding environment and make alterations in the plan of care when needed.

valuable accessories, if used as such; otherwise what is in the book stays in the book" (Nightingale, 1954b, p. 355).

Using critical thinking and Nightingale's environmental theory requires use of her 13 canons (Selanders, 1998) and the nursing process. Table 5-1 illustrates the interaction of the nurse and the patient with Nightingale's environmental theory.

Although the 13 canons are central to Nightingale's theory, they are not all-inclusive. She believed that the person was a holistic individual and thus had a spiritual dimension. She believed nursing was a spiritual calling, and with that belief she assumed that nurses could help those clients who were in spiritual distress (Nightingale, 1969, 1954a). This is an assumption because of the time period in which Nightingale lived; it was expected that Christians would help other Christians. She identified nursing of the sick (nursing proper) and nursing of the well (nursing general) (Nightingale, 1969). She believed the two to be almost identical, with the outcome being the major difference.

Because Nightingale believed in nursing well persons—or health promotion—it is logical that she assumed her nurses would do some health teaching as they were caring for the sick or for those who were already well. In using Nightingale's theory, the nurse must consider the 13 canons as well as health promotion and spiritual distress.

CASE HISTORY OF DEBBIE

Debbie is a 29-year-old woman who was recently admitted to the oncology nursing unit for evaluation after sensing pelvic "fullness" and noticing a watery, foul-smelling vaginal discharge. A Papanicolaou smear revealed class V cervical cancer. She was found to have a stage II squamous cell carcinoma of the cervix and underwent a radical hysterectomy with bilateral salpingooophorectomy.

Her past health history revealed that physical examinations had been infrequent. She also reported that she had not performed breast self-examination. She is 5 feet, 4 inches tall and weights 89 pounds. Her usual weight is about 110 pounds. She has smoked approximately two packs of cigarettes a day for the past 16 years. She is gravida 2, para 2. Her first pregnancy was at age 16, and her second was at age 18. Since that time, she has taken oral contraceptives on a regular basis.

Debbie completed the eighth grade. She is married and lives with her husband and her two children in her mother's home, which she describes as less than sanitary. Her husband is unemployed. She describes him as emotionally distant and abusive at times.

She has done well following surgery except for being unable to completely empty her urinary bladder. She is having continued postoperative pain and nausea. It will be necessary for her to perform intermittent self-catheterization at home. Her medications are (1) an antibiotic, (2) an analgesic as needed for pain, and (3) an antiemetic as needed for nausea. In addition, she will be receiving radiation therapy on an outpatient basis.

Debbie is extremely tearful. She expresses great concern over her future and the future of her two children. She believes that this illness is a punishment for her past life.

NURSING CARE OF DEBBIE WITH NIGHTINGALE'S THEORY

In Nightingale's environmental theory, Debbie is the person seeking care. She needs nature's reparative process. The nurse's goal is to assist nature in that process. The nursing process and Nightingale's theory can be used together to provide care for Debbie. This care starts with a review of the environment.

Physical Environment

Assessment. Debbie speaks of her living area as being less than sanitary. To start the nursing care of Debbie, a visit to her home environment is necessary. Assess the environment for pure air and water, light, drainage, and cleanliness. The air that Debbie breathes should be clean and free from odors. The house should have an adequate heat and air system; the filters should be free of dirt; and the system should be able to maintain the house at a comfortable temperature. Garbage should be disposed of away from the house to stop odors from polluting the air or water. The water should be evaluated for cleanliness. It may be a good idea to enlist the help of the local water company to ensure that the water is not contaminated from outside pollutants. Assess the cleanliness of the house for waste or other contaminants, such as dirt, rodents, insects, mildew, and mold. Assess the environment for artificial and natural lighting. The light fixtures should be in working order and there should be windows that allow natural light to filter in during the daytime. Assess the area around the house for adequate drainage. Water should not be under the house or in areas standing around the house.

Plan. Enlist the aid of the local water and electric companies in the assessment of the heat and air system, the water system, and the drainage of water and wastes at Debbie's house. Develop a plan to correct any deficiencies that may be found. Educate Debbie and her family on the importance of cleanliness inside the house and of the benefits of both natural and artificial lighting. Check into financial assistance from county and state resources.

Psychological Environment

Assessment. Debbie has several psychological concerns. She is worried about her family and her own health. She believes this illness is a form of punishment for her past life. She complains of continued pain and nausea. She describes her husband as emotionally distant and sometimes abusive. She admits to not having regular physical examinations and to not performing breast self-examinations.

Plan. Continue to talk to Debbie in an attempt to gather more information about her fears and concerns. Listen to her concerns and offer factual information to help alleviate her fears. Nightingale (1969) believed that talking would be helpful to the client if it was sincere and did not involve giving an opinion. Investigate the possibility of arranging for psychological help from both a psychologist and a member of the clergy. Educate Debbie on preventive health maintenance for herself and her family. Educate Debbie on self-catheterization and personal cleanliness. People usually feel better if their physical appearance improves. Discuss with Debbie the benefits of an exercise program that could be performed at least 3 times per week. Help Debbie to discover other means of pain management, such as meditation, imagery, and relaxation techniques. Encourage Debbie to speak to her physician about the inadequate pain relief with her current pain medicine. Encourage her to speak freely about all of her concerns and feelings, and be sure to include her family in these discussions. Encourage her family to provide Debbie with variety in her daily routine and around the house. This could include activities such as games, watching TV together, coloring with her kids, going on walks, or engaging in any other family activities.

Nutrition

Assessment. Debbie states she still suffers from nausea and that she has lost 21 pounds. Assess nausea in relation to timing, quality, quantity, interference with nutrition, and alleviating and aggravating symptoms. Assess her diet with a 3-day diet recall. Determine her food likes and dislikes.

Plan. Start Debbie on a well-balanced diet that includes her food preferences, and educate her on the importance of following this diet. Work meal times around the periods of nausea to facilitate eating, or, if necessary, allow for frequent, small meals. Allow for snacks to help decrease the periods of nausea. Discuss Debbie's medications with her, particularly the one for nausea, to be sure she takes it correctly and is aware of its possible side-effects. Remind her that she should not operate machinery while she is under the influence of the medication. Educate Debbie in other techniques designed to relieve nausea such as relaxation or imagery.

The remaining canons of Nightingale's theory deal with nursing management and observation. Debbie's plan of care needs to be documented so that the plan continues even in the absence of the nurse. In Debbie's case, she will be at home and undergoing outpatient therapy. Debbie and her entire family need to be aware of the nursing plan and need education to enable them to assist the nurse with the plan. Other caregivers will need access to her plan when the nurse is gone, and documentation is the best point of reference. Accurate documentation ensures that everyone who may have contact with Debbie will be aware of her nursing care plan and will be able to assist her as well as the nurse and nature.

Observation is essential to both the nursing process and Nightingale's environmental theory. Nightingale (1954a) states, "The trained power of attending to one's own impressions made by one's own senses, so that these should tell the nurse how the patient is, is the *sine qua non* of being a nurse at all" (pp. 320-321). Observation is used to provide essential information about the client's progress with the plan of care and whether the plan needs modification. Debbie's family should be taught observation techniques that would assist the nurse in modifying the plan. Nightingale (1954a) believed, "Observation may always be improved with training-will seldom be present without training; for otherwise the nurse does not know what to look for" (p. 321).

• • •

A second example of the utilization of Nightingale's theory can be illustrated in the case study of Michelle, a 25-year-old who has presented to her practitioner for preconceptual counseling. It will illustrate how sick nursing and health nursing are essentially congruent except in their differing outcomes.

CASE HISTORY OF MICHELLE

Michelle, a 25-year-old white female, presents to her nurse practitioner for preconceptual counseling. She states that she and her husband have been married for 4 years and have decided to begin their family. She desires to be as healthy as she can be before becoming pregnant. Her past medical history and family history are unremarkable. She denies smoking and states she may have a drink about once a month. She is currently employed as a computer programmer for a large computer company. She works 40 hours a week and has the weekends off. She and her husband enjoy each other's company and spend their free time outdoors as much as possible. She has been taking oral contraceptives for 6 years.

NURSING CARE OF MICHELLE WITH NIGHTINGALE'S THEORY

Preconceptual counseling is on the increase among married couples who have decided to begin raising a family. The main goal of preconceptual counseling is to place the intended mother in the best health possible before she conceives. The nurse practitioner, in order to achieve this goal, must complete a thorough assessment into the client's lifestyle and environment. Nightingale's environmental theory can be a useful tool in this endeavor.

Physical Environment

Assessment and plan. The home, workplace, and community environment should be assessed according to the 13 canons. The main areas of assessment include ventilation and warming, noise, light, and health of houses (Nightingale, 1969). Health of houses includes pure air, water, drainage, cleanliness, light, and bed and bedding. Assess both the home and the workplace with the items included under health of houses (see Table 5-1). Assess the community and neighborhood with all of the canons regarding physical environment.

Home and workplace assessment

1. Light. Assess for adequate windows and working light fixtures.
2. Pure air. Assess for ventilation, offensive odors, drafts, and a working heat and air unit.
3. Pure water. Assess for working water system that is free from contamination.
4. Drainage. Assess the area for drainage of rain water away from the house.
5. Cleanliness. Assess the home for the means to keep the house clean and for freedom from mold, mildew, excessive dust, offensive odors, and pet droppings.
6. Bed and bedding. Assess the beds for quality and comfort. Assess the bedding for cleanliness and a working washing machine (for home assessment only).
7. Noise. Assess the area for loud, offensive, and unnecessary noise.

Home and workplace plan

1. Light. Enlist the help of Michelle and the electric company in assessment of the light fixtures. Suggest replacing incandescent light fixtures with fluorescent lighting since the latter allow for better and cheaper lighting. Ensure that the windows are in working condition and that there are at least two windows in every room. Educate Michelle on the benefit of light to one's health and suggest keeping blinds or curtains open during the daytime hours.

2. Air. Enlist the help of Michelle and the electric company in assessment of the heat and air unit for working order and efficiency. The unit should be able to maintain the area at a comfortable temperature. Check the windows and doors for drafts, and ensure that the windows can be opened to allow natural air into the area.

3. Educate Michelle about changing or cleaning the air filters in the heat and air unit about once a month and of the benefit of opening the windows occasionally to allow outside air into the area. The open windows will allow for cross-ventilation and will air out the house or workplace.

4. Water. Enlist the help of Michelle and the water company to assess the plumbing for working order and freedom from contamination. Have the water checked for levels of lead and other metals that could contaminate it. Discuss the possibility of a water filtering or purification system in the house or workplace. Educate Michelle on the benefit of pure water for drinking and eating. Advise Michelle to keep garbage and other refuse away from the water supply or any parts of the water system.

5. Drainage. Enlist the help of the water company to assess for adequate drainage. Educate Michelle about removing hazards that allow standing water to remain too close to the house or the workplace.

6. Cleanliness. Talk with Michelle about using environmentally safe cleaning products that kill most common germs. Educate Michelle about mold and mildew and the potential problems both could cause with air and water contamination. Ask Michelle to constantly observe the environment for hazards to the health of her family and herself.

7. Bed and bedding. Educate Michelle on cleaning, vacuuming, and airing the bedding. Discuss ways to evaluate the bed for adequate performance and to maintain the bed in proper working order, such as turning and/or replacing the mattress.

8. Noise. Discuss with Michelle the types of noises in both the home and the workplace. Discuss ways to decrease the level of the noise, such as placing bushes in front of the home or using earplugs for work.

Community and neighborhood assessment
Assess the community and neighborhood for offensive odors, garbage and refuse, adequate water and electricity, and areas for outside activities.

Community and neighborhood plan
The community water and electric companies should conform to guidelines for operation and maintenance of their systems. The community

or neighborhood should be free from garbage or other refuse. If the community or neighborhood is close to a dump or a landfill, assess the area for offensive odors. If there is an area for outside activities, assess for maintenance of equipment and cleanliness of the area. Any assessed deficiencies can be addressed by meeting with community leaders to discuss the deficiencies and any proposed solutions.

Psychological Environment

Assessment and plan

1. Variety. Assess the activities of Michelle and her husband. Develop an exercise plan for the client that includes a variety of activities. Exercise leads to healthy lifestyle and will help the client with the weight gain of pregnancy. Educate the client that exercise should be performed at least three times per week for at least 30 minutes at a time. Encourage Michelle and her husband to continue to perform their current activities and to attempt to enjoy a variety of activities. Explain to Michelle that she can also alter her work environment with fresh flowers or new pictures.
2. Chattering hopes and advices. Refrain from giving Michelle your opinion. Provide factual information about health, exercise, and other topics of importance when talking with Michelle. Praise all activities that increase the health of the client. Allow Michelle to speak to you freely and express all of her desires and concerns.
3. Personal cleanliness (health). Encourage Michelle to continue with her routine medical checkups. Encourage 8 hours of sleep per night. Discuss the timing of the pregnancy, and instruct her to discontinue oral contraceptives for 3 months before attempting pregnancy.

Taking Food and What Food: Nutrition

Assessment and plan

1. Assess the nutritional status of Michelle by asking for a 3-day diet recall. Ask her for her food likes and dislikes and for her drink preferences. Ask whether she takes over-the-counter dietary or herbal supplements.
2. Educate Michelle on maintaining a well-balanced diet. Encourage her to consume foods from the groups in the food pyramid. She needs 2 to 3 servings from the milk group (e.g., milk, yogurt, cheese) and 6 to 8 glasses of water per day. She should also increase her folic acid intake to 400 µg per day. This can be achieved by taking prenatal vitamins once a day.
3. Educate Michelle on the hazards of alcohol consumption during pregnancy, and advise her to avoid the use of tobacco and drugs as well.

Observation

The observation of Michelle will consist of keeping routine visits in place until pregnancy is achieved. Educate Michelle and her husband about what to report to you during this period before her pregnancy. Encourage her to call you whenever she needs to talk or to ask questions. If needed, return appointments can be scheduled every 3 months to allow the nurse practitioner to reevaluate Michelle and the plan.

CONCLUSION

Nightingale's environmental theory arose out of a need to reform nursing and the environment of England in the late 1800s. Her theory is simple and easy to apply to nursing practice because it contains many of the very elements that nursing students learn during their education. Utilization of Nightingale's theory will help the nurse to have a beginning focal point and allows for the nurse to view the client as an individual who interacts with and lives in an environment that may not be conducive to optimal health.

CRITICAL THINKING EXERCISES

1. Complete an environmental assessment of your living area. Develop a plan for repair of a problem or maintenance of a current situation.
2. Complete an environmental assessment of your college campus. Compile a list of potential problems and list ways to repair them.
3. Complete an environmental assessment of your community and list ways the environment has improved and how it could be further improved.
4. Consider three patients for whom you have cared recently. Identify areas of the environment that Nightingale's theory guides you to assess and that you did not consider in the framework you used to guide your practice at the time.
5. Using Nightingale's theory, compare and contrast the practice of nursing in the late 1800s with nursing as it is in the present time.

References

Brown, P. (1988). *Florence Nightingale: The tough British campaigner who was the founder of modern nursing*. Great Britain: Exley.

Chinn, P. & Jacobs, M. (1987). *Theory and nursing: A systematic approach*. St. Louis: Mosby.

deGraaf, K., Marriner-Tomey, A., Mossman, C., & Slebodnik, M. (1994). Florence Nightingale. In A. Marriner-Tomey (Ed.), *Nursing theorists and their work* (3rd ed., pp. 73-85). St. Louis: Mosby.

Dennis, K. & Prescott, P. (1985). Florence Nightingale: Yesterday, today, and tomorrow. *Advances in Nursing Science*, 7(2), 66-81.

Henry, B., Woods, S., & Nagelkerk, J. (1990). Nightingale's perspective of nursing administration. *Nursing and Health Care*, 11(4), 201-205.

Lobo, M. (1995). Florence Nightingale. In J. B. George (Ed.), *Nursing theories: The base for professional nursing practice* (4th ed., pp. 34-48). Norwalk, CT: Appleton & Lange.

McKenna, H. (1997). *Nursing theories and models.* London: Routledge.

Nightingale, F. (1954a). Nurses, training of. In L. Seymour (Ed.), *Selected writings of Florence Nightingale* (pp. 319-334). New York: MacMillan.

Nightingale, F. (1954b). Sick-nursing and health-nursing. In L. Seymour (Ed.), *Selected writings of Florence Nightingale* (pp. 353-376). New York: MacMillan.

Nightingale, F. (1969). *Notes on nursing: What it is and what it is not.* New York: Dover.

Reed, P. & Zurakowski, T. (1996). Nightingale: Foundations of nursing. In J. Fitzpatrick & A. Whall (Eds.), *Conceptual models of nursing: Analysis and application* (3rd ed., pp. 27-54). Stamford, CT: Appleton & Lange.

Selanders, L. (1998). The power of environmental adaptation: Florence Nightingale's original theory for nursing practice. *Journal of Holistic Nursing, 16*(2), 247-263.

Whall, A. (1996). The structure of nursing knowledge: Analysis of practice, middle-range, and ground theory. In J. Fitzpatrick & A. Whall (Eds.), *Conceptual models of nursing: Analysis and application* (3rd ed., pp. 13-25). Stamford, CT: Appleton & Lange.

Woodham-Smith, C. (1951). *Florence Nightingale.* London: McGraw-Hill.

Watson's Philosophy in Nursing Practice

Mary-Jean McGraw

"Caring in nursing conveys physical acts, but embraces the mindbodyspirit as it reclaims the embodied spirit as its focus of attention. It suggests a methodology through both art and aesthetics, of being as well as knowing and doing. It concerns itself with the art of being human. It calls forth from the practitioner an authentic presencing of being in the caring moment, carrying an intentional caring-healing consciousness. It concerns itself with the transpersonal and transcultural, and with the objective, subjective and the intersubjective. There is openness to another possibility of being in the world, with caring and healing as a global ontology within an expanding cosmology...Nursing becomes a metaphor for the sacred feminine archetypal energy, now critical to the healing needed in modern Western nursing and medicine." (Watson, 1999)

HISTORY AND BACKGROUND

Throughout her career, Jean Watson seems to have felt the pain of all of nursing as if it were somehow her own. She has witnessed nursing struggle to grasp its own possibility and power, its deep, feminine healing energy. She writes to deal with this pain, attempting to rewrite nursing as she also rewrites self. In this way, she continues to evolve in her own reflective process of thinking, tracing through her work the path all nurses follow as they search for the ground of being in their own practice and as they arrive hopefully at a place called *informed moral passion*. For Watson, this place—this passion of substance for nursing—has been and remains a caring ontology. Writing from this place becomes for her and for us as reader a meditation on being. Watson herself notes that the ideas and ideals associated with her philosophy and theory of human caring are concerned with spirit rather than matter, flux rather than form, inner knowledge and power rather than circumstance. These thoughts are never final, but they are embedded with persistent values and moral imperatives related to the human interaction that flows between and connects the one-caring-for and the one-cared-for (Watson, 1989, p. 219). Watson's most recent book (1999) continues to concern itself with metaphysics in that it "encompasses contemplation of both the ontology and epistemology of caring and caring consciousness in relation to a caring-healing praxis" (p. 7). She has moved beyond contemporary nursing to a view that is rooted in Nightingale's vision. She reflects, "it is both theoretical and beyond theory" (Watson, 1999, p. 89).

Watson's philosophy (1979) and theory of human science can be traced through the last 25 years, from its earliest beginnings as a textbook that was originally planned to present an integrated curriculum for undergraduate nursing programs but evolved instead into an original structure for basic nursing process. Beginning with the question of the relationship between human caring and nursing, this initial work laid the foundation for what was to become the *Theory of Human Caring* (Watson, 1997) and *Nursing: Human Science and Human Care* (Watson, 1988a). Although Watson's early writing (1979) refers to her work as a philosophy and science of nursing, she formalized the theory of human caring in her later writings (Watson, 1985; 1988a, 1997). In her most recent work Watson (1995, 1999) attempts to wed the wisdom of the ancient premodern era with the progress of nursing in the modern era and the lessons of the postmodern era.

Watson's caring theory engages thought in an evolutionary way, reminding us that all philosophy and science are always in flux. It silences thought's incessant linear flow to a well-defined end and makes room for a different kind of mental activity—an intuitive seeing—that finds kinship with playfulness and dialectical thinking. Dialect thrives on paradox and takes the reflector to the verge of seeing (Puhakka, 1998). Dialectical thinking has been described as the gateway to the transpersonal (Wilber, 1999). In Watson's thought, you will find both purpose and play, though seemingly opposites, moving together in a dialectical dance. Examples of this occur throughout Watson's writing, which engages in poetry to explore transcendence and professional moral passion; stretches contemporary and classic literature to define nursing science and doctoral education; weds Zen of consciousness with bed-making; revisits the human body as sacred ground and touch as communion; speaks of embodied spirit and transcendence as well as to immanence and nature; and plays with caring consciousness and its relation to quantum theory, holography, and physics.

Watson's work surpasses normal empirical factors and the physical, material world of nursing practice. It embraces concepts of mind, consciousness, soul, the sacred, the ancient and contemporary Yin emergence, holism, energy fields, waves, energy exchange, quantum, holography, transcendence, time and space, healing artistry, evolution, the transpersonal. However, Watson's language also speaks to more elemental grounds of our being: beauty, truth, goodness, harmony, openings, possibility, beyond, deep understanding, oneness, coming together, nurturance, honoring, authenticity, wide awakeness, human sensitivity, suffering, pain, hope, joy, spiritual, the divine, grace, the mystical, dream work, passion, poetry, metaphor, nature, I-thou, awe, dignity, reverence, ritual, light, the sacred feminine, wonder, compassion, love, blessings, peace. It is here that most practicing nurses find the theory's truest resonance and hope. Watson is an eternal optimist (Watson, 1999), and she writes from a deep place about the personal as well as the sacred. This philosophy invites us to explore our own curiosities about the origins of our call to care. Her writing encourages explorations of questions such as the following:

- What calls me to care?
- What is the root of my caring response?
- How will I respond?
- Why do I fail to respond?
- When is it hard to care?
- How will I sustain and nurture my caring consciousness?
- Who will care for me?

Watson views nursing and caring as "both a human science and an art, and as such cannot be considered qualitatively continuous with traditional, reductionistic, scientific methodology" (Talento, 1995, p. 327). Her description of the differences in human science and traditional science places her work firmly in human science that discloses the symbolic, conceptual, and linguistic world rather than the material, concrete, sensual world (Watson, 1988a; Wilber, 1999). She has continued to champion a broader definition of nursing science that develops its own concepts, relationships, and methodology, a science that provides vistas and opportunities to behold and try to understand these landscapes in the nursing view, an epic portion of human experience that includes caring (Watson, 1990). This *science with a view*

> leans toward employing qualitative theories and research methods, such as existential-phenomenology, literary introspection, case studies, philosophical-historical work, hermeneutics, art criticism, and other approaches that allow a close and systematic observation of one's own experience and that seek to disclose and elucidate the lived world of health-illness-healing experience and the phenomena of human caring (Watson, 1989, p. 221).

This broadened interpretation of science does not negate the significant contributions of objective medical and nursing science, but rather includes and restores subjective experience and values, meaning, quality, and soul-to-human phenomena and allows an integral view of the whole. It does not deny the objective components of science but instead *situates* them. As Dossey and Dossey (1999) have said,

> Watson does not discard science, she honors it, builds on it, and extends it. She asks, if we have the courage to honor all that science is telling us, what would health care look like? What would it *feel* like to be a patient and a practitioner in a system that honors our very being? (p. viii)

In Watson's *Postmodern Nursing and Beyond* (1999) she moves very clearly through her four aspects of caring: (1) as moral ideal, (2) as intentionality, (3) as ontological competencies, and (4) as healing art and healing space in the theory of transpersonal caring-healing.

OVERVIEW OF WATSON'S PHILOSOPHY OF HUMAN CARING

The following is a brief outline of Watson's ontology and its implications for caring and healing in nursing practice. It is based on a hermeneutic examination of her earlier texts (1979, 1985), her most recent writing (1999), and her personal interpretations as offered in professional forums and teaching. When possible, her own language has been retained.

Personhood

Watson's notions of personhood and life are based on the concept of human beings as *embodied spirit*. Within a transpersonal framework, the body is a living spirit that manifests one's being-in-the-world and one's way of standing and reflects how one holds oneself with respect to one's relation to self and one's consciousness or unconsciousness (Watson, 1999). This view holds respect and awe for the concept of the *human soul* (also called *spirit, geist,* or *higher sense of self)* that transcends the physical, mental, and emotional existence of a person at any given time. The soul and spirit are those aspects of consciousness that are not confined by objective space and time and that are unconstrained by linearity. By acknowledging a spiritual dimension to life, Watson is able to speculate on the human capacity to coexist with past, present, and future in the moment. She respects the dignity, reverence, chaos, mystery, and wonder of life because of the continuous yet unknown journey the soul takes, through the infinite and eternal. Watson (1999) views the soul as

> the essence of the person, which possesses a greater sense of self-awareness, a higher (ascent) degree of consciousness, an inner strength, and a power that can expand human capacities and allow a person to transcend his or her usual self. From this higher sense of consciousness (soul level), one can more fully

access the intuitive, deep imagination, the uncanny, the mystical, dream work, and feminine/masculine archetypes, and can come to 'be' utilizing modes of awareness, feeling, and experience that rational scientific cultures inhibit (p. 224).

The soul fully participates in healing. We need to continue to explore the spiritual, nonphysical, inner, and extrasensory (beyond the five senses) realms to learn of the dynamic and creative energy currents of the soul's existence and to learn of the inner healing journey toward wholeness (Watson, 1999).

Life

"Human life is defined as *being-in-the-world*, which is continuous in time and space" (Watson, 1989, p. 224). The locus of human existence is experience. Broadly defined, experience includes sensorimotor experience, mental/emotional experience, and spiritual experience. Experience is translated through multiple layers of awareness. Consciousness has the capacity to construct and create. The world as experienced is not merely reflected and interpreted by consciousness; it is *cocreated*. As persons evolve in ascending consciousness, their worldviews change. All individual consciousness arises from the clearing created by cultural or intersubjective relations. Housed in collective consciousness, a shared worldview is interpreted as culture. Collective and individual worldviews are dynamic and cocreated.

The person is a living, growing gestalt that possesses three spheres of being—body, mind and soul—which are influenced by the concept of self. The mind and the emotions are the starting point and the point of access to the subjective world. The self is the subjective center that lives within the whole of body, thoughts, sensations, desires, memories, life history, and so forth. Self is the seat of identity. We need to honor deep, subjective meanings and feelings about life, living, the natural inner processes, personal autonomy and freedom to make choices shaped by subjective intent (Watson, 1985, 1999). Watson has said that "[t]he person is neither simply an organism, nor simply spiritual. Although a person is embodied in experience in nature and in the physical world, a person can also transcend the physical world by controlling it, subduing it, changing it, or living in harmony with it" (1989, p. 225).

Intentionality is the projection of awareness or consciousness with some purpose and efficacy toward some object or outcome. The content of such consciousness can include belief, volition, expectation, attention, action, and even the unconscious (Schlitz, 1996a, 1996b). The conscious use of intention mobilizes internal and external resources to meet the intended purpose (Watson, 1999). One's intention and attention shape experiences, as parts of the evolutionary ontological process (Watson, 1999).

Watson (1999) has said, "if our conscious intentionality is to hold thoughts that are caring, open, loving, kind, and receptive, in contrast to an intentionality to control, manipulate and have power over, the consequences will be significant for our actions" (p. 121).

Watson contends that *transpersonal* "conveys a human-to-human connection in which both persons are influenced through the relationship and the *being-together in the moment.* This human connection . . . has a spiritual dimension . . . that can tap into healing" (Watson, 1999, p. 290). She continues, *"[t]ranspersonal* includes the unique individuality of each human, while extending beyond ego-self" (Watson, 1999, p. 290).

Transpersonal Caring-Healing Philosophy and Theory

Nursing's goal is to help persons gain a higher degree of harmony within the mindbodyspirit, which generates self-knowledge, self-reverence, self-healing, and self-care processes while allowing for diversity and possibility. In an ontology of relation, the nurse pursues this goal through transpersonal caring, relationship, and the human care process and responds to persons' subjective worlds in such a way that individuals can find meaning in their existence through exploring the meaning of their disharmony, suffering, and turmoil within the lived experience. This exploration promotes self-knowledge, self-control, self-love, choice based on subjective intent, and self-determination. The general goal is mental-spiritual evolution for self and others as well as discovery of inner power and self-control through caring. Achieving this goal can potentiate health, healing, and transcendence (Watson, 1999). Engaged in caring-healing praxis, the nurse demonstrates ontological and epistemological competencies and redefines technological competencies as sacred acts that are manifested with intentional caring-healing consciousness and within communal relation.

Caring in transpersonal caring-healing is both a moral ideal and an ontology. Informed moral passion and caring ontology are nursing's substance (Watson, 1990). As the essence of nursing, "caring is the most central and unifying focus for nursing practice" (Watson, 1988a, p. 33). Watson (1988a) continues, "Caring and love are the most universal, the most tremendous, and the most mysterious of cosmic forces; they comprise the primal and universal psychic energy" (p. 32). Caring, as an ethic and moral ideal, encourages the nurse to hold or attempt to hold the conscious intent to preserve wholeness; potentiate healing; and preserve dignity, integrity, and life-generating processes at the level of human nature and universe (Watson, 1999).

In this philosophy of human caring, "healing and wholeness become the starting points, the midpoints, and the open endings for the ongoing, evolving and unfolding of the human condition" (Watson, 1999, p. 97). *Health* is redefined as the unity and harmony within the body, mind, and soul—harmony between self and others and between self and nature and openness to increased possibility. Health is associated with the degree of congruence between self as perceived and self as experienced. Health focuses on physical, social, aesthetic, and moral realms and is viewed as consciousness and a human-environmental energy field as part of the new cosmology (Watson, 1999). As a state of continuous human evolution, health reflects a person's basic striving to actualize the real self and develop the spiritual essence of self (Watson, 1988a). It is a search to connect with deeper meanings and truths and to "embrace the near and far in the instant and to seize the tangible, manifestly real, and the divine" (Watson, 1999, p. 80).

Healing is redefined and related directly to the individual's evolving personhood. *Dis-ease* is associated with disharmony between body, mind, and soul of the person or disharmony between the person and environment or nature. Such disharmony makes the individual less open to diversity. Within the transpersonal caring relationship and the caring moment, there is healing potential. The agent for change in terms of healing is the person's internal, mental-spiritual consciousness, which allows the self to be healed. Such a view holds a commitment to a particular end beyond disease or pathology, to a moral ideal that embraces inner power of self, choice shaped by subjective intent, inner healing potential and preservation of harmony (Watson, 1989). Watson calls caring "the ethical principle or standard by which curing interventions are measured"(1988b, p. 2). Within this caring ontology, technical interventions commonly aimed at cure are also reframed as sacred acts conducted with a caring consciousness and completed in a way that honors the person as embodied spirit.

Healing space and environment attends to healing and promotes the intentional healing role of architecture (or surroundings) alongside conscious, intentional caring healing modalities. Conscious attention to healing spaces shifts the healthcare facility from being simply a place for bodies to be controlled, manipulated, and treated to a place in which there is conscious promotion of mindbodyspirit wholeness; attention to the relationship between stress and illness; hospital stress factors; and acknowledgment of the key role that emotions and the senses play in healing. Through the intentional introduction of art, music, color, smell, views of nature, mythology, ritual and symbol as expressions of humanity and culture, healing spaces can assist in transcending illness, pain, and suffering.

In Watson's theory, a single caring moment becomes a moment of possibility (Watson, 1989). Watson explains,

Transpersonal describes an intersubjective, human-to-human relationship that encompasses two unique individuals, both the nurse and the patient, in a given moment. Simultaneously the relationship transcends the two subjectivities, connecting to other higher dimensions of being and a higher/deeper consciousness that accesses the universal field and planes of inner wisdom: the human spirit realm (1999, p. 115).

Watson notes that the transpersonal caring moment honors the premise that

the power of love, faith, compassion, caring community and intention, consciousness and access to a deeper/higher energy source, etc . . . one's God, are as significant sources of healing as our conventional treatment approaches, and may indeed be more powerful in the long run (1999, p. 115).

The transpersonal caring relationship, in the caring moment, honors unity of being, and seeks healing through shifting consciousness levels to harmonize being for the patient and nurse by reconnecting and tapping into one's deeper/higher self in the world. Coming together in the moment provides an opportunity—an *actual occasion*—for human caring to occur. Human caring is actualized in the moment based on the actions and choices made by both the one-caring and the one-being-cared-for. The nurse and patient both determine the relationship and the use of that moment in time and space. In the moment, how the nurse chooses to be and to act will have significant impact on the opportunities of the moment and the eventual outcomes. The goal in the relationship is the protection, enhancement, and preservation of patient dignity, humanity, wholeness, and inner harmony. This outcome for the patient is achieved through heightened self-knowledge, self-control, self-care, caring, and self-healing. The nurse influences these outcomes by intentional use of caring consciousness in the moment and by holding intentionality toward wholeness as a moral ideal. Caring-healing consciousness—an intentionality of love and wholeness—is primary; it is a source and form of life energy, life spirit, and vital energy that can be communicated by the one-caring to the one-being-cared-for, potentiating healing (Watson, 1999).

These competencies of being are essential for transpersonal caring-healing. Once they are achieved, one can "naturally begin to attend to the artistry of healing work, and make the connection between these competencies and the way in which they can be translated into professional *caring-healing modalities* and the 'knowing' and 'doing' aspects of caring praxis" (Watson, 1999, p. 192). Each caring act becomes a potential act of beauty-in-relation and thus an act of healing—an art/act. It creates an opportunity for transformation and healing inside the witnessing of art or the act of making art.

The healing arts can be used to activate specific responses to promote wellness and centering, act as modes of expression and meditation, comment on healing and illness experiences, and provide psychoarchitecture for healing spaces. Watson (1999) explains that at "a deep transpersonal level, art and art making connect us through metaphor, symbol, myth, and ritual to the human soul and an experience of humanity, shared across time" (p. 197).

Advanced caring-healing arts, or *modalities,* are integral to transpersonal practice. These modalities are also extensions of the carative factors of Watson's earlier work (1985) and the art of transpersonal caring that included "movement, touch, sounds, words, color, and forms" (pp. 66-68). These advanced caring-healing modalities include the intentional conscious use of imagery and auditory, visual, olfactory, tactile, gustatory, mental-cognitive, kinesthetic, and caring consciousness, which includes psychological and therapeutic presence modalities (Watson, 1999). By exploring the integration of such therapies as music, visualization, breath work, aromatherapy, therapeutic touch, massage, caring touch, reflexology, dream work, humor, play, journaling, poetry, art making, meditation, transpersonal teaching, dance, yoga, movement, authentic presencing, and centering into caring practice as options for patient healing, the nurse acknowledges the emerging consciousness paradigm. Within this transpersonal philosophy and theory, different caring-healing modalities may be operating as sources of the patient's healing at different levels across the spectrum of consciousness.

These examples do not preclude the other practices Watson outlined as *carative factors* (Box 6-1), including emotional, expressive and relational work; comfort measures; and teaching learning (Watson, 1979, 1985, 1988a). These carative factors provide a guide to aspects of being, knowing, and doing so as to implement a caring philosophy and inquire into your own practices of human caring. According to Watson (1999), "[t]o be implemented into care, they require of the nurse intention, caring values, knowledge, a will, a relationship, actions, and commitment" (p. 227). Nurses embrace this theoretical work where they find congruence with their practice lives. Some may find the language of Watson's earlier work more compatible than the language of her 1999 work, depending on one's philosophy. The carative factors are discussed in detail in Watson's earlier publications (1979, 1985, 1988a, 1989).

In summary, Watson's works include the following:
- An expanded view of person
- The primacy of caring-consciousness and intentionality

- The reframing of all nursing acts to acknowledge sacredness and the embodied spirit
- The foundational nature of ontological competencies
- The personal transformation necessary for the nurse from ego self to transpersonal self
- The significance of the caring moment for healing
- The incorporation of the healing arts and caring-healing modalities into everyday practice

---

BOX 6-1   WATSON'S TEN CARATIVE FACTORS

1. The formation of a humanistic-altruistic system of values.
2. The instillation of faith-hope.
3. The cultivation of sensitivity to one's self and to others.
4. The development of a helping-trust relationship.
5. The promotion and acceptance of the expression of positive and negative feelings.
6. The systematic use of the scientific problem-solving method for decision making.
7. The promotion of interpersonal teaching-learning.
8. The provision for a supportive, protective, and corrective mental, physical, sociocultural, and spiritual environment.
9. Assistance with the gratification of human needs.
10. The allowance of existential-phenomenological forces.

From Watson, J. (1979). *Nursing: The philosophy and science of caring.* Boston: Little, Brown. Reprinted (1985), Boulder: University Press of Colorado.

CRITICAL THINKING IN NURSING PRACTICE WITH WATSON'S PHILOSOPHY AND THEORY

Engaging in Watson's philosophy and theory involves subjectivity and both rational and nonrational reflection. Watson suggests that you experiment with the conscious use of caring consciousness in patient relations, experience the transpersonal body in centering and meditation practices, experience your own caring through the use of art or healing therapies on yourself, and compare your experience with the theory. In Watson's frame, theory involves guiding and seeing that moves *through* being, knowing, and doing, and seeing that moves the personal *through* the professional (Watson, 1998). She emphasizes that the nurse's subjectivity and ontological competencies are critical to caring and healing. Using caring philosophy and caring science as a lens for reflective caring practice can bring wholeness to poetic fragments and fractures and begin to make some sense of the broader landscape uniting the marshes of messy "practice" and the lofty mountains of "abstract thought" (Watson, 1998, p. 215). In an integrated knowledge-in-action approach much of what is called knowing may be spontaneous and tacit, given the murky nature of clinical situations, the embedded assumptions that often direct decisions, the unique subjectivity of both the nurse and the patient, and the hectic variables that are impossible to control.

In coming to know the patient during a caring moment, the nurse always begins first in relation with self and other. Reflection is lived out both inside the caring moment as *reflection-in-action,* and retrospectively as *reflection-on-action.* In the first instance, during the caring moment, reflection begins with a genuine need to know the other with compassionate concern. Reflection assists the nurse to question what calls her to care, her responses to that call, the patient's response to the nurse's caring-consciousness and caring actions, the healing space that is being created, and most significantly, the meaning of the situation for the patient. Watson's recently revised carative factors (1998, 1999) address the patient's and the nurse's subjective worlds (Table 6-1). The nurse's subjectivity always has the intent to heal and acts as both a way of creating compassionate understanding through common human bonding with the patient and as a way of learning from each other because of each unique history. The telling of the story, in whatever form (physical symptoms, oral communications, behavior, presence, or spiritual connection) becomes a way for the patients to find their voices, own the experience as lived, and create some distance from experiencing so as to allow introspection and the seeking of meaning. The day-to-day concerns and personal worlds of the nurse and patient can become instructive for locating and understanding a deeper, more universal, more complex pattern of life. In this way, each of these revised carative factors contributes to their relationship and the meaning transpersonal caring has for the patient and the nurse.

In *retrospective reflection-on-action,* deeper personal meaning can come from looking back on a nurse's lived experience that accumulates and gathers interpretive significance as it is re-membered. Retrospective contemplation involves integrating nursing experiences—physical, mental, and spiritual—into personal history, which then becomes foreground for future caring relations. Reflection starts from a place of unique experience where uncomfortable feelings and thoughts surface, and where existing knowledge (aesthetic, personal, moral, empirical, metaphysical) seems insufficient to make sense of what is occurring. Sometimes reflection on a philosophy such as Watson's requires a sort of relaxed meditation, where you move away from the patient care issues at hand and allow thoughts to move at a much deeper level to the transpersonal, nonrational. Coming back into conscious awareness, the evolved meaning of the experience is now felt as owned, and a sense of intuitive understanding and spiritual insight can be achieved. These retrospective reflections are often life-affirming and restore purpose and meaning.

Text continued on p. 112

TABLE 6-1   Watson's Carative Factors Redefined, Patients' Subjective Worlds, and Nurses' Reflections

Carative Factors Redefined*	Patient's Subjective World†	Nurse's Reflections†
1. Practice of loving-kindness and equanimity with context of caring-consciousness	• Perception/response to caring intent • Choices of how to be in relation	Who is this person? Am I open to participate in his or her personal story? How am I being called to care? How ought I be in this situation?
2. Being authentically present and enabling and sustaining the deep belief system and subjective life world of self and the one-being-cared-for	• Conceptions of reality through storytelling • Belief system as support • Sources of faith/hope	What does this relationship mean to this patient? What health event brings this person to this health facility? What information do I need to nurse this person? Can I imagine what this experience is like? Can I encourage this person to find faith/hope?
3. Cultivation of one's own spiritual practices and transpersonal self, going beyond ego self. Being sensitive to self and other	• Aspects of soul care as part of lifestyle • Responses to one-giving-care	How am I attending to this person's spiritual needs and soul care? Does the experience of others nurture my compassionate self? Can I find new ways of caring?
4. Developing and sustaining a helping-trusting, authentic caring relationship	• Degree of trust (openness) • Signs of vulnerability in relation • Signs of invitation to relate • Willingness to disclose deep meanings • Past experiences in caring relation • Responses to nurse as subject/presence • Validation of concerns, needs, priorities • Translation of concerns to goals for care	How can I enter this person's private space? Can I establish a caring dialogue to help this person find meaning in this experience? What specific forms of caring will best acknowledge, affirm and sustain this person? What strategies can I use to help this person translate his or her concerns to me and use them as goals for his or her recovery and self-healing?

*Reference: Watson, J. (2001). Jean Watson: Theory of Human Caring. In M. E. Parker, *Nursing theories and nursing practice*, pp. 343-354. Philadelphia: F. A. Davis Co.
†References: Watson, J. (1998). A meta-reflection on reflective practice and caring theory. In C. Johns & D. Fleshwater (Eds.), *Transforming nursing through reflective practice* (pp. 214-220). London: Blackwell Science; and Watson, J. (1999). *Postmodern nursing and beyond*. Edinburgh: Churchill Livingstone/W. B. Saunders.

TABLE 6-1	Watson's Carative Factors Redefined, Patients' Subjective Worlds, and Nurses' Reflections—cont'd	
Carative Factors Redefined	**Patient's Subjective World**	**Nurse's Reflections**
5. Being present to and supportive of the expression of positive and negative feelings as a connection with deeper spirit of self and the one-being-cared-for	• Comfort level with self disclosure • Expression of feelings about experiences • Search for interpretation and meaning • Disclosure of deep search • Relation of behavior and expressions to cultural mores • Openness to others' interpretations • Clarity of current health situation and its meaning for his life/choices	How can I enable this person to express his or her concerns? How must this person be feeling? How does this person show his or her pain? What are the mores about pain in his or her culture? What are the subtle patterns that surface in this person's story? Can I use this to help him or her under-stand the deep meanings of his or her health event/moment? Am I meeting my obligation to reveal my understandings to the one-being-cared-for with a healing intent?
6. Creative use of self and all ways of knowing as part of the caring process and engagement in artistry of caring-healing practices	• Disclosure of uniqueness as person • Perceptions of pattern of experiences/responses to health situation • Perceptions of life pattern and role changes and consequences • Definition of helpful care • Responses to art/act and other caregivers • Openness to nontraditional, creative interventions and care	What is the uniqueness of this person and this situation? How has this event affected his or her usual life pat-terns and roles? How can I contextualize the theory of care for this person and situation? How does this sit-uation compare with my previous experience? What are the significant issues to attend to? How can I help this person? Which healing arts are appropriate?

Continued

TABLE 6-1	Watson's Carative Factors Redefined, Patients' Subjective Worlds, and Nurses' Reflections—cont'd	
Carative Factors Redefined	**Patient's Subjective World**	**Nurse's Reflections**
7. Engaging in genuine teaching-learning experience that attends to unity of being and meaning, and attempts to stay within other's frame of reference	• Definition of health, healing, wholeness • Understanding of experiences, self-care needs and limitations • Awareness of personal resources, strengths for healing • Identification of habitual ways of responding • Sense of freedom and commitment to action • Preferred ways of knowing • Past experiences with learning and health • Openness to self-discovery, participative learning, accessing external resources • Goals for recovery/healing	Is this person able to understand what he or she is experiencing? Is he or she aware of his or her choices, and their consequences? How does this person view the future? How can this person's concerns be translated into goals for recovery? What are his or her preferred ways of knowing? How can I share knowledge in a way that can assist with self-care and healing?
8. Creating healing environment at all levels (physical, as well as nonphysical) whereby wholeness, beauty, comfort, dignity, and peace are potentiated	• Role of emotion/senses in healing • Definition of space that is healing • Stressors in environment • Responses to stress and preferred methods of stress management • Use of healing arts in lifestyle • Sense of self-worth, dignity, peace • Responses to beauty, sources of color, movement, texture, and form	What is important to this person to make his or her stay comfortable? What meanings do the surroundings, sounds, and smells have for this person? How can the healing art be incorporated into this space? How can I use assertiveness and political action to create a healing environment for this person? How can I creatively deal with institutional imperfections, manage constraints, contin-gencies, and dilemmas with wisdom, while maintaining the goal of healing and wholeness?

References: Watson, J. (1998). A meta-reflection on reflective practice and caring theory. In C. Johns & D. Fleshwater (Eds.), *Transforming nursing through reflective practice* (pp. 214-220). London: Blackwell Science; and Watson, J. (1999). *Postmodern nursing and beyond.* Edinburgh: Churchill Livingstone/W. B. Saunders.

TABLE 6-1	Watson's Carative Factors Redefined, Patients' Subjective Worlds, and Nurses' Reflections—cont'd	
Carative Factors Redefined	**Patient's Subjective World**	**Nurse's Reflections**
9. Assisting with basic needs, with an intentional caring consciousness; administering human care essentials, which potentiate alignment of mindbodyspirit, wholeness, and unity of being in all aspects of care; attending to both embodied spirit and evolving emergence	• Perception of self as embodied spirit • Relationship of self to physical body • Willingness to assume central role in healing • Priorities for needs/goals for care • Sense of personal wholeness/fragmentation • Personal supports and involvement in care • Preferred timeline for healing • Feedback on responses to care	Am I process focused or outcome focused? Can I let go of the need to fix situations? What supports does this person have in his or her life? How involved are they in his or her care? Which caring/healing modalities are appropriate for his or her care? Am I honoring this person as embodied spirit in my actions? What is the desirable practice here that will honor caring as moral ideal?
10. Opening and attending to spiritual-mysterious, and existential dimensions of one's own life-death; soul care for self and the one-being-cared-for	• Openness to deeper self-exploration and soul care • Personal definition of spiritual needs/soul care and relation to healing • Key existential life issues in this moment/ experience • Role of dream work, deep imagination, intuitions, myth, etc. in search of meaning • View of future, purpose in life • Critical life decision areas	How does this person view the future for himself or herself and others? How can I enable this person to find meaning in this experience and make good decisions about his or her life and/or death? What are the life lessons in this situation for the patient and myself? What soul care is useful for this patient?

CASE HISTORY OF DEBBIE

Debbie is a 29-year-old woman who was recently admitted to the oncology nursing unit for evaluation after sensing pelvic "fullness" and noticing a watery, foul-smelling vaginal discharge. A Papanicolaou smear revealed class V cervical cancer. She was found to have a stage II squamous cell carcinoma of the cervix and underwent a radical hysterectomy with bilateral salpingooophorectomy.

Her past health history revealed that physical examinations had been infrequent. She also reported that she had not performed breast self-examination. She is 5 feet, 4 inches tall and weights 89 pounds. Her usual weight is about 110 pounds. She has smoked approximately two packs of cigarettes a day for the past 16 years. She is gravida 2, para 2. Her first pregnancy was at age 16, and her second was at age 18. Since that time, she has taken oral contraceptives on a regular basis.

Debbie completed the eighth grade. She is married and lives with her husband and her two children in her mother's home, which she describes as less than sanitary. Her husband is unemployed. She describes him as emotionally distant and abusive at times.

She has done well following surgery except for being unable to completely empty her urinary bladder. She is having continued postoperative pain and nausea. It will be necessary for her to perform intermittent self-catheterization at home. Her medications are (1) an antibiotic, (2) an analgesic as needed for pain, and (3) an antiemetic as needed for nausea. In addition, she will be receiving radiation therapy on an outpatient basis.

Debbie is extremely tearful. She expresses great concern over her future and the future of her two children. She believes that this illness is a punishment for her past life.

NURSING CARE OF DEBBIE WITH WATSON'S PHILOSOPHY

A Caring Moment with Debbie

I hear her first from behind the drawn curtain. It is a low muffled sob that seems to fill the room. The other patient turns quietly toward the wall, unsure how to respond or what to do. Another's vulnerability publicly displayed is awkward. The silence behind the crying is magnified off the walls. As I stand frozen, I feel myself tense up and release. I am unsure whether to disturb her, to enter her private space and offer care, or whether to retreat and let her weep alone. I didn't know her at all, other than the brief sterile comments in report—29 years old, cervical cancer, radical hysterectomy, poor social supports, kids, urinary retention, pain, nausea, radiation as outpatient. It tells you nothing, really. I know very little *about Debbie*. I remember I found myself wincing when several of the nurses described her husband as a loser and her kids as sweet and very young to be motherless. Their judging her life seemed to me to be a violation of her. I can only imagine what she must be facing right now and how she must feel alone.

This is the Watson caring occasion staring me right in the face. Either you commit at 8:02 AM and get involved, or you walk away. Why care? Why not? The word *alone* tugs at me. I quietly pull the curtain back slightly and move into her space. My stomach is in knots. This is never easy, no matter how often you do it. It requires such a delicate, tactful touch. I consciously take a deep breath in and steady myself. I have no idea what I have to offer her, not knowing her or even knowing what I will find behind the curtain. Every patient is unique. I just try to keep myself open to receive them. I have confidence that the right words will somehow find their way to me. I know I can be present for her on several levels and be authentic if I stay true to who I am. I look up and try to hold caring thoughts as intent, but I can feel I am still hesitant and my focus is still on the sobbing and on what to do. I need to find a way to connect that is real, not just a technique, and relate with Debbie the person.

She has her face turned away, but I can see enough to immediately sense the anguish written there, the despair, the frailness. She seems so young, only a few years younger than I am. I always feel compelled to engage in the person's face first. It's there that I have discovered that I first feel or see the need or call to care. Debbie's face is drawn and pale; her thin hand is at her mouth; and she holds a soggy tissue to her lips. I feel a twinge down deep, an ache for her vulnerability, caught up in those moist eyes and soggy effort at self-control. I feel myself pulled to her. There is a part of me that just wants to reach out and hold her, but I hardly know her. She is coiled tightly into a fetal position, with the sheet pulled up to her shoulders, as if to shelter herself from the world, including me. She sees the movement of the curtain and turns. She meets my concerned gaze with reddened eyes and a sob. It catches in my throat. I lean across the remaining space between us and reach for her free hand. Her hand is damp and cool and bruised from a previous venapuncture. She doesn't withdraw from my touch but keeps her eyes on my face. She is hesitant and uncertain too. There is no script for this work; it's pure nursing. I can feel myself consciously center, steady, and open. In a quiet gentle voice, almost a whisper, I ask if I can be of any help. I reach for a fresh tissue, and I offer it to her but keep my eyes on hers. I offer my self. She looks briefly away then returns my gaze. I breathe out. In between breaths she apologizes for crying and says she hopes she is not disturbing the other patient. I hesitate.

What can I say? I tell her she needs to be where she is now and to live out how she is feeling. The other patient will understand. She needs now to focus on herself and her own healing. I leave, reminding myself to check in with her roommate later in the morning, since witnesses also share pain. Debbie looks away and down for a moment, as if struggling for self-composure, for dignity. It is awkward meeting someone new in this way. I smile gently, trying unobtrusively to show her feelings are okay; she can trust me. No words pass between us. She turns to lift herself up in the bed. I extend an arm to help her gain her balance. She winces as she frees the covers from her back. Her eyes are shut tight now as she uses my arms for leverage and tries to find a more comfortable position. She is obviously in discomfort.

I ask to see her dressing, carefully pull back the covers, and see that everything seems to be intact and dry. I ask her when she last had some pain medication and continue watching her face. She is unsure. She looks over at the untouched breakfast tray and responds, "Some time during the night, I guess. Perhaps it would calm me down some if I had another shot now. I just feel so teary and weak. This just isn't me. I need to pull myself together for my kids. I am all they've got." Falling apart and pulling together, she is looking for a sense of wholeness, trying to make sense of what is happening to her. She seems to be feeling some dissonance between how she sees herself "before" and how she is now. Her hope seems anchored firmly in her relationship with her children.

She glances down to the only personal thing in the sterile, cold, gray hospital room—there are no flowers, no bathrobes here—only a small framed photo of a healthier-looking Debbie smiling up at me, her arms wrapped protectively around her two young children. She touches the photo from a happier time, as if to touch the young boy and girl there, a precious touchstone, then lays back in bed with a sigh. She gazes through the window. She seems lost and far away in thought. There is so much I want to say about the children and about the despair that I hear around the edges of her voice. I hear it all tumble in my mind—*what I could, what I should*—but instead I give her some space and remain silent. Her face, my bellwether, is blank. She has left me now and is probably with those two young faces, tracing their day. I quietly excuse myself, telling her I will be right back with some pain medication. I ask her if she will be okay alone for a few moments. She turns with a faint smile and responds, "Yes, and thank you." I look back as I return the curtain to its place of privacy. Her gaze has found its way out the window again.

Her hand is pressed slightly into her abdomen. The pain is back. I leave, sensing some unspoken urgency in the moment. Outside the room, I look down at my watch and am shocked to find only 10 minutes have passed. It felt like I was moving in slow motion with Debbie—light touch, light words softly, slowly, quietly, delicately, like a slow rhythmic waltz. But now it all floods in as a rush of experience. My mind is racing, trying to sort through what has just happened, trying to find a pattern in the words and gestures, in the look of a face, the untouched tray, the family, the pain, the dressing, the information from report. How can I make sense of this? How can I be of help to Debbie? Where is the place of healing for her? Where is the harmony in it all? So much of life has seemed to rush by the two of us in such little time. I know I can't fix it for her, but maybe I can help her find her own sources for healing. I sense strength there beneath the surface. She certainly has a strong motive to heal. I admire and am touched by the obvious love she has for her children, and her determination to parent them well, to be there for them. But who will be there for her? I sense there are many complex issues here for Debbie, not the least of which must be her very own mortality. How does she feel about what she is facing? What meaning does it have for her? Where does she get her own inner strength?

On this floor I have had to work through my own fears and come to terms with my own death so that I will be able to talk about it comfortably and honestly with patients, when and if they are ready (usually 2:00 AM when you're alone with them in the darkness). Sometimes it gets very raw, but it's beautiful too. It's odd how patients connect issues of life, love, meaning, purpose, anger, denial, failure, and guilt. They all seem processed together. My being there for them has taught me so much about my own life. In some significant ways, they give me a reason to be. The human spirit is amazing. I wonder what Debbie's hopes and dreams are. I commit myself to care for Debbie in whatever way I can, to be there for her. Her "thank you" and shaky smile make me think she may be connecting with me as well. I move quickly to get the medication for her pain. Perhaps we can continue to get to know each other later. I want to hear more of her story.

DISCUSSION

Artistry in nursing is finding the beauty in a single moment. We see in these reflections by the nurse on her moments with Debbie as just such human beauty and art. It is a human dance as both find their way slowly into relation. These caring moments have their own radiance and vividness that confirms their value for the patient and the nurse. As in all things beautiful, they require us to be truly present, in complete contact with the whole of experience, to appreciate and find their truth.

Reflecting-in-the-moment, the nurse moves along the curve of the spiral from experience, to interpretation and arrives in a very preliminary way at understanding. We see in her dialectic a struggle with the notion of caring-consciousness—that is, how to be with another in a way that is healing. How can she shape her caring intent toward Debbie in a way that is beyond technique? The answer is in returning to Debbie and the connection she feels with her, human to human. In so doing, she embraces her transpersonal self. She recognizes her own call to care, first in an echo. She is touched by the sound of a sob and hears in it the echo of herself. In the nurse's understanding at a deep transpersonal level, Debbie's sob made a claim on her that called her to respond in care. To hearken, the nurse needed to be in tune first with her own being and to listen carefully for the inner voice of her own heart echoing back a response "I am here for you." She also needed to be open to what Debbie's sobbing signified as a call to care, and here she needed to wrestle with her own hesitation in committing to care. But these limits are transcended when she faces her own moral ideals. The realization of Debbie suffering alone raised the call bar, and she surrendered to the need to be there for her.

Throughout these moments, we see the nurse being drawn into Debbie's suffering and in so doing making it her own. In Debbie's face she recognizes vulnerability as a call to woundedness, to deep inner pain, to despair, to fear. She sees in Debbie's eyes hesitation, withholding, the need for dignity and affirmation. In Debbie's hand, she touches embodied spirit. In Debbie's touchstone, she sees a mother's love, and the face of hope. In Debbie's room, she sees little healing space, save a small picture frame, a remembrance. The nurse responds lightly, in gentle acknowledgment, respect, and reverence. These are the brush strokes of an artist—touch, whisper, gaze, silence, smile, and intuitions. Consciousness is shaped to the moment, finely crafted in sensitive form to reach out to Debbie. Vital energy, or life energy, is shaped and passed as conscious intentionality. It is not a grasping, grudging, manipulative activity but a very subtle aesthetic knowing that speaks to a deeper part of Debbie, other than the body physical. We can see in these moments the technical competencies, or the doing that still needs to be an active part of caring-healing relations, and an acknowledgment of the need for empirical knowledge to interpret for care. We cannot ignore the scientific, curing aspects of the nurse's role but must situate them in a higher purpose—that is, Debbie's healing and harmony of mindbodyspirit that includes the beauty of the human spirit and the wonder and awe the soul brings to care.

In her reflection-on-action in the hall, the nurse concedes to the need for active engagement in critical thought, in pattern seeking, priority setting, and mutual planning with Debbie to identify healing modalities that would best suit her needs. She resists labeling and categorizing that would morally situate Debbie as object and seeks instead Debbie's own meaning related to care. She approaches her care in an open-ended way, recognizing the limits of human control in a universe with its own grander purposes. In all her actions, we see evidence of a reframing, a consideration of the larger consciousness in which they reside. She is able to place her own subjectivity and history-in-care as foreground for her relationship with Debbie. She is able to measure her own competencies and see the need to evolve to a higher level through her own soul care. She sees the need to animate her own spirit of being and nourish it. She envisions possibility in the coming together of herself and Debbie, consciousness to consciousness, so that a new field of possibility for choice and advanced human capacity can be realized. From this place, both have the opportunity to evolve as humans. Finally, we see that caring is something we must continually redeem, retrieve, regain, and recapture each time we are called to be in "caring occasions" (Hultgren, 1994, p. 180).

CASE HISTORY OF JIMMY

A Caring Moment with Jimmy

I am speaking to a staff member in the hallway when Cameron approaches. He seems agitated and reluctant to talk with Sally there, so I tell Sally I will meet up with her later in the afternoon and turn my full attention to Cameron. He is the life partner of one of the patients on the palliative unit, Jimmy, a 35-year-old writer who is dying of Acquired Immunodeficiency Syndrome (AIDS). Jimmy has been with us now for over 3 weeks. He has pneumocystis pneumonia (PCP) and severe Kaposi's sarcoma (KS) lesions on his lower right leg. This, coupled with severe neuropathy, has caused Jimmy intense pain. Jimmy is not a favorite on the unit; dementia has taken a most precious gift, his mind. He spends most of his day yelling out and shouting at the nurses and picking at his clothes. Cameron is beside himself with worry and is trying to arrange for Jimmy to be moved to an AIDS hospice in the community. But the waiting list is long, and Jimmy is rapidly deteriorating.

I have not cared for Jimmy for the past week, as I was busy assigned in another part of the hospital. Cameron asks me if I would relieve him from taking care of Jimmy for 30 minutes while he goes down for a break in the cafeteria. He looks tired and wasted himself, torn up trying to comfort the man he loves and running interference with the staff. He was not always welcomed at the nurses' station, so he "picked his fights carefully" and sought support where he could. For some reason, he trusts me to care. I value his trust.

I enter Jimmy's room quite unprepared for what I find there. Jimmy is propped up in bed, his spent body angled awkwardly against the pillows. His hands are agitated against the covers, and he plucks at imaginary objects in the air. These are the same hands that crafted beautiful words on paper not that long ago. Cameron had showed me some of his elegant poetry. Inside I feel my heart begin to weep at such incredible loss. I take a deep breath and shift my attention to his face, to Jimmy.

Jimmy is still with me, but barely. Before me lies an emaciated shell of a man. Now completely confined to his bed, Jimmy continuously scratches at himself. His cheeks are sunken, his temples hollow, eye sockets deepening, and eyes scattering their gaze, ricocheting in fear from object to object. His eyes are vacant, gone. His skin, normally tanned, is pale with festering sores; his hair is thin and dull; his mouth and tongue are coated; his lips move incessantly in gibberish. Jimmy doesn't talk much. He yells out in raw emotion during the night hours, but he has no urge for conversation. He sees Cameron but does not *see* him.

I am struck by the disintegration of his physical self. It is alarming; it catches the breath. The individuality of Jimmy's body, what enabled Cameron and me and others who love him to recognize Jimmy as the person that he is and no other, is dulled. It has almost become imperceptible. It is Jimmy, and it is also not Jimmy. Jimmy's loss of bodily integrity is startling and disconcerting. I need to center myself to look beyond the physical body. I sense in a very deep way that this loss is more, due not only to the ravaging changes of Jimmy's presence, but is combined somehow with a dulling of his interior life, so that his very soul is somehow lost as well. It seems like the soul and body mirror each other. This frightens me. It is a form of living death.

Jimmy's days are now numbered. His world is night sweats, fever, and diarrhea. Each breath is a struggle; to survive is a struggle. Gone from view is his most magnificent imagination. Moments from only a few minutes ago are lost to him. His gestures and facial expressions are now shallow, as if disappearing slowly from sight. It is almost as if Jimmy's body is slowly dissolving. I can only imagine Cameron's pain at seeing his lover fade away.

I walk closer to be with Jimmy in whatever way I can. I pull his hands down from the air, and, holding them in my own, I speak directly to him. "Hi, Jimmy. How are you doing? I am going to spend some time with you while Cameron gets some lunch, okay? You look a little uncomfortable. Let me help you roll over on your side for a while." I get no response. I expect none.

Very carefully I try to roll Jimmy over on his side, aware that with each touch of my hand, there may be pain. I know that Jimmy is embodied spirit and believe somewhere inside he is still there with me. I want to reach him if I can. I want to touch his spirit and get beyond and above the body that is dissolving in front of me. To do this I must get beyond my own pain. I watch it rise in thought and then slowly fade.

Once I have him comfortably on his side, I reach for the back-care lotion and, slowly warming my hands, I center my consciousness and pool my energy. In ritual and silence I prepare my hands and myself. Then, focusing on Jimmy, I begin to slowly, rhythmically move my hands along his back, rocking my body forward and back. Smoothly I rotate the flow. I move my hands rhythmically in silence, to soothe his tearing flesh. I reach and receive, as in a sacred act.

The room is silent except for Jimmy's noisy, labored breathing. The noon sun falls softly through the window onto the table by his bed. Everywhere in pictures and flowers there are remembrances of love. This is a healing space, a place of soul. I can feel my own rhythm match his. The stretching and pulling of my arms and hands are a part of the motion of his body under my touch. My own breathing rises and falls with the stretch and pull, the flow of the hands, the flow of the mind, breathing in, taking in, breathing out, flowing out. I feel Jimmy relax under my hands. Carefully, I slowly begin to disengage. The hands gently take an ever-widening spiral and then come to a stop. I walk in silence to Jimmy's side and pull up a chair into the sunrays. Jimmy's eyes are resting on the flowers at his bedside. His hands have stopped their agitation. His mouth is lax.

I begin to tell Jimmy a story, a story crafted in part by my own imagination quite spontaneously but born in the reality of the spring garden behind my home. Jimmy and I take an enchanted walk round the paths, through the dandelions, over the chipmunk's hollow, peering into birdhouses and ending up out by the old barn. I talk in color and form, in birdsong, in nature and promise, because, after all, it is spring, and spring is a walk through wonder, through the smallest of possibilities, through birth and death and rebirth. My eyes never leave Jimmy's face.

About halfway through the garden, Jimmy's eyes begin to close. His eyelashes, remarkably untouched by his disease, rest on his cheeks. It is hard to tell whether he is still listening or if he has ever heard what I have said, but at least he is calmer and more relaxed now, so I finish the garden tour. Then I quietly stand up to leave, looking a last time at Jimmy's face, now caught in the grace of light from the window, and there a gift—a single tear rolls gently down his cheek.

DISCUSSION OF NURSING CARE OF JIMMY WITH WATSON'S PHILOSOPHY

Each art has its own moves, and we see this play out in the moments of care of Jimmy. The nurse is confronted with silence and decay. She is caught up in grief and the sense of loss. Through caring for Jimmy and by serving Jimmy through caring, she finds the meaning of life in her world. She returns to her own center to find renewed self-awareness and return to the call for a caring response to a greater human need, beyond her self. In this caring moment, as she struggles to recover her center, she raises questions about the relationship between the mind and body, identity and body, and the embodied spirit. Her moral dilemma remains: "How can I serve and care for Jimmy, in this, his darkest hour? How can I *be there* for him?" "How can I help Jimmy find some sense of harmony in his final days?" "What is my purpose, my goal for Jimmy?"

To be centered in caring consciousness means finding a way through to peace and hope and preparing anew to hear and respond to the deeper call to care. The nurse intuited a deep inner need, beyond the physical body, and she responded artfully to the call. Her reframing of the back-care ritual is the recognition of the sacred nature of nursing care, the power of conscious intentionality, and an honoring of the human spirit. The nurse sensed unity of consciousness between herself and Jimmy, and out of that field of possibility came the beautiful walk in the garden—beauty and healing walking hand in hand. As artist, this nurse wisely crafted a healing space, deftly selecting the healing arts and healing modalities for that moment-in-time. It was a simple, spontaneous act, and both were changed by it.

CRITICAL THINKING EXERCISES

1. Select a caring moment in which you were recently engaged, and write about your experience. Try to examine your own consciousness inside the moment through thoughtful reflection. Can you identify the ways in which you came to know the other as subject? What were the aspects of the experience that have become significant parts of your own personal history?
2. Observe a place in a hospital and assess the environment as a healing space. How would you describe this space in terms of its potential to heal? How could you use psychoarchitecture and artistry to enhance this healing space?
3. Describe a patient situation in which you have found it difficult to care. What aspects of the situation made it difficult to care? Describe yourself as the one-who-cared-for, and describe the one-cared-for. How could you alter your own being, knowing, and doing when this situation confronts you again?
4. Create a piece of art—a poem, a painting, a dance movement, or notes of music—that illustrates a beautiful moment in your nursing practice. Describe how the piece of art expresses your experience of caring as art. Reflect on your process of performing the art of nursing in relation to Watson's theory.
5. Reflect on the caring moments with Debbie and Jimmy and describe caring in the two cases according to Watson's 10 carative factors.

References

Dossey, B. M. & Dossey, L. (1999). Forward. In J. Watson, *Postmodern nursing and beyond* (pp. vii-x). Edinburgh: Churchill Livingstone/WB Saunders.

Hultgren, F. H. (1994). Being called to care-or-caring? Being called to be: Do we have a new question? In M. E. Lashley, M. T. Neal, E. T. Slunt, L. M. Berman, & F. H. Hultgren (Eds.), *Being called to care* (pp. 179-209). New York: State University of New York.

Puhakka, K. (1998). Contemplating everything: Wilber's evolutionary theory in dialectical perspective. In D. Rothberg & S. Kelly (Eds.), *Ken Wilber in dialogue* (pp. 283-304). Wheaton, IL: Quest.

Schlitz, M. (1996a). Intentionality and intuition and their implications: A challenge for science and medicine. *The Journal of Mind-Body Health, 12*(2), 58-66.

Schlitz, M. (1996b). Intentionality: A program of study. *The Journal of Mind-Body Health, 12*(3), 31-32.

Talento, B. (1995). Jean Watson. In J. B. George (Ed.), *Nursing theories* (3rd ed.). East Norwalk, CT: Appleton & Lange.

Watson, J. (1979). *Nursing: The philosophy and science of caring.* Boston: Little, Brown. Reprinted (1985), Boulder: Colorado Associated Press.

Watson, J. (1985). *Nursing: Human science and human care.* Norwalk, CT: Appleton & Lange.

Watson, J. (1988a). *Nursing: Human science and human care.* New York: National League for Nursing.

Watson, J. (1988b). Introduction: An ethic of caring/curing/nursing qua nursing. In J. Watson and M. A. Ray (Eds.), *The ethics of care and the ethics of cure: Synthesis in chronicity* (pp. 1-3). New York: National League for Nursing.

Watson, J. (1989). Watson's philosophy and theory of human caring in nursing. In J. Riehl-Sisca (Ed.), *Conceptual models for nursing practice* (3rd ed., pp. 219-236). Norwalk, CT: Appleton & Lange.

Watson, J. (1990). Caring knowledge and informed moral passion. *Advances in Nursing Science, 13*(1), 15-24.

Watson, J. (1995). Postmodernism and knowledge development in nursing. *Nursing Science Quarterly, 8*(2), 60-64.

Watson, J. (1997). The theory of human caring: Retrospective and prospective. *Nursing Science Quarterly, 10*(1), 49-52.

Watson, J. (1998). A meta-reflection on reflective practice and caring theory. In C. Johns & D. Fleshwater (Eds.), *Transforming nursing through reflective practice* (pp. 214-220). London: Blackwell Science.

Watson, J. (1999). *Postmodern nursing and beyond.* Edinburgh: Churchill Livingstone/W. B. Saunders. Copyright Harcourt Health Sciences.

Wilber, K. (1999). *The collected works of Ken Wilber, volume 4.* Boston: Shambhala.

Benner's Philosophy in Nursing Practice

Karen A. Brykczynski

"Nursing is an integrative science that studies the relationships between mind, body, and human worlds. It is concerned with far more than the cognitive structure of formal mental properties, such as attitudes and belief systems of the mind-brain, and the physiology and pathophysiology of the body as a system of cells, tissues and organs. Nursing is concerned with the social sentient body that dwells in finite human worlds: that gets sick and recovers; that is altered during illness, pain, and suffering; and that engages with the world differently upon recovery." (Benner, 1999)

HISTORY AND BACKGROUND

Benner began what she describes as an articulation project of the knowledge embedded in nursing practice some 25 years ago (Benner, 1999). Her initial thrust toward further understanding of the theory/ practice gap in nursing (Benner, 1974; Benner & Benner, 1979) became transformed during the conduct of the Achieving Methods of Intraprofessional Consensus, Assessment and Evaluation (AMICAE) project, during which she uncovered profound exemplars of caring practices from observations and interviews with clinical nurses (Benner, 1984). This research showed that knowledge could not only be applied in practice but also could be developed.

The author gratefully acknowledges comments by Patricia Benner, RN, PhD, FAAN on an earlier draft of this manuscript. Jackie Carlson, administrative secretary at the University of Texas—Galveston School of Nursing, is gratefully acknowledged for her assistance with formatting parts of this manuscript.

123

Two direct outcomes of the AMICAE research project were: (1) validation and interpretation of the Dreyfus model of skill acquisition for nurses and (2) description of the domains and competencies of nursing practice. Benner's ongoing research studies have continued the development of these two components and have been applied extensively in clinical practice development models (CPDMs) for nursing staff in hospitals around the world (Alberti, 1991; Balasco & Black, 1988; Brykczynski, 1998; Dolan, 1984; Gaston, 1989; Gordon, 1986; Hamric, Whitworth, & Greenfield, 1993; Huntsman, Lederer, & Peterman, 1984; Nuccio, 1996; Silver, 1986). It has also been used for preceptorship programs (Neverveld, 1990) and symposia on nursing excellence (Ullery, 1984).

From Novice to Expert (Benner, 1984) and *Expertise in Clinical Nursing Practice* (Benner, Tanner, & Chesla, 1996) were both studies of skill development in nursing and research-based interpretations of the nature of clinical nursing knowledge. The ongoing development of interpretive phenomenology as a narrative qualitative research method is described and illustrated in each of Benner's knowledge development publications. The growing body of research that this work has generated is highlighted in the book *Interpretive Phenomenology: Embodiment, Caring, and Ethics in Health and Illness* (Benner, 1994b). In this book, Benner and colleagues delineate the historical background, philosophical foundations, and methodological processes of interpretive phenomenological research and examine aspects of the moral dimensions of living with a chronic illness.

Benner's thesis (1984) that caring is central to human expertise and to curing and to healing was extended in *The Primacy of Caring: Stress and Coping in Health and Illness* (Benner & Wrubel, 1989). The meaning of caring in this work is that persons, events, projects, and things matter to people. This work examines the relationships between caring, stress and coping, and health. It claims that caring is primary for the following reasons: (1) what matters to people sets up not only what counts as stressful but also what options are available for coping; (2) it enables a person to notice salient aspects of a particular situation, to discern problems, and to recognize potential solutions; and (3) it sets up possibilities for giving and receiving help (Benner & Wrubel, 1989). This book articulates the nursing perspective of approaching persons in their lived experiences of stress and coping with health and illness. It is based on "the notion of the good inherent in the practice and the knowledge embedded in the expert practice of nursing" (Benner & Wrubel, 1989, p. xi). The primacy of caring has been used as a framework for nursing curricula in several schools of nursing including the University of Toronto in Ontario and McMurray College in Illinois (P. Benner, personal communication, January 12, 2000).

Benner's work is research-based and derived from actual practice situations. Darbyshire (1994) proposed that her "work is among the most sustained, thoughtful, deliberative, challenging, empowering, influential, empirical (in true sense of being based on data) and research-based bodies of nursing scholarship that has been produced in the last 20 years" (p. 760). Benner's work has been developed and applied in general staff nursing, critical care nursing, community health nursing, and advanced practice nursing.

Benner's research offers a radically different perspective from the cognitive rationalist quantitative paradigm prevalent during the 1970s and 1980s (Chinn, 1985; Webster, Jacox, & Baldwin, 1981). Her research constitutes an interpretive turn—a move away from epistemological, linear, analytic, and quantitative methods toward a new direction of ontological, hermeneutic, holistic, and qualitative approaches. Benner (1992) has stated that "the platonic quest to get to the general so that we can get beyond the vagaries of experience was a misguided turn. . . .We can redeem the turn if we subject our theories to our unedited, concrete, moral experience and acknowledge that skillful ethical comportment calls us not to be beyond experience but tempered and taught by it" (p. 19).

OVERVIEW OF BENNER'S PHILOSOPHY

The original domains and competencies of nursing practice (Benner, 1984) were identified and described from clinical situation interviews and observations of novice and expert staff nurses in actual practice. This interpretive phenomenological study used a situational approach to the study of the knowledge and meanings embedded in the everyday practice of nurses. A holistic perspective such as this provides details of the situational contexts that guide interpretation. Thirty-one competencies (or interpretively-defined skills) were identified and described from the narrative data. These competencies were grouped according to similarities of function, intent, and meaning to form seven domains of nursing practice (Box 7-1).

BOX 7-1 | BENNER'S DOMAINS OF NURSING PRACTICE

- The helping role
- The teaching-coaching function
- The diagnostic and patient-monitoring function
- Effective management of rapidly changing situations
- Administering and monitoring therapeutic interventions and regimens
- Monitoring and ensuring the quality of health care practices
- Organizational and work-role competencies

From Benner, P. (1984). *From novice to expert: Excellence and power in clinical nursing practice*. Menlo Park, CA: Addison-Wesley. Reprinted by permission of Pearson Education, Inc. Upper Saddle River, NJ 07458.

The *helping role* domain includes competencies related to establishing a healing relationship, providing comfort measures, and inviting active patient participation and control in care. Timing, readying patients for learning, motivating change, assisting with lifestyle alterations, and negotiating agreement on goals are competencies in *the teaching-coaching function* domain. The *diagnostic and patient-monitoring function* domain refers to competencies in ongoing assessment and anticipation of outcomes. Competencies in the *effective management of rapidly changing situations* domain include the ability to contingently match demands with resources and to assess and manage during crisis situations. The domain *administering and monitoring therapeutic interventions and regimens* incorporates competencies related to preventing complications during drug therapy, wound management, and hospitalization. *Monitoring and ensuring the quality of healthcare practices* domain includes competencies with regard to maintenance of safety, continuous quality improvement, collaboration and consultation with physicians, self-evaluation, and management of technology. The domain *organizational and work-role competencies* refers to competencies in priority setting, team building, coordinating, and providing for continuity.

The domains and competencies of nursing practice are nonlinear, with no precise beginning or endpoint. Instead, the nurse enters the hermeneutic circle of caring for the patient by way of whichever competency is needed at the time. One competency in one domain may be more prominent at a particular point in time, but all seven domains and numerous competencies (some not yet identified) will perhaps overlap and come into play at various times in the transitional (ongoing) process of caring for a patient.

The domains and competencies of nursing practice (Benner, 1984) were initially put forth as an open-ended interpretive framework for enhancing understanding of the knowledge embedded in nursing practice. They are always expected to be interpreted in the context of the situations from which they arise along with articulation of notions of the good or ends of nursing practice. Narrative text must accompany the identification and description of domains and competencies. They are not mutually exclusive, jointly exhaustive categories that can be abstracted from their narrative sources. Because of the socially embedded, relational, and dialogical nature of clinical knowledge, the domains and competencies need to be adapted for each institution. This is achieved through study of clinical practice at each specific locale. An individualized clinical practice development model (CPDM) can be designed specifically for the particular setting (Benner & Benner, 1999).

Benner's work focuses on developing perceptual acuity, clinical judgment, skilled know-how, and ongoing experiential learning. Benner's proposal (1994b) that narrative data be interpreted as text rather than being coded with formal criteria is useful for understanding her work, specifically with regard to expertise, practical knowledge, and intuition. These terms sometimes have been mistakenly considered as formal, explicit criteria (Cash 1995; English, 1993). Therefore each term is discussed in detail in the following sections.

The Dreyfus (1986) model of skill acquisition maintains that expert practice is holistic and situational. Qualitative distinctions between the levels of competence, from the novice to expert skill acquisition model (Benner, Tanner, & Chesla, 1996) reflect "the situational and relational nature of common-sense understanding and developing expert practice" (Darbyshire, 1994, p. 757). According to this model, which Benner (1984) validated for nursing practice, expert practice develops over time through committed, involved transactions with persons in situations.

Clinical nursing expertise is embodied—that is, the body takes over the skill. Embodied expertise means that as human beings, we know things with our feelings, and bodily senses (sight, sound, touch, smell, intuition), not just our rational minds. According to Brykczynski (1998),

> To say that expertise is embodied is to say that, through experience, skilled performance is transformed from the halting, stepwise performance of the beginner—whose whole being is focused on and absorbed in the skilled practice at hand—to the smooth, intuitive performance of the expert. The expert performs so deftly and effortlessly that the rational mind, feelings, and perceptions are available to notice the patient and others in the situation and to perceive salient aspects of the situational context (p. 352).

Because expertise in this model is situational and is not defined as a trait or talent, one is not expert in all situations. When a novel situation arises or the usually expert nurse incorrectly grasps a situation, his or her performance in that particular situation relates more to competent or proficient levels. This experience then becomes part of the nurse's repertoire of background experiences. As a result, another similar situation will be approached more expertly. This variable nature of expertise is very troublesome for those seeking abstract, objective, mutually exclusive, jointly exhaustive categories. However, it is quite compatible with the holistic, interpretive phenomenological approach.

Next, an understanding of distinctions between practical and theoretical knowledge is essential for grasping this perspective (Kuhn, 1970; Polanyi, 1958). Embodied knowledge is the kind of global integration of knowledge that develops when theoretical concepts and practical know-how are refined through experience in actual situations (Benner, 1984). The more tacit knowledge of experienced clinicians is uniquely human. It is the kind of knowledge that computers do not have (Dreyfus, 1992). It requires a living person, actively involved in a situation with all the complexity of the background and context. This distinction between human and computer capabilities can aid in clarifying aspects of the theory-practice gap so widely discussed in practice disciplines, as follows:

> All of knowledge is not necessarily explicit. We have embodied ways of knowing that show up in our skills, our perceptions, our sensory knowledge, our ways of organizing the perceptual field. These bodily perceptual skills, instead of being primitive and lower on the hierarchy, are essential to expert human problem-solving which relies on recognition of the whole (Benner, 1985b, p. 2).

Theoretical knowledge can be acquired in a decontextual fashion through reading, observing, or discussing, whereas the development of practical knowledge requires actual experience in a situation because it is contextual and transactional. Clinical nursing requires both types of knowledge. Table 7-1 provides definitions and examples of aspects of practical knowledge based on Benner (1984).

The examples of aspects of practical knowledge described in Table 7-1 should be self-explanatory. The maxims are one possible exception. The maxim "When you hear hoofbeats in Kansas, think horses, not zebras" reminds clinicians that for common occurrences, most time-consuming, extensive searches for rare conditions are usually not warranted. This maxim surfaces frequently in both acute care and primary care. The maxim "Follow the body's lead" relates to the perceptual acuity developed by nurses to tune into the direction the patient's body is going. It appears, for example, in situations in which patients are being assessed for readiness to be weaned from ventilator assistance and nurses evaluate comfortable positions preferred by a particular infant.

In this interpretive phenomenological perspective, the body is indispensable for intelligent behavior rather than getting in the way of thinking and reasoning. According to Dreyfus (1992), three areas that underlie all intelligent behavior include the following: (1) the role of the body in organizing and unifying our experience of objects, (2) the role of the situation in providing a background against which behavior can be orderly without being rule-like, and (3) the role of human purposes and needs in organizing the situation so that objects are recognized as relevant and accessible.

Finally, intuition is defined as immediate situation recognition (Dreyfus & Dreyfus, 1986). It is based on background understanding of prior similar and dissimilar situations. Benner (1996) argues that "[c]linical reasoning is necessarily reasoning in transition, and the intuitive powers of understanding and recognition only set up the condition

TABLE 7-1   Aspects of Practical Knowledge

Aspect	Definition	Examples
Qualitative distinctions	Perceptual, recognitional clinical judgment that refers to accurate detection of minute alterations that cannot be quanitified and that are often context-dependent.	• Discrete alterations in skin color. • Meanings of changes in mood. • Different manifestations of anxiety.
Maxims	Cryptic statements that guide action and require deep situational understanding to make sense.	• When you hear hoofbeats in Kansas, think horses, not zebras. • Follow the body's lead.
Assumptions, expectations, and sets	Knowledge from past experience that helps orient and provide a frame of reference for anticipatory guidance along the typical trajectory. Assumptions are often taken for granted as tacit beliefs that something is true. Expectations are notions that something can be reasonably anticipated following a certain scenario. Sets are inclinations or tendencies to respond to anticipated situations.	• Assumptions include the ability to maintain and communicate hope in situations based on possibilities learned from previous similar situations. • One expects that an obese person with essential hypertension who loses weight and engages in aerobic exercise 3 times a week will experience a decrease in BP. • A set can be illustrated by thinking about the difference in the way a nurse would approach a woman in labor for whom everything seemed to be going normally and the way a nurse would approach the woman if there was a known fetal demise.
Common meanings	Shared, taken-for-granted, background knowledge of a cultural group that is transmitted in implicit ways.	• It is often better to know even bad news than not to know.

Developed from Benner, P. (1984). *From novice to expert: Excellence and power in clinical nursing practice.* Menlo Park, CA: Addison-Wesley.

Continued

TABLE 7-1	Aspects of Practical Knowledge—cont'd	
Aspect	**Definition**	**Examples**
Paradigm cases	Clinical experiences that stand out in one's memory as having made a significant impact on the nurse's future practice and profoundly alter perceptions and future understanding.	• A nurse's first patient who stops smoking. • The first patient with a breast lump whom a nurse refers for evaluation.
Exemplars	Robust clinical examples that convey more than one intent, meaning, or outcome and can be readily translated to other clinical situations that may be quite different. An exemplar might constitute a paradigm case for a nurse depending on its impact on personal knowledge and future practice.	• Helping a patient and his or her family experience a peaceful death. • Teaching/coaching a patient or family to live with a chronic illness.
Unplanned practices	Knowledge that develops as the practice of nursing expands into new areas.	• Experience gained with available alternative therapies and patient responses to them.

Developed from Benner, P. (1984). *From novice to expert: Excellence and power in clinical nursing practice.* Menlo Park, CA: Addison-Wesley.

of possibility for confirmatory testing or a rapid response to a rapidly changing clinical situation" (p. 673).

Interfacing with Practice

Practice and theory are seen as interrelated and interdependent. They form a dialogue between practice and theory that creates new possibilities (Benner & Wrubel, 1989). In Benner's work, practice is viewed as a way of knowing in its own right (Benner, 1999). As noted earlier, Benner's approach to articulating nursing practice is developmental and interpretive. She locates it in "the feminist tradition of consciousness raising that seeks to name silences and to bring into public discourse poorly articulated areas of knowledge, skill, and self-interpretations in clinical nursing practice" (Benner, 1996, p. 670).

Articulation is defined as "describing, illustrating, and giving language to taken-for-granted areas of practical wisdom, skilled know-how, and notions of good practice" (Benner, Hooper-Kyriakidis, & Stannard, 1999, p. 5). Since the publication of *From Novice to Expert* in 1984, which involved staff nurses from various clinical areas, Benner and her colleagues have focused on articulating the skill acquisition processes and competencies of nurses in critical care areas (Benner, Tanner, & Chesla, 1996; Benner, Hooper-Kyriakidis, & Stannard, 1999). The domains and competencies have also been useful for ongoing articulation of the knowledge embedded in advanced nursing practice (Fenton, 1985; Fenton & Brykczynski, 1993; Lindeke, Canedy, & Kay, 1997; Martin, 1996) as well as in basic nursing practice (Brykczynski, 1998).

The following discussion summarizes selected studies that furthered Benner's work and continued the articulation of the competencies of nursing practice. Fenton's study (1985) indicated that all the original domains were present in the practice of the clinical nurse specialists (CNSs) studied. She identified additional competencies for three of Benner's original domains and one additional domain (Figure 7-1). For example, Fenton described the competency *making the bureaucracy respond* in her study of CNSs. This skill involved knowing how and when to work around bureaucratic roadblocks in the system so patients and families could receive the care they needed.

Brykczynski (1985) developed an additional domain from her study of nurse practitioner (NP) practice. This new domain consolidated and replaced two of Benner's domains that had been more typical of inpatient nursing practice (see Figure 7-1). The remaining five of Benner's seven domains were interpreted as valid for the practice of the NPs studied. An illustration of the cumulative nature of this body of qualitative research is demonstrated by Brykczynski's initial identification (1985) of *managing the system* as a competency in her study of NPs. Further interpretation of the data revealed that this competency was identical to that described by Fenton with CNSs. Fenton's term *making the bureaucracy respond* (Fenton, 1985) was used because that description had been labeled previously. This competency involves negotiating and interpreting for patients so that they can fit into the system and get what they need. It demands flexibility in the nurse's stance toward the system and requires not getting involved in interpersonal conflicts; instead, the nurse uses knowledge of the bureaucracy and interpersonal communication skills to provide the care the patient needs.

Several years later, Fenton and Brykczynski (1993) compared the findings from their earlier studies to uncover the commonalties and distinctions between the practice of NPs and CNSs. This comparative analysis indicated that there was "a shared core of advanced practice competencies as well as distinct differences between the practice roles" (Fenton & Brykczynski, 1993, p. 313). For example, *making the bureau-*

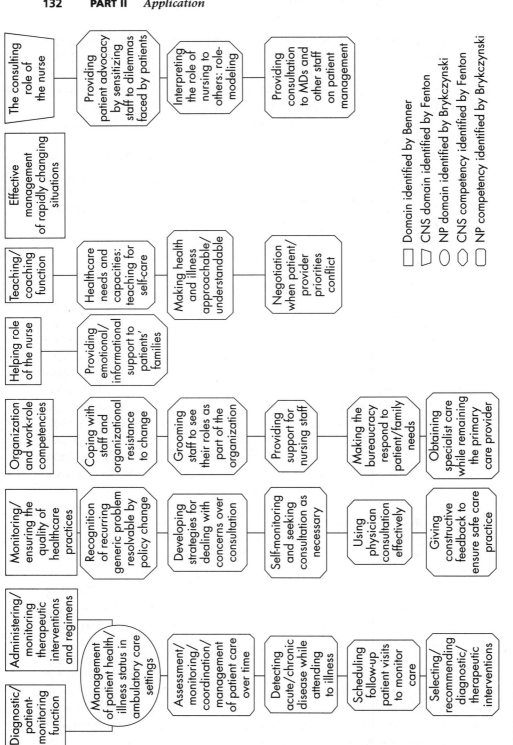

FIGURE 7-1

Expert practice domains of the clinical nurse specialist and the nurse practitioner. (From Fenton, M. V. & Brykczynski, K. A. [1993]. Qualitative distinctions and similarities in the practice of clinical nurse specialists and nurse practitioners. *Journal of Professional Nursing, 9*(6), 317. Used with permission.)

cracy respond was shared by both groups, whereas the *organizational and work-role* competencies were more prominent in the practice of the CNSs. NPs practiced more as direct providers of care, whereas CNSs functioned more as facilitators of care. The new domain, *the consulting role of the nurse,* was evidenced in the practice of both CNSs and NPs. The competencies in this domain represent an initial articulation of skills and knowledge more typical of advanced practice nurses.

Lindeke, Canedy, and Kay (1997) followed up this work with a study of similarities and differences between CNS and NP roles among CNSs who completed a postmaster's NP program. They found that although practice domains were similar, there was distinct expression of the domains in each advanced practice nurse (APN) role. The post-master's participants "stated that they experienced significant role change in the transition from CNS to NP roles" (Lindeke, Canedy, & Kay, 1997, p. 287). These findings have implications for curriculum planning for advanced practice roles.

Excerpts from Brykczynski's study (1998) of peer-identified expert staff nurses can be used to illustrate the connections between descriptions of practical knowledge and descriptions of competencies of nursing practice. There is overlap between these two types of interpretive descriptions. New competencies described in this study were *debriefing after rounds* and *managing frustrations when limited options constrain the ability to help* (Box 7-2). *Debriefing after rounds* can also be interpreted as an example of practical knowledge called *common meanings* (Benner, 1984). Nurses have long recognized that physician rounds can be traumatic and incomprehensible experiences for patients. Over the years, nurses have learned to incorporate clarification of what transpired during rounds into their care as a matter of course—what nurses often call common sense. They translate the "medicalese" so that patients and their families can relate this information to their particular situations. Naming this practice a competency brings it to public recognition so that nurses, physicians, and others can become aware of it.

The competency *managing frustrations when limited options constrain the ability to help* (see Box 7-2) can also be interpreted as an example of practical knowledge when new knowledge is developed as a result of expanded practice. With the advent of heart transplants, cardiac care unit (CCU) nurses faced the situation of long-term chronic patients who were too unstable to be transferred to step-down units. They were radically different from the unstable, acute patients they accustomed to caring for and who typically either recovered or expired in a fairly circumscribed period of time. For example, a CCU nurse in Brykczynski's study (1998) described a situation with a 50-year-old male with severe cardiomyopathy who became depressed while awaiting a cardiac transplant in CCU

BOX 7-2	DOMAINS AND COMPETENCIES OF PEER-IDENTIFIED EXPERT STAFF NURSES[a]

DOMAIN: THE DIAGNOSTIC AND MONITORING FUNCTION
Areas of Skilled Practice

Detecting and documenting significant changes in a patient's condition

Providing an early warning signal:

   Anticipating breakdown and deterioration prior to explicit confirming diagnostic signs

   Anticipating problems: Future think

Understanding the particular demands and experiences of an illness: Anticipating patient care needs

Assessing the patient's potential for wellness and for responding to various treatment strategies

Thinking critically about data collection[b]

DOMAIN: THE HEALING ROLE OF THE NURSE[c]
Areas of Skilled Practice

The healing relationship: Creating a climate for and establishing a commitment to healing, *establishing rapport, managing conflict*[d]

Providing comfort measures and preserving personhood in the face of extreme breakdown

Presencing: Being with a patient

Maximizing the patient's participation and control in his/her own health/illness care, *existential advocacy*[d] (Gadow, 1980)

Interpreting kinds of pain and selecting appropriate strategies for pain management and pain control

Providing comfort and communication through touch

Providing emotional and informational support to patients' families

Maximizing the family's role in care[b]

Normalizing the situation[b]

Managing frustrations when limited options constrain the ability to help[b]

Participating in significant intimate life events[b]

Healing through communicating[b]

DOMAIN: ORGANIZATION AND WORK-ROLE COMPETENCIES
Areas of Skilled Practice

Coordinating, ordering, and meeting multiple patient needs and requests: Setting priorities

Orchestrating the whole situation, contingency management[b]

From Brykczynski, K. A. (1998). Clinical exemplars describing expert staff nursing practices. *Journal of Nursing Management, 6,* 354. Used with permission.

[a]Areas of skilled practice are adapted from Benner (1984) unless otherwise noted.

[b]Indicates competencies identified in this project.

[c]Domain: The Helping Role of the Nurse changed to the Healing Role of the Nurse. In Zimmer, P. A., Brykczynski, K. A., Martin, A. C., Newberry, Y. G., Price, M. J., & Warren, B. (1990). *Advanced nursing practice: Nurse practitioner curriculum guidelines.* Washington, D.C.: National Organization of Nurse Practitioner Faculties.

[d]*Indicates competency expanded in this project.*

Gadow, S. (1980). Existential advocacy: Philosophical foundation of nursing. In S. F. Spicker & S. Gadow (Eds.), *Nursing images and ideals* (pp. 79-101). New York: Springer.

BOX 7-2   DOMAINS AND COMPETENCIES OF PEER-IDENTIFIED EXPERT STAFF NURSES—cont'd

DOMAIN: ORGANIZATION AND WORK-ROLE COMPETENCIES—cont'd
Areas of Skilled Practice—cont'd

Providing for continuity and discharge planning[b]

Building and maintaining a therapeutic team to provide optimum therapy, *conflict management*[d]

Coping with staff shortages and high turnover:

- Contingency planning
- Anticipating and preventing periods of extreme work overload
- Using and maintaining team spirit; gaining social support from other nurses
- Maintaining a caring attitude towards patients even in absence of close and frequent contact
- Maintaining a flexible stance towards patients, technology, and bureaucracy

Making the bureaucracy respond to patients' and families' needs[e]

Coaching other nurses; role-modeling[b,e]

DOMAIN: ADMINISTERING AND MONITORING THERAPEUTIC INTERVENTIONS AND REGIMENS
Areas of Skilled Practice

Starting and maintaining intravenous therapy with minimal risks and complications

Administering medications accurately and safely: Monitoring untoward effects, reactions, therapeutic responses, toxicity, and incompatibilities

Combating the hazards of immobility: Preventing and intervening with skin breakdown, ambulating and exercising patients to maximize mobility and rehabilitation, preventing respiratory complications

Creating a wound management strategy that fosters healing, comfort, and appropriate drainage

DOMAIN: MONITORING AND ENSURING THE QUALITY OF HEALTHCARE PRACTICES
Areas of Skilled Practice

Providing a back-up system to ensure safe medical and nursing care

Formulating own perspective on what should be done and using this as a yardstick for interpreting the course of events[b]

Maintaining environmental safety: attending to principles of asepsis, infection control, body mechanics, general safety[b]

Participating in Continuous Quality Improvement monitoring and evaluation for safety, efficiency, effectiveness, and cost containment[b]

Monitoring documentation for quality and accuracy[b]

Assessing what can be safely omitted from or added to medical orders

Getting appropriate and timely responses from physicians

Using physician consultation effectively[e]

Collaborative consultation—*"Dr. shopping"*[d]

---

[e]Competency identified by Fenton, M. V. (1985). Identifying competencies of clinical nurse specialists. *Journal of Nursing Administration, 15*(12), 31-37.

Continued

BOX 7-2 DOMAINS AND COMPETENCIES OF PEER-IDENTIFIED EXPERT STAFF NURSES—cont'd

DOMAIN: MONITORING AND ENSURING THE QUALITY OF HEALTHCARE PRACTICES—cont'd

Areas of Skilled Practice—cont'd

Self-monitoring and seeking consultation as necessary[f]

Giving constructive feedback to physicians and other care providers to ensure ensure safe care practices[f]

Critically evaluating and incorporating relevant research into practice[b]

Managing technology, preventing unnecessary technological intrusions[b,h]

DOMAIN: THE TEACHING-COACHING FUNCTION OF THE NURSE

Areas of Skilled Practice

Timing: Capturing a patient's readiness to learn

Motivating a patient to change[f]

Assisting patients to integrate the implications of their illnesses and recovery into their lifestyles

Assisting patients to alter their lifestyles to meet changing healthcare needs and capacities: Teaching for self-care[f]

Eliciting an understanding of the patient's interpretation of his/her illness

Negotiating agreement about how to proceed when priorities of patient and provider conflict[f]

Providing an interpretation of the patient's condition and giving a rationale for procedures

The coaching function: Making culturally avoided and uncharted health and illness experiences approachable and understandable[g]

Guiding a patient through emotional and developmental change:[i]

Providing new options, closing off old ones: Channeling, teaching, mediating:

* Acting as a psychological and cultural mediator
* Using goals therapeutically
* Working to build and maintain a therapeutic community

Debriefing with patient after rounds[b]

DOMAIN: EFFECTIVE MANAGEMENT OF RAPIDLY CHANGING SITUATIONS

Areas of Skilled Practice

Skilled performance in extreme life-threatening emergencies: Rapid grasp of a problem

Contingency management: Rapid matching of demands and resources in emergency situations

Identifying and managing a patient crisis until physician assistance is available

From Brykczynski, K. A. (1998). Clinical exemplars describing expert staff nursing practices. *Journal of Nursing Management, 6*, 354. Used with permission.

[f]Competency identified by Brykczynski, K. A. (1999). An interpretive study describing the clinical judgment of nurse practitioners. *Scholarly Inquiry for Nursing Practice: An International Journal, 13*(2), 75-104.

[g]Competency expanded by Brykczynski (1999).

[h]Benner, P., Tanner, C. A., & Chesla, C. A. (1996). *Expertise in clinical nursing practice: Caring, clinical judgment, and ethics.* New York: Springer.

[i]Indicates competency moved from Benner's Domain: The Helping Role to the Domain: The Teaching-Coaching Function, NONPF (1990) Curriculum Guidelines.

Gadow, S. (1980). Existential advocacy: Philosophical foundation of nursing. In S. F. Spicker & S. Gadow (Eds.), *Nursing images and ideals* (pp. 79-101). New York: Springer.

for 2 months. The nurse related that both nurses and physicians found this situation to be disheartening and frustrating. The nurses learned to cope with this challenge by doing the following:

- Establishing a core group of nurses to work with this patient to provide consistency in care
- Normalizing the situation as much as possible by relaxing visiting restrictions and giving the wife kitchen privileges
- Keeping the door to the patient's room closed and knocking on entry
- Suspending vital sign checks during the night to allow for 4 hours of uninterrupted sleep
- Arranging for regularly scheduled ventilation sessions with a psychologist attended by nursing and medical staff.

CRITICAL THINKING IN NURSING PRACTICE WITH BENNER'S APPROACH

Benner addresses critical thinking in a developmental and interpretive way that differs from the more common use of this term in nursing. Formal definitions of critical thinking tend to signify abstract, rational calculation along with analysis and weighing of options and factors to arrive at decisions. For Benner, such a thinking process would be typical of beginning nurses, whereas a more interpretive process based on past-whole-concrete-cases would characterize expert nurses. Benner's perspective is inclusive, incorporating the formal, analytic definition at novice and advanced beginner levels of practice and the more qualitative definition at proficient and expert practice levels.

Benner, Hooper-Kyriakidis, & Stannard (1999) identified six aspects of clinical judgment and skillful comportment that can be viewed as interpretive aspects of critical thinking (Table 7-2). These six aspects were identified and described through study of critical care nursing practice. They constitute components of the thinking-in-action approach required in critical care. *Reasoning in transition* involves the thinking-in-action demanded as an ongoing situation evolves over time. *Skilled know-how* refers to embodied knowing described earlier. *Response-based practice* involves the ability to read a situation and respond flexibly and proactively to changing needs and demands. *Agency* is the nurse's ability to function within a given situation. *Perceptual acuity* and *involvement* refer to acquiring a good grasp of the situation through emotional engagement with the problem and interpersonal involvement with patients and families. "Notions of good guide the actions of nurses and help them notice clinical and ethical threats to patients' well-being" (Benner, Hooper-Kyriakidis, & Stannard, 1999, p. 17), thus *linking clinical and ethical reasoning.*

TABLE 7-2   Critical Thinking in Nursing Practice with Benner's Theory

Aspects of Clinical Judgment and Skillful Comportment	Definition
Reasoning in transition	Practical reasoning in an ongoing clinical situation.
Skilled know-how	Embodied intelligent performance which involves knowing what to do, when to do it, and how to do it.
Response-based practice	Adapting interventions to meet changing needs and expectations of patients.
Agency	One's sense of and ability to act upon or influence a situation.
Perceptual acuity and involvement	Ability to tune in to a situation and hone in on the salient issues by engaging with the problem(s) and the person(s).
Links between clinical and ethical reasoning	Understanding of good clinical practice cannot be separated from ethical notions of good outcomes for patients and families.

Developed from Benner, P., Hooper-Kyriakidis, P., & Stannard, D. (1999). *Clinical wisdom and interventions in critical care: A thinking-in-action approach.* Philadelphia: W. B. Saunders.

In this recent work, Benner, Hooper-Kyriakidis, and Stannard (1999) have sought to generate "a dialogue with practice and theory to create an enlarged view of rationality that is dialogic, relational, and cumulative rather than a collection of decisions and facts" (p. 22). Clinicians need to understand the distinctions and commonalties within the clinical situation as it takes place. According to Benner, Hooper-Kyriakidis, and Stannard (1999), "[c]linical reasoning requires reasoning-in-transition (or reasoning about the changes in a situation) about particular patients and families" (p. 10). The term *thinking-in-action* is intended to convey "the innovative and productive nature of the clinician's active thinking in ongoing situations" (Benner, Hooper-Kyriakidis, & Stannard, 1999, p. 5). According to Benner and Benner (1999),

> clinical practice is a socially embedded knowledge that draws on theoretical and scientific empirical knowledge but also on the practical know how, compassionate meeting of the other, and front-line knowledge work of practitioners. . . .The practitioner, whether nurse, physician, lawyer, teacher, or social worker, reasons about the particular across time, observing transitions in the client's condition, and also transitions in his or her own understanding of the clinical situation (p. 22).

Benner (1994a) has suggested that both practical clinical knowledge and caring practices have been minimized in modern healthcare. It is her hope that identification and description of these practices on which healthcare institutions depend will promote their recognition and legitimacy (Benner, 1994a).

Benner's work portrays nursing practice as an interpretive (hermeneutic) rather than a linear process. She agrees with Good and Good (1981) that "all clinical encounters have a hermeneutic dimension; clinicians and patients interpret one another's meanings to bring to light an underlying coherence or sense" (Good & Good, 1981, p. 208). Benner maintains agreement with Good and Good (1981) that "the negotiation by the healer and the patient of a common understanding of the cause of suffering, the construction of a shared illness reality, provides the basis for the therapeutic efficacy of many healing transactions" (Good & Good, 1981, p. 193). Thus for Benner, nursing practice is constituted by a circular or hermeneutic process between the nurse and the patient.

CASE HISTORY OF DEBBIE

Debbie is a 29-year-old woman who was recently admitted to the oncology nursing unit for evaluation after sensing pelvic "fullness" and noticing a watery, foul-smelling vaginal discharge. A Papanicolaou smear revealed class V cervical cancer. She was found to have a stage II squamous cell carcinoma of the cervix and underwent a radical hysterectomy with bilateral salpingooophorectomy.

Her past health history revealed that physical examinations had been infrequent. She also reported that she had not performed breast self-examination. She is 5 feet, 4 inches tall and weights 89 pounds. Her usual weight is about 110 pounds. She has smoked approximately two packs of cigarettes a day for the past 16 years. She is gravida 2, para 2. Her first pregnancy was at age 16, and her second was at age 18. Since that time, she has taken oral contraceptives on a regular basis.

Debbie completed the eighth grade. She is married and lives with her husband and her two children in her mother's home, which she describes as less than sanitary. Her husband is unemployed. She describes him as emotionally distant and abusive at times.

She has done well following surgery except for being unable to completely empty her urinary bladder. She is having continued postoperative pain and nausea. It will be necessary for her to perform intermittent self-catheterization at home. Her medications are (1) an antibiotic, (2) an analgesic as needed for pain, and (3) an antiemetic as needed for nausea. In addition, she will be receiving radiation therapy on an outpatient basis.

Debbie is extremely tearful. She expresses great concern over her future and the future of her two children. She believes that this illness is a punishment for her past life.

NURSING CARE OF DEBBIE WITH BENNER'S APPROACH

This case is presented in a factual outside-in way that Foucault (1963) called *the clinical gaze*—that is, we observe but do not meet Debbie. Presumably, the nurse would meet Debbie and discover her concerns to develop a shared understanding of how to proceed. A clinical herme- neutic takes place in interpreting nursing care.

Domain: The helping role. The helping role domain is a good place to start in thinking about Debbie's care. In establishing a healing relationship with Debbie, you would begin by getting to know her as a person. By coming to know Debbie's unique life situation, beliefs, values, needs, and goals, you develop an understanding of the meanings this illness experience has for her. At the same time, who the nurse is, what his or her background experiences have been, and what his or her level of competence in caring for women with cancer happens to be influences how the particular nurse-patient transaction develops over time. Debbie's relationship with each of the nurses involved in her care will vary in some ways according to each nurse's competence, unique personality, and approach to care.

Benner, Tanner, and Chesla (1996) describe the experiential learning associated with learning the skill of involvement. Learning how to be engaged in the clinical situation and how to be connected with patients and families in helpful ways is ongoing. This skill requires attunement to the situation and to the individuals involved because what is an appropri- ate level of involvement at one phase may be inappropriate at another. Also, different individuals have different comfort zones and expectations, and these may change during the course of an illness experience. By engaging in ongoing dialogue about the situated meanings of Debbie's illness experience, you can personalize her care and help Debbie discover her own situated possibilities. Debbie and you can plan her care together and modify it according to transitions as the situation evolves.

Other salient issues might emerge in the helping relationship, includ- ing maximizing Debbie's participation and control in her recovery, interpreting kinds of pain, and selecting appropriate strategies for pain management and control. Guiding Debbie through the emotional, phys- iological, social, and developmental change of losing her uterus and ovaries at 29 years of age is also important here. No general techniques can be offered because it depends on what Debbie's concerns are and her openness and readiness to discuss them. The patient-nurse relationship opens up situated possibilities. For example, Debbie may be fearful that she might die, but such fears are best discussed when she indicates that she is ready. You can follow Debbie's lead by asking well-timed questions.

To do this, however, you must address your own fears of dying to be open to Debbie's.

Domain: The teaching-coaching function. Teaching-coaching functions may be relevant in Debbie's situation depending on your assessment of her readiness to learn. For example, her tears might signal a readiness to engage in discussion of her fears, and/or they may point to sadness and depression. Understanding the meaning of Debbie's tears requires attentive listening and open-ended questioning to make the necessary qualitative distinctions. If Debbie appears to be receptive to learning, coaching her about the implications of her illness and recovery in her unique life situation can proceed in an individualized way.

Domain: The diagnostic and monitoring function. At all points, you will anticipate future problems and attempt to understand the particular demands of Debbie's illness. For example, you will anticipate care needs related to Debbie's catheterizing herself at home, managing her pain, and controlling her nausea. Based on your and Debbie's assessments of her potential for wellness and responses to various treatment strategies, you will develop a discharge plan and discuss this plan with the home-care nurse.

Domain: Organizational and work-role competencies. *Building and maintaining a therapeutic team to provide optimum therapy* for Debbie is a relevant competency from this domain. There is no information available on the staffing situation in Debbie's nursing unit, so the significance of the other competencies in this domain is unknown. However, communicating Debbie's concerns will be crucial.

CASE HISTORY OF ROSA

This case is a narrative exemplar shared by two of the nurses in Brykczynski's peer-identified nurse expert project (1998 & 1993-1995). It illustrates the development of new clinical knowledge and skill when nurses expand into new practice areas. A group of eight obstetric (OB) nurses who had recently received training in critical care took care of Rosa in the labor and delivery (L&D) unit during her hospital stay. This training in critical care was provided to enable these nurses to care for the increasingly high-risk maternity patients who were having babies at their institution. Previously, obstetric patients requiring critical care were transferred to the intensive care units (ICUs).

Rosa is a pseudonym for a 22-year-old young woman from South America who spoke only Spanish. She had moved to the southwestern United States and was admitted to our institution for the birth of her first baby. She was a full-term prima para. The father of the baby was Mexican-American and had family who lived approximately 5 hours from the hospital. Rosa was not married to the baby's father; however, he was identified as the father before the baby's birth.

Rosa became comatose secondary to acute fatty liver of pregnancy following delivery of her healthy baby. She was intubated, placed on a ventilator, and required hemodialysis. Her electroencephelograms (EEGs) showed minimal brain wave activity. At one point, Rosa had been considered a possible candidate for a liver transplant but, because of multi-system failure, she was eventually designated a "do not resuscitate" (DNR), and the transplant was not pursued further. In fact, the family was asked to consider donating her organs.

In contrast to the physicians' hopeless prognosis for Rosa's recovery, the nurses sensed possibility in this extreme situation. In following what they perceived as the lead of Rosa's body, the nurses sought to put her body in the best condition for healing. For example, they provided an environment enriched with sound and touch. They spoke to her in Spanish whenever possible and placed her baby across her chest where she could hear her and feel her presence. They provided ongoing supportive care while her liver regenerated itself. The supportive nursing care included nutrition via tube feedings, passive range-of-motion exercises, pulmonary toileting, care of the mouth and skin, and frequent position changes. They also provided (in Spanish, whenever possible) updates about her baby and explanations of what was happening. The nurses also included the baby's father in their care.

A photo of Rosa and her baby, taken just before her discharge from the hospital and showing her swollen jaundiced body, and another, taken during a return visit to the hospital clinic and showing her as a tiny attractive woman, are posted in the nurses' station and serve as a reminder to recognize situations in which it is imperative to buy time while the patient's body heals itself.

NURSING CARE OF ROSA WITH BENNER'S APPROACH

Domain: The helping role. The holistic interpretive perspective of the nurses enabled them to perceive Rosa's situation very differently from the objective clinical gaze of the physicians (Foucault, 1963). As one of the nurses narrates,

> Neuro came in and looked at her head—that was what they saw, her head and lack of neurological function. GI came in and they saw just the liver. Renal came in and saw her kidneys. OB came in and saw a comatose postpartum woman. Anesthesia came in and so on (Brykczynski, 1998, pp. 355-356).

This excerpt illustrates that the objective clinical gaze is depersonalizing and divides the person into the separate organs and systems of interest to different specialties.

The nurses recognized that Rosa was a young, healthy woman before developing this rare pregnancy-induced illness, and they had developed the perceptual acuity to follow the lead of Rosa's body toward restoration of health. In understanding how the nurses worked out establishing a healing climate for Rosa, it is important to know that no mother had ever been declared a DNR in this L&D unit before. Having no prior experience with such a situation, the nurses did what they had to do to maintain and support her so that her body could heal itself—if that was to be. This is an example of the common meaning Benner (1984) calls *situated possibility*, in which nurses learn that even the most deprived illness circumstance has its own possibility. Knowing that the hormonal stress response associated with giving up hope can influence the course of an illness (Benner, 1985a), the nurses never gave up hope, nor did the family members. They stayed close by and prayed for Rosa throughout her hospital stay. The power of prayer in influencing healing is recently receiving more research attention as complementary therapies are becoming more widely accepted (Byrd, 1997).

Two obvious aspects that clearly impacted the development of a collaborative relationship between Rosa and her nurses were that Rosa was comatose and unable to communicate in any obvious way with the nurses caring for her and the fact that the majority of the nurses spoke only English and knew few, if any, words in Spanish. In striving to create a healing climate for Rosa, the nurses realized that she probably could hear but was unable to acknowledge this. For this reason, they spoke to her while they provided her care. If an interpreter was not available, they spoke to her in English, hoping to convey their feelings and concern by the tone of their voices. The nurses reported that when Rosa returned to the conscious state, she recognized those who had cared for her by their voices.

Domain: The teaching-coaching function. The nurses reported that they described what they were doing while they cared for Rosa and consistently provided ongoing feedback about her condition and her family in order to promote her participation in care as much as possible. They were involved with the father of the baby, who was struggling with this very difficult situation. The nurse reported,

> At times he would cry if he was holding the baby and not want to cry—especially being a Hispanic male. This was not something he wanted to do and tried not to. We encouraged him to hold the baby himself. We realized that this was not something he had planned on—you know basically the woman is expected to help with the baby and integrate the baby into the household. It was kind of like, "here's the baby," and it was really hard for him.

He had a lot of mixed emotions. He wasn't sure what he was going to do (Brykczynski, 1993-1995).

In coaching the father through this uncharted illness experience, the nurses got a lot of support from a social worker who was fluent in Spanish.

Domain: The diagnostic and monitoring function. Understanding the particular demands and experiences of Rosa's illness was crucial in anticipating her care needs. The nurses reported reading everything they could find about Rosa's rare condition (acute fatty liver of pregnancy) to increase their understanding of her illness and enhance their ability to assess her potential for wellness and for responding to various treatment strategies.

Domain: Administering and monitoring therapeutic interventions and regimens. All the competencies in this domain were significant in this situation. In an effort to normalize the situation as much as possible—for the nurses as well as Rosa—they continued to bring Rosa's baby in to her and place the baby on her chest. One of the critical care nurses participating in the interviews recalled a postpartum woman in ICU for whom the nurses played a tape of her baby's sounds during her stay in the ICU. Rosa was fortunate that she could be cared for by these OB nurses who had recently received critical care training and that she did not have to be transferred to the ICU. One of the nurses describes how bringing the baby in to the mother helped them as well as Rosa:

> Part of it I think initially when we were bringing the baby in was it helped us in a way too because we didn't want the baby staying in the nursery for 4 or 5 days without really being nurtured (Brykczynski, 1993-1995).

The nurses came up with the idea of providing nutritional support for Rosa. They reported approaching every specialty physician team involved in Rosa's care, including OB, neurology, renal, and GI, until one specialty service agreed to order a nutritional consult so that Rosa could receive tube feedings. Based on their assessment of the physiological parameters and the past experience of one of the physicians who had prior experience with patients with this rare condition who did not do well, the physicians' prognosis was bleak. Their attitude toward the nurses was one of humoring them. They reasoned that "if it makes the nurses feel better, they can feed her," because they felt it would not do her any harm. As it turned out, nutritional support was essential to her recovery, particularly for her liver regeneration.

Domain: Organizational and work-role. *Building and maintaining a therapeutic team to provide optimum therapy* was an important competency in this situation. As noted earlier, the group of eight OB nurses who had recently participated in critical care training experiences, which prepared them to care for high-risk women during labor and delivery, formed the team of nurses who cared for Rosa. Their obstetric nursing background and recent critical care experience made them uniquely capable of individualizing Rosa's care. By expanding into a new area of nursing practice the nurses opened up the opportunity to develop new knowledge in high-risk OB nursing. For example, as OB nurses they were acutely aware that not hearing the sounds of her baby could make Rosa feel that her baby was not alive. An interesting aspect of this situation was that, as OB nurses, nutrition was not generally a particularly salient issue for them. One nurse related:

> It's real common for us not to feed our patients. When they are on mag [magnesium sulfate] they may go for three days without food. Or even postpartum for PIH [pregnancy-induced hypertension], so we're used to starving our patients because it really is in the back of our minds that it is okay not to feed a patient because they are usually normal, healthy people who are pregnant. [The idea of feeding her] developed from our experiences rotating through the critical care units where we came in contact with TPN (total parenteral nutrition) and Hepatic A tube feedings and that made us more aware of nutrition as a support for this patient (Brykczynski, 1998, p. 356).

Domain: Monitoring and ensuring the quality of healthcare practices. The group of specially trained OB nurses had ready access to the critical care nurses with whom they had recently worked, thereby providing a readily accessible backup system for safe care. This combination of obstetric and critical care knowledge and skill enabled them to ensure that optimal supportive care was provided. They made adjustments in the care plan over and above that recommended by the physicians. Examples included bringing the baby in to the mother and providing nutritional support.

One of the two nurses who described this exemplar in Brykczynski's study (1998) reported caring for Rosa as she regained consciousness. This nurse related that she was doing the neuro check as usual and noticed a slight change in Rosa's pupil reaction where there had been none before. She rechecked the pupils and had another nurse verify that there was a slight response. The physician who was summoned did not detect any pupillary reaction. Gradually, however, Rosa became more and more alert throughout this nurse's shift and was able to be extubated. Rosa's baby was crying in the room when she became conscious. Remarkably, Rosa's liver had regenerated itself; she recovered with no residual brain damage; and she went home to be with her baby and the baby's father. This case history constitutes an exemplar of nursing provided in an open, receptive, adaptive, creative, and hermeneutic manner as described by

Benner and colleagues as a reasoning-in-transition approach (Benner, Hooper-Kyriakidis, & Stannard, 1999).

CRITICAL THINKING EXERCISES

1. Describe a memorable situation from your beginning practice as a nurse that taught you to modify, refine, and embody knowledge in a very practical way.
2. Using the novice to expert model, describe why a nurse functioning primarily at a competent level of expertise might be preferable for precepting a new graduate than a nurse functioning in most situations at the expert level.
3. Using Benner's approach, explain how you would respond to a nurse administrator's request to revise your institution's nursing service clinical ladder.
4. As a student representative to the curriculum committee in your school of nursing, describe how you would proceed to suggest using Benner's work for planning and evaluating the curriculum at your school.
5. Contrast the differences between the approach the physicians followed in caring for Rosa (i.e., *the formal scientific problem solving process* that yielded the absolute judgment that she be designated a DNR with no hope for recovery) with *the reasoning-in-transition approach* followed by the nurses in their care of Rosa, which was open-ended and created possibilities for recovery. Referring to Benner, Hooper-Kyriakidis, and Stannard (1999) may be useful for responding to this exercise.

References

Alberti, A. M. (1991). Advancing the scope of practice of primary nurses in the NICU. *Journal of Perinatal and Neonatal Nursing, 5*(3), 44-50.

Balasco, E. M. & Black, A. S. (1988). Advancing nursing practice: Description, recognition, and reward. *Nursing Administration Quarterly, 12,* 52-62.

Benner, P. (1974). Reality testing a "Reality Shock" program. In M. Kramer (Ed.), *Reality shock: Why nurses leave nursing* (pp. 191-215). St. Louis: Mosby.

Benner, P. (1984). *From novice to expert: Excellence and power in clinical nursing practice.* Menlo Park, CA: Addison-Wesley.

Benner, P. (1985a). The oncology clinical nurse specialist: An expert coach. *Oncology Nurse Forum, 12*(2), 40-44.

Benner, P. (1985b, January). Heideggerian phenomenology. Abstract of presentation delivered at The Third Annual Research in Nursing Education Conference, San Francisco.

Benner, P. (1992). The role of narrative experience and community in ethical comportment. *Advances in Nursing Science, 12*(2), 1-21.

Benner, P. (1994a). The role of articulation in understanding practice and experience as sources of knowledge in clinical nursing. In J. Tully & D. M. Weinstock (Eds.), *Philosophy in an age of pluralism. The philosophy of Charles Taylor in question* (pp. 136-155). Cambridge, UK: Cambridge University.

Benner, P. (Ed.). (1994b). *Interpretive phenomenology: Embodiment, caring and ethics in health and illness.* Thousand Oaks, CA: Sage.

Benner, P. (1996). A response by P. Benner to K. Cash (1995), Benner and expertise in nursing: A critique. *International Journal of Nursing Studies, 33*(6), 669-674.

Benner, P. (1999). Claiming the wisdom and worth of clinical practice. *Nursing and Health Care Perspectives, 20*(6), 312-319.

Benner, P. Personal Communication, January 12, 2000.

Benner, P. & Benner, R. V. (1979). *The new nurses' work entry: A troubled sponsorship.* New York: Tiresias.

Benner, P. & Benner, R. V. (1999). The clinical practice development model: Making the clinical judgment, caring and collaborative work of nurses visible. In B. Haag-Heitman (Ed.), *Clinical practice development, using novice to expert theory* (pp. 17-42). Gaithersburg, MD: Aspen.

Benner, P., Hooper-Kyriakidis, P., & Stannard, D. (1999). *Clinical wisdom and interventions in critical care: A thinking-in-action approach.* Philadelphia: W. B. Saunders.

Benner, P., Tanner, C. A., & Chesla, C. A. (1996). *Expertise in clinical nursing practice: Caring, clinical judgment and ethics.* New York: Springer.

Benner, P. & Wrubel, J. (1989). *The primacy of caring: Stress and coping in health and illness.* Menlo Park, CA: Addison-Wesley.

Brykczynski, K. A. (1985). Exploring the clinical practice of nurse practitioners. Doctoral dissertation, University of California—San Francisco School of Nursing. *Dissertation Abstracts International, 46,*3789B (University Microfilms No. DA8600592).

Brykczynski, K. A. (1998). Clinical exemplars describing expert staff nursing practices. *Journal of Nursing Management, 6,* 351-359.

Brykczynski, K. (1999). An interpretive study describing the clinical judgment of nurse practitioners. *Scholarly Inquiry for Nursing Practice: An International Journal, 13*(2), 141-166.

Brykczynski, K. A. Principal Investigator, "Developing a Profile of Expert Nursing Practice," Project of the UTMB Nursing Service Task Force Studying Expert Nursing Practice, supported by UTMB Joint Ventures, 1993-1995.

Byrd, R. C. (1997). Positive therapeutic effects of intercessory prayer in a coronary care unit population. *Alternative Therapies, 3*(6), 87-90.

Cash, K. (1995). Benner and expertise in nursing: A critique. *International Journal of Nursing Studies, 32*(6), 527-534.

Chinn, P. L. (1985). Debunking myths in nursing theory and research. *Image, 18*(2), 45-49.

Darbyshire, P. (1994). Skilled expert practice: Is it "all in the mind"? A response to English's critique of Benner's novice to expert model. *Journal of Advanced Nursing, 19,* 755-761.

Dolan, K. (1984). Building bridges between education and practice. In P. Benner (Ed.), *From novice to expert: Excellence and power in clinical nursing practice* (pp. 275-284). Menlo Park, CA: Addison-Wesley.

Dreyfus, H. L. (1992). *What computers still can't do: A critique of artificial reason.* Cambridge, MA: MIT Press.

Dreyfus, H. L. & Dreyfus, S. E. (1986). *Mind over machine: The power of human intuition and expertise in the era of the computer.* New York: Free Press.

English, I. (1993). Intuition as a function of the expert nurse: A critique of Benner's novice to expert model. *Journal of Advanced Nursing, 18,* 387-393.

Fenton, M. V. (1985). Identifying competencies of clinical nurse specialists. *JONA, 15*(12), 31-37.

Fenton, M. V. & Brykczynski, K. A. (1993). Qualitative distinctions and similarities in the practice of clinical nurse specialists and nurse practitioners. *Journal of Professional Nursing, 9*(6), 313-326.

Foucault, M. (1963). In A. M. Sheridan Smith (Trans.), *The birth of the clinic: An archeology of medical perception.* New York: Vintage.

Gadow, S. (1980). Existential advocacy: Philosophical foundation of nursing. In S. F. Spicker & S. Gadow (Eds.), *Nursing images and ideals* (pp. 79-101). New York: Springer.

Gaston, C. (1989). Inservice education: Career development for South Australian nurses. *Australian Journal of Advanced Nursing, 6*(4), 5-9.

Good, B. J. & Good, M. D. V. (1981). The semantics of medical discourse. In E. Mendelsohn, & Y. Elkana (Eds.), *Sciences and cultures: Sociology of the sciences, Volume 5* (pp. 177-212). Holland: D. Reidel Publishing Co.

Gordon, D. R. (1986). Models of clinical expertise in American nursing practice. *Social Science and Medicine, 22*(9), 953-961.

Hamric, A. B., Whitworth, T. R., & Greenfield, A. S. (1993). Implementing a clinically focused advancement system. *JONA, 23*(9), 20-28.

Huntsman, A., Lederer, J. R., & Peterman, E. M. (1984). Implementation of staff nurse III at El Camino Hospital. In P. Benner (Ed.), *From novice to expert: Excellence and power in clinical nursing practice* (pp. 244-257). Menlo Park, CA: Addison-Wesley.

Kuhn, T. (1970). *The structure of scientific revolutions* (2nd ed.). Chicago: University of Chicago Press.

Lindeke, L. L., Canedy, B. H., & Kay, M. M. (1997). A comparison of practice domains of clinical nurse specialists and nurse practitioners. *Journal of Professional Nursing, 13*(5), 281-287.

Martin, L. L. (1996). Factors affecting performance of advanced nursing practice. Doctoral dissertation, Virginia Commonwealth University, School of Nursing. (University Microfilms No. 9627443).

Neverveld, M. E. (1990). Preceptorship: One step beyond. *Journal of Nursing Staff Development, 6*(5), 186-189.

Nuccio, S. A., Lingen, D., Burke, L., Kramer, A., Ladewig, N., Raaum, J., & Shearer, B. (1996). The clinical practice developmental model: The transition process. *JONA, 26*(12), 29-37.

Polanyi, M. (1958). *Personal knowledge.* Chicago: University of Chicago Press.

Silver, M. (1986). A program for career structure: A vision becomes a reality. *The Australian Nurse, 12*(2), 44-47.

Ullery, J. (1984). Focus on excellence. In P. Benner (Ed.), *From novice to expert: Excellence and power in clinical nursing practice* (pp. 258-261). Menlo Park, CA: Addison-Wesley.

Webster, G., Jacox, A., & Baldwin, B. (1981). Nursing theory and the ghost of the received view. In J. C. McCloskey & H. K. Grace (Eds.), *Current issues in nursing* (pp. 26-35). Boston: Blackwell Scientific.

Zimmer, P. A., Brykczynski, K. A., Martin, A. C., Newberry, Y. G., Price, M. J., & Warren, B. (1990). *Advanced nursing practice: Nurse practitioner curriculum guidelines.* Washington, DC: National Organization of Nurse Practitioner Faculties.

Johnson's Behavioral System Model in Nursing Practice

Bonnie Holaday

Nursing is "an external regulatory force that acts to preserve the organization and integration of the patient's behavior at an optimal level under those conditions in which the behavior constitutes a threat to physical or social health or in which illness is found." The goal of nursing is to "restore, maintain or attain behavioral integrity, system stability, adjustment and adaptation, efficient and effective functioning of the system." (From Johnson, D. [1980]. The Behavioral Systems Model for nursing. In J. Riehl & C. Roy [Eds.], Conceptual models for nursing practice [2nd ed., pp. 207-216]. New York: Appleton-Century-Crofts. Reprinted by permission of Pearson Education, Inc. Upper Saddle River, NJ 07458.)

HISTORY AND BACKGROUND

The Johnson Behavioral System Model (JBSM) was conceived and developed by Dorothy Johnson while she was a professor of nursing at the University of California, Los Angeles (UCLA). The process of developing this model began in the late 1950s as she examined the explicit goal of action of patient welfare that was unique to nursing. The task was to clarify nursing's social mission from the perspective of a theoretically sound view of the client. The conceptual model that resulted was presented at Vanderbilt University in 1968 (Johnson, 1968). Since that time other noteworthy presentations of the model have been offered (Auger, 1976; Derdiarian, 1990, 1993; Dee, 1990; Grubbs, 1974; Johnson, 1980, 1990). Johnson retired from UCLA in 1978, but she maintained her interest in "systems" through her hobby ·of shell collecting. She traveled extensively to collect shells, and later donated them to a museum in Sanibel, Florida. Johnson died in February, 1999. Johnson's papers, documents, and letters, per her request, are available at the Eskind Biomedical Library Special Collections at Vanderbilt University in Nashville, Tennessee.

The JBSM offers useful guidelines for nursing practice. Used in conjunction with the nursing process, it has provided a useful conceptual map to plan patient care. Poster, Dee, and Randell (1997) provided evidence supporting the efficacy of the JBSM as a tool for evaluating patient outcomes. Auger and Dee (1983) developed the UCLA Neuropsychiatric Institute and Hospital Classification System, which is based on the JBSM. This system was integrated with the nursing process and is used as a clinical measure of patient progress.

The work of Auger and Dee led to the development of behavioral indices, with each subsystem operationalized in terms of critical adaptive and maladaptive behaviors. The behaviors were ranked into categories according to their assumed level of adaptiveness. Nurse clinicians can rate each behavior for compliance with an activity rating scale of one to four. This scale provided a basis for allocating nursing resources at the UCLA Neuropsychiatric Institute (Dee & Randell, 1989).

Derdiarian used the JBSM to develop the Derdiarian Behavioral System Model (DBSM) instrument (Derdiarian, 1983, 1988; Derdiarian & Forsythe, 1983). The DBSM's 22-category interview generated data pertaining to the major changes in the behavioral systems as a result of illness as well as the positive or negative effects of these changes. Specifically, two types of subjective data were generated. This included the "set"-related variables (the variables that potentially predict or influence the patient's usual behavior) and the behavior resulting from illness. Overall, research findings suggested that the DBSM instrument improved the focus, comprehensiveness, and quality of nursing assessment, diagnoses, interventions and evaluation of outcomes of adult patients with cancer, Acquired Immunodeficiency Syndrome (AIDS), and myocardial infarction (Dediarian, 1983, 1988).

Other studies have also documented the utility of the JBSM for nursing practice. Holaday (1980) used the model to assess health status and to develop nursing interventions for children undergoing surgical procedures. Rawls (1980) used the model to develop a nursing care plan for an adult amputee with a body image problem. Dee, van Servellen, and Brecht (1998) found that the JBSM could be used to derive meaningful conclusions about the impact of managed care on nursing care problems, and Turner-Henson (1993) demonstrated that the JBSM could be used to identify the functional requirements of mothers caring for chronically ill school-age children. Riegel (1989) operationalized the JBSM to examine social support and adjustment to coronary heart disease.

Holaday's work demonstrated that subsystem disorders can be identified, validated the notion of behavioral subsystems and their utility and usefulness in nursing practice, broadened the understanding of the role of "set," and most recently examined the relationship between sustenal imperatives and action (Holaday 1974, 1981, 1982, 1987; Holaday, Turner-Henson, & Swan, 1996). Derdiarian's research demonstrated the factor-isolating and categorizing potential of the JBSM, validated the notion of behavioral subsystems, and provided empirical descriptions of central concepts in the theory (Derdiarian, 1983, 1988, 1990; Derdiarian & Forsythe, 1983). Meleis (1991) described the body of research related to nursing practice that the JBSM has generated and noted that it has provided "significant developments in the conceptualization of the nursing client" (p. 269).

OVERVIEW OF JOHNSON'S BEHAVIORAL SYSTEM MODEL

Johnson's model for nursing presents a view of the client as a living open system. The client is seen as a collection of behavioral subsystems that interrelate to form a behavioral system. Therefore the behavior is the system, not the individual. This behavioral system is characterized by repetitive, regular, predictable, and goal-directed behaviors that always strive toward balance (Johnson, 1968).

Johnson (1968) proposed that the nursing client is a behavioral system with behaviors of interest to nursing and is organized into seven subsystems of behavior: achievement, affiliative, aggressive, dependence, eliminative, ingestive, and sexual. Nurses using the model believed that an additional area of behavior needed to be addressed (Grubbs, 1974; Auger, 1976; Derdiarian, 1990; Holaday, 1980). They added an eighth subsystem, restorative. Each subsystem has its own structure and function. Each subsystem comprises a goal based on a universal drive, set, choice, and action. Each of these four factors contributes to the observable activity of a person. Boxes 8-1 and 8-2 provide examples of how one might operationalize the function and structure of each subsystem. Grubbs (1980) provides excellent definitions of the concepts and terms used in the JBSM.

The goal of a subsystem is defined as "the ultimate consequence of behaviors" (Grubbs, 1974, p. 226). The basis for the goal is a universal drive, the existence of which is supported by existing theory or research. The goal of each subsystem is the same for all people when stated in general terms; however, variations among individuals occur and are based on the value placed on the goal and drive strength.

The second structural component is set, which is a tendency to act in a certain way in a given situation. Once they are developed, sets are relatively stable. Set formation is influenced by such societal norms and variables as culture, family, values, perception, and cognitive abilities. Set can be divided into two types: preparatory and perseverative sets. The

---

BOX 8-1   AFFILIATIVE SUBSYSTEM

Function

To form cooperative and interdependent role relationships within human social systems

To enjoy interpersonal relationships

To belong to something other than oneself

To share

To achieve intimacy and inclusion

Structural Components

Goal: To relate or belong to something or someone other than oneself, to achieve intimacy and inclusion.

Perseveratory Set: A consistent approach (or pattern of behavior) to establishing affiliative relationships; a consistent tendency to select a certain individual or group for the purpose of affiliation; inherited generic characteristics that determine the influence affiliative behaviors; development of self-identity and self-concept to a group; cultural beliefs and customs.

Preparatory Set: Perception of a situation as requiring particular role behaviors required by the interaction setting; selective inattention to social behaviors; mood.

Choice: Selection from among the alternatives available in the situation as perceived through set, the behaviors considered appropriate to meet the goal. Within the context of the situation, the behaviors range from affiliation, avoidance, nonreciprocated relationships, noncontingent social relationships, maintenance of a relationship, and affiliation with animals or other objects.

Acts: Any directly observable behavior that facilitates movement toward others in the environment. Specific acts include smiling, visual contact, talking (social greeting, conversation, extending invitations), facial expression, motor behaviors (touching, holding, hugging), and other actions that establish or maintain a reciprocal relationship between two or more individuals.

Sustenal Imperatives: Conditions that serve to protect, stimulate, and mature behaviors related to affiliation. Included are learned behaviors to initiate and maintain a social exchange: presence of an environment where these skills can be taught and nurtured; development of trust; kinship; awareness of one's self-identity; self-esteem; ability to communicate verbally and nonverbally; membership in groups; knowledge of formal and informal guidelines for interpersonal processes; and secure parent-infant attachment.

---

preparatory set describes one's focus in a particular situation. The perseverative set, which implies persistence, refers to the habits one maintains. The flexibility or rigidity of the set varies with each person. Set plays a major role in determining the choices a person makes and actions eventually taken.

Choice refers to the alternate behaviors the person considers in any given situation. A person's range of options may be broad or narrow. Options are influenced by such variables as age, sex, culture, and socioeconomic status.

BOX 8-2 INGESTIVE SUBSYSTEM

Function

To sustain life through the intake of food and fluids and oxygen
To obtain knowledge or information useful to the self
To obtain pleasure or gratification through taking in nonfunctional materials such as smoking, alcohol, or drugs
To restore a felt deficiency within the self system
To relieve pain or other psychophysiological symptoms

Structural Components

Goal: To internalize the external environment.

Perseveratory Set: Status of sensory modalities digestive system, respiratory system, fluid and electrolyte balance; oral cavity condition; socialization into food types; drinking habits; smoking use; oral medications; subcutaneous, intravenous and intramuscular injections; sensory assistance, such as hearing aids, glasses, and dentures.

Beliefs and values about times and places for eating and drinking; types of foods and beverages preferred by the social group, attitudes toward alcohol and smoking, beliefs about efficiency of oral, intravenous, and subcutaneous medication. Perception of self as fat or thin; abstainer or alcoholic, addict, smoker, asthmatic.

Preparatory Set: Awareness of being hungry or thirsty, in need of a drink, wish to be high, relief of pain, time for eating, availability of food, fluid, or medication resources; barriers to respiration, desire for information, awareness of ignorance.

Choice: Behavioral options available for food and fluid, medications, air supply, tobacco, alcohol, marijuana, narcotics; supplies available in the environment selections are made on the basis of set and situation. Choice includes deferred gratification and overindulgence. Options available for taking in information.

Acts: Behaviors may include visual, auditory, olfactory, and gustatory acts or overindulgences (or less than optimal) and preferences for particular substances. Ingestive acts may be directed toward goals other than ingestion. Sensory acts (seeing, hearing, smelling, tasting, and sensations) are used in all other subsystems to serve other goals. When sensory acts are directed toward getting information, the acts are ingestive goal-oriented. The process of hearing also requires ingestive acts. The ingestion may be for achievement goals.

The action is the observable behavior of the person. The actual behavior is restricted by the person's size and abilities. Here the concern is the efficiency and effectiveness of the behavior in goal attainment.

Each of the subsystems also functions in a manner analogous to the physiology of biological systems (e.g., the urological system has both structural and functional components). The goal of the subsystem is a part of the structure. It is not entirely separate from its function.

For the eight subsystems to develop and maintain stability, each must have a constant supply of "functional requirements" or sustenal imperatives (Johnson, 1980, p. 212). The environment must supply the functional requirements/sustenal imperatives of protection from unwanted, disturbing stimuli; nurturance through giving input from the environment (e.g., food, caring, conditions that support growth and development); encouragement; and stimulation by experiences, events, and behavior that would "enhance growth and prevent stagnation" (Johnson, 1980, p. 212).

The subsystems maintain behavioral system balance as long as both the internal and external environments are orderly, organized, and predictable and each of the subsystems' goals are met. Behavioral system imbalance arises when structure, function, or functional regimen is disturbed. The JBSM differentiates four diagnostic classifications to delineate these disturbances: insufficiency, discrepancy, incompatibility, and dominance.

Nursing has the goal of maintaining, restoring, or attaining a balance or a stability in the behavioral system or in the system as a whole. Nursing acts as an "external regulatory force" to modify or change the structure or to provide ways in which subsystems fulfill the structure's functional requirement (Johnson, 1980, p. 214). Interventions directed toward restoring behavioral system balance are directed toward repairing damaged structural units, with the nurse temporarily imposing regulatory and control measures or helping the client to develop or enhance his or her supplies of essential functional requirements.

CRITICAL THINKING IN NURSING PRACTICE WITH JOHNSON'S MODEL

Making wise choices about nursing care requires the ability to think critically—that is, to analyze the available information, make inferences, draw logical conclusions, and critically evaluate all relevant elements as well as the possible consequences of each nursing decision. From a constructivist perspective, individuals presented with complex information use their own existing knowledge and previous experience to help them make sense of the material. In particular, they make inferences, elaborate on the information by adding details, and generate relationships between and among the new information and the information already in memory. In short, they think critically about the new and old information (Pressley, 1992; Wittrock, 1990). The JBSM provides a useful framework for organizing information so that one can arrange information in a way that permits problem solving and care planning (Table 8-1).

The focus of the assessment process is to obtain knowledge of the client through interviews and observations of the patient and family to evaluate the present behavior in terms of past patterns, to determine the impact

TABLE 8-1   The Johnson Model and the Nursing Process

Framework Elements	Nursing Thought
BEHAVIORAL ASSESSMENT	
Eight subsystems	Do I understand the patient's perceptions?
Achievement	How complete are my data collections?
Affiliative	Could I have missed something?
Aggressive/protective	How do I know I have the facts right?
Dependency	What data might need to be verified?
Eliminative	How do these data compare with previously
Ingestive	collected data?
Restorative	How do my client's data compare with
Sexual	accepted standards/behaviors for someone
	of this age, culture, and disease process?
ENVIRONMENTAL ASSESSMENT	What general and specific factors supply the
Internal	functional requirements for subsystems?
Biological	
Pathological	
Psychological	
Developmental	
Level of wellness	
External	
Cultural	
Ecological	
Familial	
Sociological	
DIAGNOSTIC ANALYSIS	
Behavior subsystem (e.g., achievement)	What subsystem(s) is involved?
Structural unit	What structural unit(s) is involved?
Goal, set, choice, action	Is behavioral succeeding or failing to achieve
	the goal?
	Is there a clear relationship between the stated
	goal of the person, set, and chosen
	behavior?
	Does the set of the person result in
	misperception of the information?
	Are the choices appropriate?
	Is the sequence of action orderly and
	purposeful?
Sustenal imperatives	Which of the sustenal imperatives are causing
Variables from the environment	or influencing the behavior(s)?
(e.g., familial)	What regulating and control mechanisms are
	present?
	What is the quality and quantity of sustenal
	imperatives?

Continued

TABLE 8-1   The Johnson Model and the Nursing Process—cont'd

Framework Elements	Nursing Thought
DIAGNOSTIC ANALYSIS—cont'd	

Diagnostic label
  Insufficiency
  Discrepancy
  Incompatibility
  Dominance
	Questions to guide determination of diagnosis:
	  What is the meaning of _____?
	  What are the implications of _____?
	  What do we already know about _____?
	  How does _____ affect _____?
	  Explain why _____?
	  Explain how _____?
	  Why is _____ important?
	  What do you think causes _____?
	    Why?
	  What are the relationships
	    between _____ and _____?

PLANNING AND INTERVENTION	

Mutual goal setting
Identify focus of intervention
Identify mode of intervention
Identify technique
	Questions to guide development of
	  intervention:
	What would happen if _____?
	What are some possible interventions for
	  the diagnosis of _____?
	What are possible unintended consequences
	  of the intervention?

EVALUATION	

Establish long-term goals
Establish short-term goals
Develop behavioral objectives to
  measure progress toward goals
	Are goals socially, culturally, and biologically
	  appropriate?
	Are the goals reasonable?
	Are the goals client centered?
	Are the objectives measurable and theory
	  based?

of the present illness or perceived health threat and/or hospitalization on behavioral patterns, and to establish the maximum possible level of health toward which an individual can strive. The behavioral systems analysis approach provides a comprehensive framework in which various types of data can be organized into a cohesive structure.

The assessment gathers specific knowledge regarding the structure and function of the eight subsystems (behavioral assessment) and those general and specific factors that supply the subsystems' functional requirements/sustenal imperatives (environmental assessment). Interview questions in both areas need to be theory-based. For example, Piagetian theory can be used to develop questions to assess the child's ability to express knowledge about illness—eliminative subsystem (Holaday, 1980).

Once the interview has been completed, data analysis (diagnostic analysis—see Table 8-1) is necessary to identify patterns of behavior that are adaptive and functional for the client and those that are maladaptive and indicate behavioral systems imbalance. One component of the analysis seeks to determine congruency among all structural units. Congruency is expressed as stable, patterned behavior, whereas discrepancy among the various components is expressed as unstable and disorganized behavior. The second component examines how the functional requirements/sustenal imperatives influence subsystem behavior. For example, how does family interaction style affect the client's affiliative subsystem? The latter analysis is critical because it plays an important role in determining how the nurse needs to function as an "external regulator" (Johnson, 1980, p. 214).

The nursing diagnosis is a summary of the results for the analysis and describes the current level of behavioral system function. It serves as a guide for intervention planning by the nursing team. The overall objective of the nursing intervention is to establish regularities in the client's behavior to meet the goal of each subsystem. The focus of the intervention will be on either a structural part of the subsystem or on the supply of sustenal imperatives/functional requirements.

Identifying goals is essential for evaluating client outcomes and for professional nursing care. To evaluate, the nurse must first predict expected client outcomes. This helps to ensure a purposeful, predictable course of client responses. To evaluate effectively, the nurse sets both long-term and short-term goals and behavioral objectives that will indicate progress toward achieving these goals.

CASE HISTORY OF DEBBIE

Debbie is a 29-year-old woman who was recently admitted to the oncology nursing unit for evaluation after sensing pelvic "fullness" and noticing a watery, foul-smelling vaginal discharge. A Papanicolaou smear revealed class V cervical cancer. She was found to have a stage II squamous cell carcinoma of the cervix and underwent a radical hysterectomy with bilateral salpingooophorectomy.

Her past health history revealed that physical examinations had been infrequent. She also reported that she had not performed breast self-examination. She is 5 feet, 4 inches tall and weights 89 pounds. Her usual weight is about 110 pounds. She has smoked approximately two packs of cigarettes a day for the past 16 years. She is gravida 2, para 2. Her first pregnancy was at age 16, and her second was at age 18. Since that time, she has taken oral contraceptives on a regular basis.

Debbie completed the eighth grade. She is married and lives with her husband and her two children in her mother's home, which she describes as less than sanitary. Her husband is unemployed. She describes him as emotionally distant and abusive at times.

She has done well following surgery except for being unable to completely empty her urinary bladder. She is having continued postoperative pain and nausea. It will be necessary for her to perform intermittent self-catheterization at home. Her medications are (1) an antibiotic, (2) an analgesic as needed for pain, and (3) an antiemetic as needed for nausea. In addition, she will be receiving radiation therapy on an outpatient basis.

Debbie is extremely tearful. She expresses great concern over her future and the future of her two children. She believes that this illness is a punishment for her past life.

NURSING CARE OF DEBBIE WITH JOHNSON'S MODEL
Behavioral Assessment

The relevant behavioral assessment data are the following. ***Achievement:*** Debbie has an eighth grade education, feels a loss of control of her future and that of her children, and has lost the ability to achieve the developmental outcomes of young adulthood. ***Affiliative:*** Debbie is married but describes her husband as emotionally distant and abusive at times; there may be a possible impairment of emotional endurance. ***Aggressive/ Protective:*** Her emotional endurance may be impaired. Debbie is not protective of herself (she smoked, sought healthcare infrequently, did not perform breast self-examination). With the loss of her health, she is protective of her children, but her husband is unemployed. Who will provide for family? ***Dependency:*** Because she lives with her mother, self-sufficiency may decrease. ***Ingestive:*** Debbie has experienced weight loss and nausea. ***Eliminative:*** Debbie is unable to empty her bladder. She is tearful, expressing concern about the future. ***Sexual:*** Because Debbie has had a hysterectomy, her sexual relationship with her husband may change, and she may have concerns about her feminine identity. ***Restorative:*** Debbie is experiencing fatigue, pain, and possible sleep disturbance.

Diagnosis and intervention. The JBSM provides a perspective for nursing practice by viewing Debbie as a biopsychosocial being represented in a behavioral system. The subjective and objective data indicate a problem in the achievement subsystem. *Objective data:* Debbie has class V cervical cancer—stage II squamous cell carcinoma of the cervix with an uncertain prognosis at this time. *Subjective data:* The patient is tearful and expresses concern about her ability to fulfill personal and family needs and responsibilities.

Environmental Assessment

The environmental assessment examines the sources of sustenal impera-tives (functional requirements) to determine whether they provide the functional requirements needed to maintain behavioral system balance. If these are present (or have been present in sufficient quantity and quality over time), then the subsystems, and subsequently the entire system, operate at the same level of efficiency and effectiveness and are able to maintain overall balance and stability. If they are not present, the nurse will act as an external regulatory force to provide protection, stimulation, or nurturance; change structural units; or impose external regulatory mechanisms. The critical component of the environmental assessment is to identify the factors that cause or influence behavioral system problems.

The environmental assessment identifies several key factors. From a developmental perspective, Debbie is relatively young, and thus many of the developmental tasks of young adulthood, such as raising her children and establishing a career and other future plans, could be impaired. The cancer diagnosis raises questions about her physical ability to achieve personal goals, and the pain, fatigue, and anxiety may impair her mental ability to achieve personal goals. During the first 3 months following diagnosis, Debbie needs to address issues related to the diagnosis, in-cluding dying, the future, and the meaning life has had (Weisman, 1979). During this same time, Debbie will be presented with a treatment plan and will simultaneously and learn to cope with recovery from surgery and side-effects of cancer therapy and plan for the future. The signifi-cance of this initial period cannot be overemphasized as Debbie attempts to regain control over herself and the environment.

Diagnosis and intervention. In examining Debbie's perseveratory set, one would note that Debbie's perception of herself as an independent agent generally capable of accomplishing her tasks and goals has been sub-stantially altered. In terms of the preparatory set, her situational context is also substantially altered. She is most likely uncertain about her choices. The diagnosis is insufficiency in the achievement subsystem. In terms of intervention, the nurse may protect Debbie from noxious stimuli because she is not presently able to cope with all situations. The nurse can provide nurturance in terms of providing counseling and help with goal setting. Stimulation in terms of teaching new self-care behaviors can also help. The biological disease process is unique for each person, and the psychosocial response to mastering the situation will be equally unique. Thus frequent reassessment and revision of the care plan will be needed.

Most patients faced with a diagnosis of cancer experience a life crisis. Although death is often the first fear, the potential for other stressors exists. Surgery, adjuvant therapy (radiation), the possible spread of malignancy, and an uncertain prognosis are all stressors. Surgery may lead to an altered body image with accompanying feelings of lost femininity. It is reasonable to assume that Debbie is experiencing some sexual concerns, and the sexual subsystem should be thoroughly examined because objective data indicate the potential for behavioral system imbalance.

The objective data identify that Debbie had a radical hysterectomy, which means the vaginal canal has been shortened. Because the trigone of the bladder and sigmoid colon may be closely associated with the new vaginal apex, sexual intercourse may be uncomfortable. Debbie will receive radiation therapy. Side-effects from this therapy may include fatigue, nausea and vomiting, impaired vaginal membrane integrity, bleeding, sexual dysfunction, and infection. The subjective data indicate that Debbie's husband is emotionally distant and sometimes abusive and that Debbie is tearful and worried about the future. The perseveratory set reveals that the current physiological functioning of the sex organs has been disrupted. Past socialization and experience in sex role behaviors may no longer seem applicable to Debbie. Within the context of the present situation (preparatory set), Debbie is most likely unsure where to direct her attention. The selection of a sexual behavior (choice) to meet goals is unclear.

Because the subsystem is not functioning to its fullest capacity, the nurse could diagnose insufficiency. If Debbie takes actions that do not meet the intended goal of the subsystem, a diagnosis of discrepancy could also be made.

Evaluation

Debbie has a knowledge deficit regarding radiation therapy and needs nurturance in terms of education to help her understand and cope with the situation. A careful assessment to determine Debbie's understanding of the purpose and goal of treatment is needed. Debbie must be taught preventive health practices that decrease the risk of impaired vaginal membrane integrity and comfort measures such as sitz baths and compresses to the perineum. Alternative methods of sexual intercourse can be discussed, especially because sexual intercourse during treatment is encouraged to prevent adhesions and to prevent shortening of the vagina. Counseling Debbie and her husband can help them create their own special intimacy, sense of affection, and physical gratification. The nurse's goal of helping to restore the patient's sexual function is tied in closely with goals of restoring or maintaining self-image and self-esteem.

CASE STUDY OF MARK

Mark is a 12-year-old boy with myleomeningocele and neurogenic bladder. He was also diagnosed with diabetes at age 9. He is admitted for a bladder augmentation and placement of an artificial sphincter. Mark has been hospitalized many times for surgical procedures (shunt revisions and orthopedic procedures). His mother and father are both present during the interview, and his mother does most of the talking. Mark is also interviewed alone. Mark's brothers, ages 17 years and 15 years, will visit him in the evenings but are not present during the admission interview.

NURSING CARE OF MARK WITH JOHNSON'S MODEL
Behavioral Assessment

Achievement: Mark looked at the nurse with a great little smile when he described his school and how it is different. He describes it as a "handicap school." He likes it because there are only "16 kids and two teachers and I get lots of help." He is also proud of what he can do on the computer. Mark attributes his success to the presence or absence of ability and attributes little to motivational factors. He enjoyed the Piagetian testing, which placed him in the concrete operations period. Both the nursing staff and his mother note that he requires verbal prompts to perform self-care activities. His mother notes that he has missed a lot of school during the past 2 years, which is why she and her husband removed Mark from regular public school and placed him in a special education school. The classes are ungraded, but his mother says he has made great progress at this school and now reads at a sixth-grade level and has math skills at a fifth-grade level. Mark is worried about "getting behind" while he is in the hospital. Mark has no idea what he wants to be when he grows up. He has not been to camp, nor has he ever spent the night at another child's home. Mark has never been home alone; a parent or sibling is always present.

Affiliative: Mark seems emotionally more attached to his mother than his father. He likes and admires his older brothers and wishes he "could ride dirt bikes with them." He spends a lot of time at home with his mother and alone watching TV or "messing around on the computer." He watches football games and other sports on TV with his father on the weekends. Mark cannot name a friend at his school or in his neighborhood. His mother states he likes to be "with other kids" and likes when his brothers' friends are at the house. She also could not name a child who was a friend. The nursing staff and his mother describe Mark as shy, and the nurse's observation in the playroom confirms this. He is more talkative when his mother is absent. When she is present, Mark lets his mother answer questions or asks her to do so.

Aggressive/Protective: His mother and the nursing staff describe him as passive and more likely to sulk than get angry. When the nurse asked what he would do if someone took something of his or hit him, Mark said he "wouldn't like it."

Dependency: Mark refused to answer questions about self-care. The nursing staff state that they saw little evidence of self-care activity during previous admissions. He lets the nursing staff or his mother maintain his blood sugar, inject his insulin, select his menu, and perform his bowel and bladder care. Mark's mother states that he has become more dependent on her during the past year. He asks for help to dress in addition to his other requests. The staff has noted more independent behavior when the mother and grandmother are absent. Nurses noticed a tremendous difference between the way he acted with them when his mother and grandmother were not present (adult/child to adult/parent with the nurse and child/parent with mother and grandmother).

Ingestive: Mark states, "I like to eat." His mother also describes Mark as "loving food" and "eating too much." The switch to the "diabetic diet has been difficult for him." The family eats meals together. Postoperatively, he usually has nausea and vomiting, and fluid and food intake are poor. Mark is very observant of what goes on around him. He likes to "have tests and things explained" to him when he is in the hospital.

Eliminative: Mark has minimal bowel and bladder control. He has frequent problems with dribbling of urine. Mark himself admits this bothers him. His mother suspects he does not perform intermittent self-catheterization regularly at school because he is embarrassed about sexual changes and about the fact that he must wear sanitary protection pads. As for his communication pattern, Mark tucks his head to his chest and mumbles when he is talking about his feelings or his parents. Sometimes he simply refuses to answer or looks away. The nurse suspects the mumbling and shyness is a means of coping with his overtalkative and overprotective mother and grandmother.

Sexual: Mark looked away when the nurse asked about changes in his body and "becoming a man." He did not answer questions. He said he did not like "wearing special pants." When asked who he was most like in his family, he said his mother, who admits that she and her husband have not talked with Mark about sex. "We don't know what to tell him because of his birth defect." His father has told him the changes "are part of growing up and becoming a man." His mother is concerned because

Mark "hasn't asked any questions like the other boys." Mark is Tanner Stage 3. She adds, "I think his brothers have talked with him because they joke around about making out."

Restorative: Mark sleeps 8 hours a night but sleeps less in the hospital "because they wake you up all the time." He usually gets up around 7 AM on school days and 8:30 AM on the weekends. He has a somewhat restricted repertoire of interests and activities. He watches a lot of television and rental videos and plays computer games. He participates in no groups, clubs, or regular physical activity. He enjoys family weekend trips to the lake and dune buggy and boat rides.

Environmental Assessment

Familial: Structure: Mark is the youngest of three boys. His mother works part-time as a secretary and is home in the afternoon when Mark returns from school. His father works as a manager of a large department store. The maternal grandparents live nearby. The grandmother visits frequently. *Dynamics:* Mark is included in all family activities, and Mark and his brothers are involved in home activities and chores. It appears that the parents do not fully discuss all aspects of Mark's illness (sexuality issues, compliance, approaching adolescence), nor do they discuss all issues with Mark. The mother is overresponsible for Mark's treatments; she encourages Mark's overdependency. In turn, the mother assumes more responsibility for care.

Social/Cultural: Mark is part of a Protestant, middle-class family that does not attend church regularly. Both parents place a high value on home and family. The father has assumed the patriarchal provider role in the family. The family has lived in the same house for 17 years and has several close friends in the neighborhood who will help whenever needed. The parents have also maintained social relationships with several of his father's business associates. They belong to no outside social clubs or groups. Insurance covers 90% of Mark's expenses, and they sometimes face financial troubles. Currently, however, there are no major financial problems.

Developmental: Mark laughed when the nurse said he was about to become a "terrible teen." He said he has heard adults talk about it but he would not elaborate. Mark enjoys heavy metal rock, computer games, and watching television. When asked about girls, he shrugged and looked away. Mark attends a special education school and is behind his grade level. His social skills are not age-appropriate. Medical treatments, parental overprotectiveness, and physical disability all seem to be reinforcing dependence while diminishing any sense of self-control over health. Self-care responsibility is less than we would expect of a 12-year-old.

Pathological and Biological: Mark stated that he hates "everything about hospitals." He acknowledged that the increase in restrictions of activity bothered him. The "tests" and "surgery" worry him. He knows the surgery is to try to stop the "leaking" of urine, but Mark is uncertain about where they will operate and exactly what will be done. Mark doesn't like diabetes because he can no longer "eat whatever I want." Mark has a poor understanding of diabetes. He could not explain the role of insulin and diet in the management of the illness. Mark better understands myelomeningocele and how that affects his walking and bowel and bladder control. On admission, Mark's vital signs are normal. He is in the 25th percentile for height for his age and 90th percentile for weight. His BUN, creatinine, and blood-sugar levels are slightly elevated. His glycohemoglobin level is elevated, indicating poor long-term control.

Ecological: The family owns a home in the suburbs. A park is located about a mile from their home, and a school and playground are located about one-half mile from home. The parents describe the neighborhood as safe. No public transportation is available in the area.

Psychological: As a preadolescent, Mark is concerned about body image and is anxious about any bodily disruption or change. He seems self-conscious about his early sexual maturation. His mother has noted Mark's childlike behaviors and increasing dependency during the past year (e.g., wants help dressing). He is socially isolated from peers, and interaction with his brothers has decreased during the past 2 years. He also needs more emotional support from his mother. His mother calls Mark shy, and the nursing staff's observations support this assessment. His scores on the self-esteem interview were low. He copes by withdrawing from situations that make him uncomfortable. He does not like to discuss his feelings about sensitive issues (e.g., parents, sexuality, illness). However, he wants information about specific events that are stressful for him (e.g., surgery).

• • •

This case study is presented because it reflects both acute and long-term problems associated with managing a chronic illness. It also demonstrates that children's developmental domains (behavioral subsystems) are often significantly influenced by their illness. One of the strengths of JBSM is that it not only identifies current acute problems but also identifies chronic subsystem alterations that lead to behavioral system disturbances. These alterations involve a disturbance in normal developmental sequences. Without intervention, these alterations may lead to more serious problems as the child matures. This analysis applies the nursing process to an acute problem related to this admission and to a long-term problem.

Diagnostic analysis. The essential characteristic of human beings is their purposefulness. This purposefulness is based on their ability to select their goals and make choices for achieving them. To successfully intervene in a clinical situation, it is necessary to consider people's choices and to understand how people make their choices. The JBSM directs the nurse's attention to human choice phenomena. The degree to which the nurse can help the client restore behavioral system balance depends on the extent to which the client understands behavioral actions. Once an explanation has been found, the client can obtain behavioral system balance by changing his or her goals or by changing the environmental conditions in such a way that previously established goals can be obtained through changes in behavior. To accomplish this, nurses need to adopt an input-oriented approach to their case-model building. To focus on the proper inputs, nurses need to develop an assessment strategy that allows them to thoroughly understand small segments of behavior at the subsystem level and to integrate that understanding for the entire system.

An output-oriented approach describes only the person's choices, and the description provides only knowledge of the behavior. This information is of some use. However, to understand the behavioral elements in the system, nurses must seek an explanation for a person's action, and this comes only from an input focus. The JBSM's focus on environmental assessment as well as behavioral assessment provides input-focused data as well as output-focused data. The two diagnoses addressed in this section provide insight about the process.

Acute problem. Mark has been admitted to the hospital for a bladder augmentation and placement of an artificial sphincter. He is behind his grade level at school. Piagetian testing places him at the concrete operations level of cognitive development. The subjective data inform the nurse that Mark is worried about "tests" and "surgery" and is unsure about specific aspects of the surgery. He has some understanding of myelomeningocele and little understanding of diabetes. However, he does like to have "tests and things" explained to him. Also contributing to this problem is the mother's overprotection of Mark and the apparent failure of the family to openly discuss aspects of the illness.

The goal of the ingestive subsystem is to internalize the external environment, and one of the functions is to obtain knowledge or information useful to the self (Grubbs, 1974). The perseveratory set refers to usual status or habits. All of Mark's sensory modalities—speech, sight, hearing, and touch—are intact, and he values being informed about tests. In terms of the preparatory set, Mark is in the period of concrete operations. He can assimilate new experiences, has developed an awareness of conservation, is capable of seeing the relationships of the part to the whole, and also has developed a concept of causality. *Choice* refers to the alternate behaviors Mark sees himself as available to him in this situation. Since little preoperative teaching has been done, Mark's choice and actions are limited. The diagnosis is insufficiency of the ingestive subsystem. The major stressor is functional—a lack of information. The nurse's goal is to protect the basic goal of the subsystem by providing information. A successful intervention will inform Mark about the surgery to clarify the range of choices and actions.

Planning and intervention. Given the complexity of this case, the intervention needs to be planned carefully. The intervention could also impact the dependency subsystem (self-care), achievement subsystem (sense of mastery), affiliative subsystem (socialization), and eliminative subsystem (expression of feelings). It was mutually agreed that the preoperative teaching would be done with both Mark and his parents together and alone with Mark. Diagrams and pictures will be used to explain the surgery, and postoperative treatments and procedures would also be explained and demonstrated. Thus the nurse will provide the functional requirements of protection and nurturance.

The immediate goal of the intervention is to inform Mark about his surgery and postoperative care. The intermediate goal is for Mark to maintain his health physiological system through the intake of food, fluids, and medicine during the postoperative period. This will occur as a result of his understanding the surgical procedure and the postoperative care needed for recovery (e.g., internalizing the external environment). The long-term objective is that the intervention will restore Mark's sense of mastery and of autonomy.

Nursing interventions need to be theory-based. These theories need to be compatible with systems theory and the assumptions of the JBSM. For example, the technique selected for this intervention is based on Vygotsky's Zone of Proximal Development (ZPD) (Vygotsky, 1962). One of the strengths of the JBSM is the ease with which theories can be incorporated into all phases of the plan of care.

Wertsch and Rogoff (1984) have defined the ZPD as "the phase in development in which the child has only partially mastered a task but can participate in its execution with assistance and supervision of an adult or more capable peer" (p. 1). There are two important dimensions of the ZPD—joint collaboration and transfer of responsibility—in which both the child and the adult actively participate and contribute to some aspect of task performance or problem solution. Joint collaboration is based on the child being guided to actively define and redefine the task situation in terms of the adult's definition (Holaday, LaMontague, & Marciel, 1994).

The second dimension is the transfer of responsibility, which refers to the adult's decreasing role in regulating and managing behavior task performance. This gradual relinquishment and transfer of adult responsibility is described as "guided participation" (Wertsch & Rogoff, 1984, pp. 1-6). Thus as a child's competence increases, effective scaffolders gradually withdraw their support in accord with the child's efforts. Scaffolding refers to the gradual decrease and eventual withdrawal of adult control and support as a function of the child's increasing mastery of a given task or problem.

Thus the preoperative teaching plan developed by the nurse, as an external regulator, is a scaffold for Mark. The nurse structures the situation, but Mark decides about his degree of involvement in the program and later about his role in postoperative care. Mark is supported and rewarded for his independent actions and efforts to regulate his care. This intervention also permits the nurse to role-model new behaviors for the parents.

Chronic problem. It is helpful to think of parenting in terms of the JBSM as a set of environmental actions performed by the parents or a set of environmental conditions arranged by parents that assists or impedes the child in carrying out his/her functions. It is important to make clear that in this examination of parenting actions and conditions as elements external to the child, the independence of the child and environment are not implied. Rather, the examination occurs only for the purposes of assessment and the convenience of organization.

From a JBSM perspective, the idea of an external regulator of growth and development is also useful. The idea of nursing care as a set of regulatory acts aimed at successful adaptation and goal attainment for the child (behavioral system) is consistent with most ecological developmental models and with the general precepts of control systems theory. However, as potentially useful as the concept of an external regulator might be in classifying the actions and conditions of nursing care (i.e., in terms of adjusting parenting actions or environmental conditions arranged by the parent), it carries with it a practical paradox—external regulation is unlikely to be a simple matter for a complex organism. The JBSM provides a means to approach this issue, but much work remains in building theory in this area. The next care problem clearly addresses the complexity involved.

The data from the environmental assessment identify Mark's mother as overprotective and highly responsible for Mark's care. Mark spends a good deal of time with his mother and seems to be more emotionally attached to her than to his father. Mark takes little responsibility for self-care activities. He is described as shy and cannot name a friend. The goal of the dependency subsystem is to maintain environmental resources needed for obtaining help, assistance, attention, reassurance, and security—in other words, to gain trust and reliance. The primary diagnosis is dominance of the dependency subsystem. The behaviors in the dependency subsystem are being used more than any other subsystem regardless of the situation, to the detriment of other subsystems (Grubbs, 1974). A number of secondary diagnoses could also be made in terms of incompatibility between the dependency subsystem (set, choice, action, and goal) and other subsystems (most notably achievement and affiliative). Problems for both child and parent are evident in terms of set, choice, and action. In terms of the perseveratory set, both parents and child are unsure about the appropriate age at which a child with a chronic health problem should be expected to meet his or her own needs and at which times and places assistance with tasks should be sought. Mark does not perceive himself as self-sufficient and independent. The preparatory set shows that Mark and his parents have difficulty perceiving whether a situation requires task-oriented assistance. Given the problems with set, it is not surprising that the range of choice is narrow and that actions are not always appropriate.

The major stressors are both functional and structural. The functional stressors arise from the environment and are related to parenting style. The structural stressors involve internal control mechanisms and reflect inconsistencies between the subsystem goal and set, choice, and action.

The short-term goals in this case are to help the parents gain some insight into their behavior and its impact on Mark's behavior and to facilitate a change in Mark's behavior (an increase in independent behaviors while hospitalized). The long-term goal is to promote Mark's optimal development by designing an external regulatory system to do the following: (1) sustain Mark's current level of independence, (2) stimulate activity directed at more independent behaviors, and (3) control the amount and pattern of experience (inputs) that reach Mark to achieve an optimal fit between Mark's current abilities and his projected goals. This family-centered intervention would be best carried out by a nurse with sustained contact with Mark and his parents.

The central goal for the nurse, as an external regulatory force, is to construct a system of caregiving episodes the parents can use to integrate the functional requirements for the environmental/developmental relationship. The nurse helps the parents provide protection and nurturance to maintain Mark's current level of behavior (his internal organizational coherence and environmental relationships) so he can continue to function. The nurse maintains whatever stability is present to avoid encouraging more dependent behaviors. The nurse stimulates incremental change (alter set, choice, and action) for both the parents and Mark through a process of self-construction. New information and new experiences will be introduced in a controlled fashion, which will lead to successive changes in existing structures. Goal setting is one technique that can accomplish this. People can cognitively construct representations of potential future states. By personal goal setting, individuals disrupt their status quo or disorganize themselves and then organize their behavior to resolve the disruption or create a new coherent organization. They become "producers of their own development" (Lerner, 1982, p. 342). Thus in goal setting, negative feedback reduces a discrepancy, but it does so by altering the system through incremental change.

Evaluation. The JBSM directs the nurse's attention toward areas that need to be addressed in practice. Currently no specific interventions delineate this system of caregiving episodes for parents of chronically ill children. What broad, basic regulatory functions of the nurse need to be included in this system of caregiving episodes? The actual episodes and conditions of parenting entail numerous physical/structural properties, not just broad abstractions. From the standpoint of understanding the development of a chronically ill child, what are the most salient dimensions of these real acts and conditions for each of the subsystems? How does the nurse function as an external regulator of chronically ill children's health and development with the goal of a good fit between the child's characteristics, environmental opportunities, and constraints? Using the JBSM, the nurse learns that a chronically ill child's developmental pathways do not unfold along a predetermined course; they are constructed through processes of living that involve continuities, discontinuities, and uncertainties. The nurse as an external regulator and source of functional requirements plays a critical role in helping a family achieve optimal development outcomes for a special-needs child.

CRITICAL THINKING EXERCISES

1. Considering the assessment of Debbie according to the achievement subsystem, how might different goals (drive) or set have altered her choices or actions? How would this difference have altered the structure of Debbie as a behavioral system?
2. What other two subsystems would have been altered by different goals or set? How might these different goals alter the structure of Debbie's behavioral system?
3. Think back to the last health problem you experienced. Recall your behaviors and assess their structure (drive, set, choice, and action) according to the behavioral assessment of the subsystems as outlined in Table 8-1.
4. Recall your environment at a time when you were ill and assess your sustenal imperatives using the guide in Table 8-1.
5. Based on the assessments carried out in critical thinking exercises 3 and 4, conduct a diagnostic analysis on the data and determine what nursing diagnosis might have been used to guide the planning of nursing interventions for you according to Johnson's Behavioral Systems Model.

References

Auger, J. (1976). *Behavioral systems and nursing.* Englewood Cliffs, NJ: Prentice Hall.

Auger, J. & Dee, V. (1983). A patient classification system based on the Behavioral System Model of nursing: Part 1. *Journal of Nursing Administration, 13*(4), 38-43.

Dee, V. (1990). Implementation of the Johnson model: One hospital's experience. In M. E. Parker (Ed.), *Nursing theories in practice* (pp. 33-44). New York: National League for Nursing.

Dee, V. & Randell, B. (1989). *NPH patient classification system: A theory-based nursing practice model for staffing.* Los Angeles: Nursing Department, UCLA Neuropsychiatric Institute and Hospital.

Dee, V., van Servellen, G., & Brecht, M. (1998). Managed behavioral health care patients and their nursing care problems, level of functioning, and impairment on discharge. *Journal of the American Psychiatric Nurses Association, 4*(2), 57-66.

Derdiarian, A. K. (1983). An instrument for theory and research development using the Behavioral System Model for nursing: The cancer patient: Part I. *Nursing Research, 32,* 196-201.

Derdiarian, A. K. (1988). The sensitivity of the DBSM instrument to age, site and stage of cancer: A preliminary validation study. *Scholarly Inquiry for Nursing Practice, 2,* 103-120.

Derdiarian, A. K. (1990). The relationships among the subsystems of Johnson's Behavioral System Model. *Image, 22,* 219-225.

Derdiarian, A. K. (1993). The Johnson Behavioral System Model: Perspectives for nursing practice. In M. E. Parker (Ed.), *Patterns of nursing theories in practice* (pp. 267-284). New York: National League for Nursing.

Derdiarian, A. K. & Forsythe, A. W. (1983). An instrument for theory and research development using the Behavioral System Model for nursing: The cancer patient: Part II. *Nursing Research, 32,* 260-266.

Grubbs, J. (1974). The Johnson Behavioral System Model. In J. Riehl & C. Roy (Eds.), *Conceptual models for nursing practice* (pp. 217-249). New York: Appleton-Century-Crofts.

Grubbs, J. (1980). The Behavioral Systems Model for nursing. In J. P. Riehl & C. Roy (Eds.), *Conceptual models for nursing practice* (pp. 207-216). New York: Appleton-Century-Crofts.

Holaday, B. (1974). Achievement behavior in chronically ill children. *Nursing Research, 23,* 25-30.

Holaday, B. (1980). Implementing the Johnson model for nursing practice. In J. P. Riehl & C. Roy (Eds.), *Conceptual models for nursing practice* (2nd ed., pp. 255-263). New York: Appleton-Century-Crofts.

Holaday, B. (1981). Maternal response to their chronically ill infants' attachment behavior of crying. *Nursing Research, 30,* 343-348.

Holaday, B. (1982). Maternal conceptual set development: Identifying patterns of maternal response to chronically ill infant crying. *Maternal Child Nursing Journal, 11*(1), 47-59.

Holaday, B. (1987). Patterns of interaction between mothers and their chronically ill infants. *Maternal Child Nursing Journal, 16,* 29-36.

Holaday, B., LaMontague, L., & Marciel, J. (1994). Vygotsky's Zone of Proximal Development: Implications for nurse assistance of children's learning. *Issues in Comprehensive Pediatric Nursing, 17,* 15-27.

Holaday, B., Turner-Henson, A., & Swan, J. (1996). Explaining activities of chronically ill children: An analysis using the Johnson Behavioral System Model. In P. Hinton-Walker & B. Newman (Eds.), *Blueprint for use of nursing models: Education, research, practice and administration* (pp. 33-63). New York: National League for Nursing Publications.

Johnson, D. (1968). One conceptual model for nursing. Paper presented at Vanderbilt University, Nashville, TN. (Copy available at Eskind Biomedical Library, Vanderbilt University; Nashville, Tennessee. Contact Mary Teloh, Special Collections Librarian, (615) 936-1406).

Johnson, D. (1980). The Behavioral Systems Model for nursing. In J. Riehl & C. Roy (Eds.), *Conceptual models for nursing practice* (2nd ed., pp. 207-216). New York: Appleton-Century-Crofts.

Johnson, D. (1990). The Behavioral System Model for nursing. In M. E. Parker (Ed.), *Nursing theories in practice* (pp. 23-32). New York: National League for Nursing.

Lerner, R. M. (1982). Children and adolescents as producers of their own development. *Developmental Review, 2,* 342-370.

Meleis, A. I. (1991). *Theoretical nursing: Development and progress.* Philadelphia: J. B. Lippincott.

Poster, E. C., Dee, V., & Randell, B. P. (1997). The Johnson Behavioral Systems Model as a framework for patient outcome evaluation. *Journal of the American Psychiatric Nurses Association, 3*(3), 73-80.

Pressley, M. (1992). Encouraging mindful use of prior knowledge: Attempting to construct explanatory answers facilitates learning. *Educational Psychologist, 27,* 91-109.

Rawls, A. G. (1980). Evaluation of the Johnson behavioral model in clinical practice. *Image, 12,* 13-16.

Riegel, B. (1989). Social support and psychological adjustment to chronic coronary heart disease: Operationalization of Johnson's Behavioral System Model. *Advances in Nursing Science, 11*(2), 74-84.

Turner-Henson, A. (1993). Mothers of chronically ill children and perceptions of environmental variables. *Issues in Comprehensive Pediatric Nursing, 16,* 63-76.

Vygotsky, L. S. (1962). *Thought and language.* Cambridge, MA: MIT Press.

Weisman, A. D. (1979). *Coping with cancer.* New York: McGraw-Hill.

Wertsch, J. V. & Rogoff, B. (1984). Editor's notes. *New Directions for Child Development, 23,* 1-6.

Wittrock, M. C. (1990). Generative processes of comprehension. *Educational Psychologist, 24,* 345-376.

King's Interacting Systems Framework and Theory in Nursing Practice

Diane M. Norris and Maureen A. Frey

"Knowledge used by nurses has been derived from natural and behavioral sciences. More recently, nurses have been discussing nursing science and studying ways in which an organized body of knowledge essential to nursing practice can be identified." (From King, I. M. [1968]. A conceptual frame of reference. Nursing Research, *17[1], 27-31.)*

HISTORY AND BACKGROUND

In the mid-1960s, Imogene King wrote of the need for focus, organization, and use of nursing's knowledge base (King, 1968). Knowledge for nursing results from the systematic use and validation of knowledge about concepts relevant to nursing situations. In discussing the role of concepts in knowledge development, King stated, "Concepts offer a way of thinking about nursing: a way of observing behavior and a way of collecting specific information essential for decision making based on knowledge available to meet some of the needs of individuals at a particular point in time" (King, 1968, p. 30). Use of knowledge in critical

---

To be true to the original sources cited in this text, the terminology for King's theory used in this text reflects the terminology in most of the applications of King's theory to date. However, King (personal communication, February 8, 2001) has indicated that she prefers her work now be called King's Conceptual System and Theory of Goal Attainment.

thinking results in decisions that are implemented in professional nursing practice.

In 1971, King proposed a conceptual framework for nursing around four concepts she considered universal to the discipline of nursing: social systems, health, perception, and interpersonal relationships. These areas were identified from the synthesis and reformulation of concepts using inductive and deductive reasoning and critical thinking and from extensive review of nursing and literature from other health-related disciplines. Concepts were organized around individuals as personal systems, small groups as interpersonal systems, and larger social systems such as community and school (King, 1971). Role, status, social organization, communication, information, and energy were identified as basic concepts of functions of systems. King proposed that concepts were interrelated and could be used across systems to identify the essence of nursing.

King expanded the conceptual framework during the 1970s by further explicating the nature of persons and environment, strengthening the general systems orientation, and expanding the concepts. A more formalized conceptual framework of personal, interpersonal, and social systems was presented in 1981. Concepts in the personal system were perception, self, growth and development, body image, time, and space. Concepts in the interpersonal system were human interaction, communication, transactions, role, and stress. Concepts in the social system were organization, authority, power, status, and decision making.

Also presented in the 1981 text was the Theory of Goal Attainment, derived from the personal and interpersonal systems. The Theory of Goal Attainment specifically addressed how nurses interact with patients to achieve health goals. The initial concepts of the theory (perception, communication, interaction, transaction, self, role, and decision making) represented the essence of nursing (King, 1981, 2000). Since 1981, King has provided clarification, explanation, and some additional concepts. The concepts of learning and coping were added; the concept of space was redefined as personal space; and the concept of stress was expanded to include stressors (Frey, 1996; King, 1990, 1991).

Although King's *A Theory for Nursing: Systems, Concepts, Process* (1981) is 20 years old, King has provided ongoing clarification and theoretical discussion of the systems framework and Theory of Goal Attainment— including middle-range theories derived from the systems framework by others—through journal publications and presentations. Although there have been no major changes in the conceptual/theoretical structures, King has explicated the philosophical basis and enduring nature of the framework and theory for nursing with an emphasis on the twenty-first century and world as community (King, 1990, 1994, 1995a, 1995b, 1996,

1997, 1999, 2000). Contemporary themes include the information explosion, technological advances, and changes in organization and delivery of healthcare. For example, King (1999) recently reiterated and explicated the importance of knowledge of ethical theories and principles for decision making.

In addition, King has addressed issues raised by others who have analyzed her framework (Gonot, 1989; Fawcett, 1989; Magan, 1987; Meleis, 1991, 1997). King (1990) clarified her definition of health as a dynamic process rather than a linear concept suggested by her use of the word *continuum* in earlier writings. By illustrating the use of concepts from the interpersonal and social systems to guide nursing practice in the care of neurologically compromised patients, Carter and Dufour (1994) responded to the challenge that King's framework had limited applicability in caring for patients who were unable to communicate.

The ongoing work with the interacting systems framework for nursing, Theory of Goal Attainment, and theories derived by others (Frey & Sieloff, 1995) greatly facilitated the application of King's framework and theory to practice. In a recent review, Sieloff, Frey, and Killeen (2000) found that the systems framework and theory had been used with patients across the life span, nursing specialties, care settings, models of care delivery, cultures, and types of care (i.e., primary, secondary and tertiary) as well as for multidisciplinary research. The King International Nursing Group was founded in 1997 to further this important work.

OVERVIEW OF KING'S SYSTEMS FRAMEWORK AND THEORY

King's systems framework is based on the assumption that human beings are the focus of nursing. The goal of nursing is health: its health promotion, maintenance, and/or restoration; care of the sick or injured; and care of the dying (King, 1992). King (1996) states that "nursing's domain involves human beings, families, and communities as a framework within which nurses make transactions in multiple environments with health as a goal" (p. 61). King (1992) identified relevant concepts within each system to organize knowledge about individuals, groups, and society but noted that these concepts are often interrelated. According to King (1981, 1988, 1991), concepts are critical because they provide knowledge that is applicable to practice. Systems and concepts within King's framework are described and defined in the following sections.

Personal Systems

Individuals are personal systems (King, 1981). Each individual is an open, total, unique system in constant interaction with the environment. Interactions between and among personal systems are the focus of King's conceptual framework. Patients, family members, friends, other health-care professionals, clergy, and nurses are just a few examples of individuals who interact in the nursing practice environment. The following concepts provide foundational knowledge that contributes to understanding individuals as personal systems:

- *Perception:* "A process of organizing, interpreting, and transforming information from sense data and memory" (King, 1981, p. 24).
- *Self:* "The self is a composite of thoughts and feelings which constitute a person's awareness of his/her individual existence, his/her conception of who and what he/she is. A person's self is the sum total of all he/she can call his/hers. The self includes among other things, a system of ideas, attitudes, values and commitments. The self is a person's total subjective environment. It is a distinctive center of experience and significance. The self constitutes a person's inner world as distinguished from the outer world consisting of all other people and things. The self is the individual as known to the individual. It is that to which we refer when we say 'I'" (Jersild, 1952, pp. 9-10).
- *Growth and development:* "The processes that take place in an individual's life that help the individual move from potential capacity for achievement to self-actualization" (King, 1981, p. 31).
- *Body image:* "An individual's perceptions of his/her own body, others' reactions to his/her appearance which results from others' reactions to self" (King, 1981, p. 33).
- *Learning:* "A process of sensory perception, conceptualization, and critical thinking involving multiple experiences in which changes in concepts, skills, symbols, habits, and values can be evaluated in observable behaviors and inferred from behavioral manifestation" (King, 1986, p. 24).
- *Time:* "Duration between the occurrence of one event and occurrence of another event" (King, 1981, p. 24).
- *Personal space:* "Existing in all directions and is the same everywhere" (King, 1981, p. 37).
- *Coping:* Although King (1981) used the term *coping* in her discussion of the concept of stress in the interpersonal system and in later discussions of the Theory of Goal Attainment (King, 1992, 1997), coping was not identified as a concept in the interacting systems framework. Doornbos (1995) selected Lazarus and Folkman's definition of coping for a middle-range theory of family health in the families of the young, chronically mentally ill. Following a review of perspectives of coping, Lazarus and Folkman's definition (1984) seemed very consistent with King's view of stress and individuals. Lazarus and Folkman (1984) define

coping as "the constantly changing cognitive and behavioral efforts to manage specific external and internal demands that are appraised as taxing or exceeding the resources" (p. 141).

Interpersonal Systems

Two or more individuals in interaction form interpersonal systems (King, 1981). As the number of individuals increase, so does the complexity of the interaction. These groups may range in size from two or three interacting individuals to small or large groups. King's process of nursing occurs primarily within the interpersonal systems between the nurse and patient. Concepts critical to understanding interactions between individuals are defined as follows:

- *Communication:* "Information processing, a change of information from one state to another" (King, 1981, p. 69).
- *Interaction:* "Acts of two or more persons in mutual presence" (King, 1981, p. 85).
- *Role:* "Set of behaviors expected when occupying a position in a social system" (King, 1981, p. 93).
- *Stress:* "Dynamic state whereby a human being interacts with the environment to maintain balance for growth, development, and performance which involves an exchange of energy and information between the person and the environment for regulation and control of stressors" (King, 1981, p. 98).
- *Stressors:* Events that produce stress (King, 1981).
- *Transaction:* "Observable behaviors of human beings interacting with their environment" (King, 1981, p. 147).

Social Systems

Social systems are composed of large groups with common interests or goals. A social system is defined as "an organized boundary system of social roles, behaviors, and practices developed to maintain values and the mechanisms to regulate the practice and rules" (King, 1981, p. 115). Examples of social systems include healthcare settings, workplaces, educational institutions, religious organizations, and families (King, 1981). Interactions with social systems influence individuals throughout the life span. Concepts that are useful to understand interactions within social systems and between social and personal systems are defined as follows:

- *Organization:* "A system whose continuous activities are conducted to achieve goals" (King, 1981, p. 119).
- *Authority:* "Transactional process characterized by active, reciprocal relations in which members' values, backgrounds, and perceptions play a role in defining, validating, and accepting the [directions] of individuals within an organization" (King, 1981, p. 124).

- *Power:* "The capacity or ability of a group to achieve goals" (King, 1981, p. 124).
- *Status:* "The position of an individual in a group or a group in relation to other groups in an organization" (King, 1981, p. 129).
- *Decision making:* "Dynamic and systematic process by which a goal-directed choice of perceived alternatives is made, and acted upon, by individuals or groups to answer a question and attain a goal" (King, 1981, p. 132).

• • •

The framework provides both structure and function for nursing. Clearly stated assumptions about persons, environment, health, nursing, and systems provide a conceptual orientation of holism and dynamic interaction, identify health as the goal of nursing, and actively include the patient (individual, family, or community) in decisions about setting and working toward health goals.

Theory of Goal Attainment

The Theory of Goal Attainment specifically addresses nursing as a process of human interaction. Indeed, King (1981) claims that the Theory of Goal Attainment is a normative theory—that is, it should set the standard of practice for nurse-patient interactions. King (1997) recalled finding an index card on which she had written the following 15 years ago, "King's law of nurse-patient interaction: Nurses and patients in mutual presence, interacting purposefully, make transactions in nursing situations based on each individual's perceptions, purposeful communication, and valued goals" (p. 184).

The nurse and patient form an interpersonal system in which each affects the other and in which both are affected by situational factors in the environment. Drawn from both the personal and interpersonal system concepts, the Theory of Goal Attainment comprises perception, communication, interaction, transaction, self, role, growth and development, stress/stressors, coping, time, and personal space. King (1981, 1991) identified that perception, communication, and interaction are essential elements in transaction. When transactions are made, goals are usually attained. The human interaction and conceptual focus dimensions of the theory guide the nursing process dimension (Figure 9-1).

King has demonstrated linkages between the Theory of Goal Attainment and the traditional nursing process as shown in Table 9-1 (King, 1992). King (1993) views the traditional nursing process as a system of interrelated actions—the method by which nursing is practiced. In contrast, knowledge of the interrelated concepts in the Theory of Goal

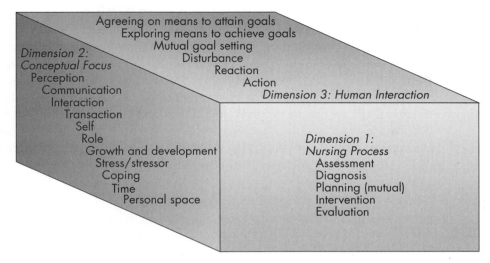

FIGURE 9-1

Three-dimensional nursing process based on King's theory. (Modified from M. A. Frey & C. L. Sieloff [Eds.], *Advancing King's systems framework and theory for nursing,* p. 212, copyright © 1995 by Sage Publications, Inc. Reprinted by permission of Sage Publications, Inc.)

Attainment (King, 1992) provides the theoretical basis for nursing practice. King (1995b) underscored the importance of nursing process as both method *and* theory when she stated, "Nurses are first, and foremost, human beings who perform their functions in a professional role. It is the way in which nurses, in their role, do with and for individuals that differentiates nursing from other health professionals" (p. 26).

TABLE 9-1 Nursing Process: Theory and Method	
Nursing Process as Method*	**Nursing Process as Theory†**
A system of interrelated actions	A system of interrelated concepts
Assess	Perception of nurse and client
	Communication of nurse and client
	Interaction of nurse and client
Plan	Decision making about goals
	Agree to means to attain goals
Implement	Transactions made
Evaluate	Goal attained (if not, why not)

From King, I. M. (1992). *Nursing Science Quarterly,* 5(1), 23, copyright © 1992 by Sage Publications, Inc. Reprinted by permission of Sage Publications, Inc.
*Yura, H. & Walsh, M. (1983). *The nursing process.* Norwalk, CT: Appleton-Century-Crofts.
†King, I. M. (1981). *A theory for nursing: Systems, concepts, process.* New York: John Wiley. (Now published by Delmar, Albany, NY).

CRITICAL THINKING IN NURSING PRACTICE WITH KING'S FRAMEWORK

It is generally agreed that critical thinking is knowing how to think, how to apply, how to analyze, how to synthesize, and how to evaluate. Whereas the traditional nursing process of "assess, plan, implement, and evaluate" provides a method, the critical thinking process emphasizes the intellectual skills of apprehension, judgment, and reasoning.

Rubenfeld and Scheffer (1999) conducted a study to define critical thinking in nursing. They formulated the following consensus statement to reflect the essence of critical thinking in nursing:

> Critical thinking in nursing is an essential component of professional accountability and quality nursing care. Critical thinkers in nursing exhibit these habits of the mind: confidence, contextual perspective, creativity, flexibility, inquisitiveness, intellectual integrity, intuition, openmindedness, perseverance, and reflection. Critical thinkers in nursing practice the cognitive skills of analyzing, applying standards, discriminating information seeking, logical reasoning, predicting, and transforming knowledge (Rubenfeld & Scheffer, 1999, p. 5).

The development and use of critical thinking in nursing has received considerable attention both in nursing education and in practice during the last decade. However, critical thinking has always been an integral component in King's perspective of nursing. In an early publication, Daubenmire and King (1973) presented a diagram (Figure 9-2) entitled "Methodology for the Study of Nursing Process." Critical thinking is illustrated by the use of terms such as *analyze, synthesize, verify,* and *interpret.* King explicitly links critical thinking to the mental acts of judgment that are implicit in perception, communication, and interactions that lead to transaction (King, 1992) and the concept of decision making (King, 1999). More recently, King (1999) identified that ethical theories and principles, along with the nursing process, have structured critical thinking and its pedagogy in most nursing programs.

The delivery of nursing care to patients is a process of thinking as well as doing. In contrast to the traditional approach to nursing process as a system of interrelated actions, King's perspective of the process of nursing reflects the science of nursing—the activities of critical thinking that provide the rationale for actions taken. The following discussion illustrates critical thinking questions that are based on concepts within King's systems framework and are essential in carrying out activities of assessing, planning, implementing, and evaluating.

At the first step of King's process of nursing, the nurse meets the patient and communicates and interacts with him or her. Assessment is

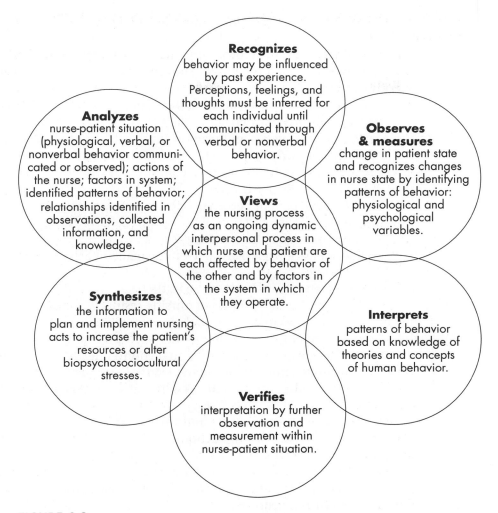

FIGURE 9-2

Methodology for the study of the nursing process. (From Daubenmire, M. J. & King, I. M. [1973]. Nursing process: A system approach. *Nursing Outlook, 21*[8], 515.)

conducted by gathering data about the patient based on relevant concepts. The nurse considers the following questions:

- What are the patient's perceptions of the situation?
- What are my perceptions of the situation?
- What other information do I need to assist this patient to achieve health?
- What does this information mean to the situation?
- What conclusion (judgment) does the patient make?
- What conclusions (judgments) do I make?

The end result of these critical thinking activities is a comprehensive patient assessment tailored to the patient and his or her situations.

The next step of King's process of nursing is identifying goals and planning to achieve those goals. The nurse considers the following questions:

- What goals do I think will serve the patient's best interest?
- What are the patient's goals?
- Are the patient's goals and professional goals congruent?
- If the goals are not congruent, what further communication and interaction is needed to achieve congruence?
- What are the priority goals?
- What does the patient perceive as the best way to achieve the goals?
- What do I perceive to be the best way to achieve the goals?
- Are the goals short-term or long-term?
- What modifications in plans need to be made to achieve goals based on mutuality?

This step is congruent with planning in the traditional nursing process.

The third step of King's process of nursing results in transactions being made. Transactions occur as a result of perceiving the other person(s) and the situation, making judgments about those perceptions, and taking some action in response. Reaction to action(s) leads to interaction between the nurse and patient, which leads to transactions that reflect a shared view and commitment. The nurse considers the following questions:

- Am I doing what the patient and I have agreed upon?
- How am I carrying out the actions?
- When do I carry out the action?
- Why am I carrying out the action?
- Is it reasonable to think that the identified goals will be reached by carrying out the action?

This step reflects implementation in the traditional nursing process.

The fourth step of King's process of nursing is goal attainment or failure to attain the goal. During the process of doing, the nurse considers the following questions:

- Are my actions helping the patient to achieve mutually defined goals?
- How well are the goals being met?
- What actions are working?
- What actions are not working?
- What is the patient's response to my actions?
- What other information do the patient and I need to modify the plan?
- Are there other barriers hindering goal achievement?
- How should the plan be changed to achieve goals?

This exercise in critical thinking is comparable to the evaluation step in the traditional nursing process.

Although nurses are expected to exercise critical thinking, King (1999) emphasizes that patients also engage in the critical thinking process. The nurse has a responsibility to communicate and interact with the patients to ensure that their thinking is transparent to one another. Goals cannot be mutually achieved unless the nurse and the patient share their perceptions, feelings, values, and conclusions. King (1999) recently used the term *participative decision making* to make explicit the active role of the patient.

In summary, the traditional nursing process is a system of interrelated actions, the methods by which nursing is practiced. The critical thinking process reflects highly developed thinking skills essential for nursing practice in the twenty-first century. The transaction process (goal attainment) requires knowledge of concepts from King's General Systems Framework as well as knowledge of professional interactions identified in the Theory of Goal Attainment. King (1999) recently drew comparisons between the process of ethical decision making, the nursing process, and the transaction process to illustrate the use of her theory for dealing with ethical issues in present-day nursing practice. Relationships between the nursing process, the critical thinking process, the transaction process, and the ethical decision making process are shown in Table 9-2.

The applicability of these interrelated processes in contemporary professional nursing practice is illustrated in the case studies of Debbie and Clare that follow.

CASE HISTORY OF DEBBIE

Debbie is a 29-year-old woman who was recently admitted to the oncology nursing unit for evaluation after sensing pelvic "fullness" and noticing a watery, foul-smelling vaginal discharge. A Papanicolaou smear revealed class V cervical cancer. She was found to have a stage II squamous cell carcinoma of the cervix and underwent a radical hysterectomy with bilateral salpingooophorectomy.

Her past health history revealed that physical examinations had been infrequent. She also reported that she had not performed breast self-examination. She is 5 feet, 4 inches tall and weights 89 pounds. Her usual weight is about 110 pounds. She has smoked approximately two packs of cigarettes a day for the past 16 years. She is gravida 2, para 2. Her first pregnancy was at age 16, and her second was at age 18. Since that time, she has taken oral contraceptives on a regular basis.

Debbie completed the eighth grade. She is married and lives with her husband and her two children in her mother's home, which she describes as less than sanitary. Her husband is unemployed. She describes him as emotionally distant and abusive at times.

TABLE 9-2 Relationship Among the Four Processes			
Nursing Process	**Critical Thinking Process**	**Transaction Process**	**Ethical Decision Making Process**
Assess and apply knowledge of relevant concepts	Conceptualize	Patient and nurse perceive each other and situation, make judgments, mental actions, and reactions. Interaction is an ongoing process characterized by communication. The nurse:	Identify ethical issues.
		• Gathers additional information	Gather information about ethical issues.
		• Validates perception	
		• Delineates and validates patient concerns	
		• Establishes mutuality and trust	
Identify goals and plans to achieve	Analyze and synthesize	Make decisions about goals. Goal must be mutually set. Make decisions for actions to meet goals	Incorporate ethical decision making into a plan of action related to goals and means to achieve goals.
Implement actions to meet goals		Transactions made Not directly observed Inferred from interactions	Take action to resolve ethical issues.
Evaluate goal attainment	Evaluate	Goals attained; if not, why not? Unmet goals can result from:	Ethical issues resolved? If not, why not?
		• Identification of incorrect or incomplete data	
		• Incorrect interpretation as the result of perceptual error, lack of knowledge, or goal conflict	
		• Contributing nurse, patient, system barriers	

Modified from I. M. King. *Nursing Science Quarterly, 12*(4), p. 295, copyright © 1999 by Sage Publications, Inc. Reprinted by permission of Sage Publications, Inc.

She has done well following surgery except for being unable to completely empty her urinary bladder. She is having continued postoperative pain and nausea. It will be necessary for her to perform intermittent self-catheterization at home. Her medications are (1) an antibiotic, (2) an analgesic as needed for pain, and (3) an antiemetic as needed for nausea. In addition, she will be receiving radiation therapy on an outpatient basis.

Debbie is extremely tearful. She expresses great concern over her future and the future of her two children. She believes that this illness is a punishment for her past life.

NURSING CARE OF DEBBIE WITH KING'S FRAMEWORK

In King's framework, Debbie is conceptualized as a personal system in interaction with other systems. Many of these interactions influence her health. In addition, her recent diagnosis of class V cervical cancer influences her health. Together, Debbie and the nurse communicate, engage in mutual goal setting, and make decisions about the means to achieve goals.

Nursing care for Debbie begins with assessment that includes collection, interpretation, and verification of data. Sources of data are Debbie herself—primarily her perceptions, behavior, past experiences, knowledge of concepts in the systems framework, critical thinking skills, ability to use the nursing process, and medical knowledge about the treatment and prognosis of class V cervical cancer. Care for Debbie may well cover the full range of nursing practice: promotion of health, maintenance and restoration of health, care of the sick, and care of the dying (King, 1981).

In nursing situations, the nurse forms an interpersonal system with Debbie. The transaction process begins with perception, judgments, mental actions, and reactions of both individuals. The nurse assesses and applies knowledge of concepts and processes. Although all of the concepts in King's framework will likely contribute to the nursing care of Debbie, the critical concepts are perception, self, coping, interaction, role, stress, power, and decision making.

The nurse's perception serves as a basis for gathering and interpreting information. Debbie's perceptions influence her thoughts and actions and are assessed through verbal and nonverbal behaviors. Because perceptual accuracy is important to the interaction process, the nurse validates with Debbie her own perceptions and interpretation of Debbie's perceptions. Debbie's perceptions might be influenced by her emotional state, stress, or pain. The nurse's perceptions are influenced by culture, socioeconomic status, age, and diagnosis of the patient (King, 1981). Perceptions form the basis for development of the self.

According to King (1981), the self is the conception of who and what one is and includes one's subjective totality of attitudes, values, experiences, commitments, and awareness of individual existence. Debbie reveals important information about self. She is tearful and expresses fear, concern, uncertainty, and blame. Debbie's past neglect of her health influences her present feelings.

Feelings about self and situation are clearly psychological stressors. Debbie has physical and interpersonal stressors as well. Physical stressors result from the illness and surgery. Bladder function, pain, and nausea are identified as immediate problems, and radiation treatment may result in other changes in physical status.

In the interpersonal system, Debbie identifies a distant and sometimes abusive husband, which constitutes a major lack of emotional support during this very difficult time. He is unemployed and she is unable to work; therefore financial troubles and lack of other basic resources are likely to be stressors as well. Her husband's inability to provide basic emotional and material support most likely contributes to Debbie's concern for her children, especially with changes that are likely to occur in her own role with them. Her living situation is another stressor. It is unsanitary and seems quite crowded. Further nursing assessment of the situation can clarify whether her home situation truly will interfere with necessary postoperative care. It is also possible that the lack of personal—and perhaps family—space contributes to stress. Coping with personal and interpersonal stressors is likely to influence both health and illness outcomes. Debbie may need additional resources to help her cope with the immediate situation and the future.

Communication is the key to establishing mutuality and trust between Debbie and the nurse and is the means to validating perceptions, establishing patient priorities, and moving the interaction process toward goal setting. Debbie is expected to participate in identifying goals. However, Debbie's overwhelming needs and lack of resources likely may necessitate direction from the nurse. Nurses can find direction for assisting patients to identify goals based on the assumptions that underlie King's systems framework. For example, the overall goal of nursing is to assist persons to function in their roles (King, 1981). Debbie has expressed major concerns about her children. These concerns may involve the maternal role. However, Debbie is also in the patient role—one that may change based on the recovery process and/or progression or remission of cancer. Another basic assumption is that nurses assist patients to adjust to changes in their health status. Decisions about goals must be based on the capabilities, limitations, priorities of the patient, and situation. In this situation, the immediate goal seems to be control of postoperative pain and nausea, although this needs to be validated with

Debbie. Debbie also will need to perform self-catheterization when necessary at home.

It is not clear from the data available about Debbie whether her fears, worries, and anxieties are interfering with her ability to participate in prioritizing goals or to identify and participate in actions to meet goals. If these problems interfered, the first nursing action would be to obtain psychological assessment and crisis intervention as necessary. Other important goals and actions might be directed toward mobilizing resources, especially family support. Although Debbie's mother may not be a very good housekeeper, she may be a good source of emotional support and direct aid and service such as transportation to and from outpatient treatments. It is possible that professional goals and patient goals may be incongruent. Continuous analysis, synthesis, and validation are critical to keep on track.

In addition to decisions about goals, Debbie is expected to be involved in decisions about actions to meet goals. Involving Debbie in decision making may be a challenge because of her sense of powerlessness over the illness, treatment, and ability to contribute to family functioning. Yet empowering Debbie is likely to increase her sense of self, which in turn can reduce stress, improve coping, change perceptions, and lead to changes in her physical state.

Goal attainment needs ongoing evaluation. Follow-up with Debbie on pain, nausea, and bladder function soon after discharge will be necessary. One way to do this might be to arrange for in-home nursing services, which would constitute a nursing action meeting a goal. Having a professional in the home also contributes to further assessment of the family, validation of progress toward goals, and modifications in plans to achieve goals.

According to King, if transactions are made, goals will be attained. Goal attainment can improve or maintain health, control illness, or lead to a peaceful death. If goals are not attained, the nurse needs to reexamine the processes of nursing, critical thinking, and transaction. Unmet goals can result from an incorrect or incomplete data base, perceptual errors, lack of knowledge, lack of mutuality in the relationship, goal conflict, and any number of other nurse, patient, or system barriers (Kameoka, 1995).

CASE HISTORY OF CLARE

Clare was born on March 31, 1999, at 37 weeks' gestation by an emergency cesarean section because of a late deceleration pattern in fetal heart rate during labor. This was her mother's second pregnancy. She had received prenatal care, and both pregnancies were uneventful.

Clare's mother is 33 years old, and her father is 35. Their first child is a 6-year-old boy who was hospitalized at birth and now has severe developmental delays. He requires constant care but is in a special program during the daytime hours.

At birth, Clare weighed 3665 g (about 8 pounds) and had Apgar scores of 8 and 9, which indicated that she was in good condition. However, respiratory distress developed several hours after birth. Clare was intubated and placed on a ventilator, but she required increasing amounts of oxygen and pressure and showed no improvement in blood gases. At 36 hours of age she was transferred to a tertiary level NICU and within 2 hours, she was placed on extracorporeal membrane oxygenation (ECMO). During the next few days, she experienced sepsis, seizures, and renal failure. One or both of Clare's parents visited daily.

After 8 days, Clare was doing well enough to be taken off ECMO but remained intubated on ventilator support. She was stable for the next 3 days but then began to require increased ventilator support to the point that her survival was questionable. Because there were no other options to offer the family, Clare was placed on experimental nitric oxide treatment for "compassionate" support. Over the next few days, Clare's condition was very unstable, and she experienced many "ups and downs."

The family, including the paternal grandparents, talked to the neonatologist about Clare's survival, the quality of her life if she survived, and any pain or discomfort she might be experiencing at the time. They also discussed the possibility of organ donation. On the sixth day of nitric oxide treatment, Clare's condition deteriorated even further, and she was not expected to survive more than a few hours. The family asked for the hospital chaplain to perform an emergency baptism.

Amazingly, Clare began to improve over the next few days, although she remained on a ventilator. Then another setback occurred. Chest tubes to drain fluid accumulation in her chest were inserted. However, 1 week later she was tolerating gavage feedings well despite the chest tubes. Blood gas levels continued to improve, and Clare was eventually extubated. Her condition stabilized and she began to make steady progress. It was anticipated that Clare would be discharged to her family when her physiological problems were resolved and growth was adequate.

NURSING CARE OF CLARE WITH KING'S FRAMEWORK

On April 3, 1999, Anne arrives for her day shift in the NICU and finds herself assigned to Clare as her primary nurse. Concepts that King (1981) articulates in her framework and Theory of Goal Attainment provide a basis for the critical thinking that Anne uses during the process of caring for Clare and her family.

There are three time periods described in Clare's case history. The first phase covers the first 2 weeks when Clare was on ECMO and began to recover. The next period is a week when Clare's death seemed likely. The last period describes stabilization and progress toward eventual discharge. Only the first two time periods will be used to illustrate the use of King's work in nursing practice because of the complexity of the case.

The first step in the process is conceptualization and assessment that uses each of the concepts identified within each system. Anne begins to think about Clare and her family in terms of King's three interrelated systems: the personal, interpersonal, and social. The personal system in King's framework refers to the individual. In Clare's case, Anne identifies four individuals, each representing a personal system: Clare, her mother, her father, and Anne. Interpersonal systems are formed when two or more personal systems interact. Anne recognizes the presence of multiple interpersonal systems that may impact Clare. Social systems are represented by larger groups that influence the personal and interpersonal systems. Anne takes note of Clare's extended family, particularly her grandparents. She also thinks about religious systems that might play a role in this case because Clare's survival is uncertain. Anne also recognizes that the NICU is a social system with its own inherent and often overwhelming power and authority, values, patterns of behavior, and role expectations.

One value that is strongly held in this NICU is the philosophy of family-centered care, which recognizes and respects the role of families in the care of their children. Anne is aware that some would challenge the usefulness of King's framework in caring for patients who, like Clare, are incapable of expressing themselves and participating in goal planning. However, Anne believes that King's framework is useful for nursing practice in a family-centered NICU because interactions, transactions, and mutual goal setting can be achieved with Clare's parents. These activities will promote the health of the family system, which is the goal of nursing in King's framework, by assisting Clare's parents to function in their roles as parents.

Now that Anne has conceptualized Clare and her family in terms of the three interacting systems, she gathers data and applies knowledge of the concepts identified within the personal system: perception, self, growth and development, body image, time, and personal space. Anne recognizes that except that of growth and development, most of these concepts do not apply to Clare as a newborn. Anne knows that Clare's illness and its treatment will interfere with normal newborn behavior, which could impede parental interaction and, possibly, attachment. It is also possible that Clare will not meet developmental milestones, either on time or at all. It is likely that development will be less problematic for Clare at this point than for her parents. The sense of chronic sorrow that accompanies the "loss" of a perfect, healthy infant may well be magnified for these parents because of their experience with their son.

Anne then turns her attention to concepts that are important for assessing Clare's parents. Clare's father visited at least once a day and phoned often during the first 4 days of Clare's life, but Anne was not on duty when he visited. During that time he had to provide care for his son and support his wife, who was recovering from a cesarean section.

Clare's parents visited together for the first time on the fourth day of her hospitalization. It was important to assess their perceptions of her health status and the situation. Clare's mother was very upset and sobbing; her father appeared overwhelmed. After providing them an opportunity to express their emotional tensions and grief, Anne engaged them in conversation about Clare. They expressed shock over the events following her birth. They had waited 6 years to have another child until their son was in school and they felt they could handle the demands of a newborn. Despite the health status of their son and the fact that no specific causes for his delays were ever identified, they had no reason to expect anything but a normal, healthy child this time. Both parents expressed concern for Clare's survival and also for any long-term health implications. Anne perceived that they were exhibiting a normal, appropriate reaction to the present situation. Their perceptions of Clare's status were congruent with Anne's, were a fair estimation of the reality and uncertainty of the situation, and clearly were influenced by their past experience.

Another important concept is self. Clare's parents bring a unique self to this experience that defines them as individuals. They already had established themselves as mother and father with their firstborn. They also had 6 years of experience with their developmentally disabled son. Anne also considers the possibility that Clare's parents may be experiencing guilt and anger about having another child with major health problems because they repeatedly question why they could not have a normal child.

The concept of personal space is pertinent in the care of Clare and her parents. There is no personal, private space in the NICU in which Clare's parents can express themselves, interact with Clare, or interact with others. There are four other infants in the same room as Clare. Furthermore, the space around Clare's warmer is congested because of the number of life support machines in use. The unit does have several screens that Anne uses to provide some small amount of privacy for short periods of time.

Time is another concept within the personal system that affects Clare's parents. Time represents a continuous flow of events, one after the other, which leads to the future. The uncertainty surrounding Clare's medical status requires continual adjustment in terms of time. Clare's parents repeatedly asked when she could be taken off ECMO. For them, that event represented movement toward the future, to survival. When Claire finally was taken off ECMO, her parents expected that in time she would be ready to go home. Unfortunately, this time sequence was disrupted by other life-threatening crises.

Growth and development is also a relevant concept for Clare's parents. The addition of another family member signals a development change—now the family unit is expanded to four. Clare's parents will continue to grow and develop as parents as they assimilate Clare into the family. This process might be challenged by the special needs of both children.

Pertinent concepts in the interpersonal system that Anne considers include interaction, communication, transaction, role, and stressors/stress. Anne communicates with Clare's parents throughout Clare's hospitalization and provides them with the information they need to function in their parental role. This open communication with Clare's parents enables Anne to validate their perceptions and judgments and understand their actions and reactions. Such communication establishes mutuality and trust between Clare's parents and Anne, which in turn leads to interactions and ultimately transactions. One characteristic of interactions is reciprocity, an interdependence in the relationship in which there is an exchange between the persons involved. Clare's mother regularly brought cookies or doughnuts for the nursing staff as a way of giving something back to the staff in exchange for their support and care of Clare and her family.

Anne recognizes that multiple psychological and social stressors inherent in the NICU experience cause stress for Clare's parents. The uncertain outcome and prognosis of Clare's illness is a major one. Clare's parents verbalize that it is difficult to adjust to changes in Clare's condition. At one moment they feel hopeful, and the next they feel despair. Other times they do not know what they hope the outcome will be.

The NICU itself is a noisy, bustling, tension-filled environment. All kinds of alarms and buzzers send out signals of potential disaster, which heighten concerns for Clare's parents. They often comment on unexpected and unplanned stress in their day-to-day lives: they must continue to provide for their older son; they feel compelled to visit Clare daily; they must drive back and forth to the hospital; they must maintain the normal routines of washing, grocery shopping, and work.

Role is another important concept in the interpersonal system. Anne knows that parents often feel inadequate compared to the nurse who cares for their infant. An alteration in the parenting role may interfere with the ability of Clare's parents to engage in mutual goal setting that leads to transactions (Norris & Hoyer, 1993). Anne brings a strong commitment to family-centered care to her nursing practice. Initially, she defines the goal of helping Clare's parents establish their parental role and also plans to redefine that goal with them when they are ready.

The concepts of authority, power, status, and decision making are characteristics of social systems that are relevant in Clare's case. Anne knows that for most parents the NICU represents a high-tech, threatening arena unlike any other social situation they have experienced. As a social system, the NICU possesses authority and power that appears to exceed that of the parents. Parents often perceive that they have little status. Physicians and nurses have expertise and skills with which parents cannot compete in caring for their child. Unless the NICU supports a philosophy of family-centered care, parents may not be actively involved in care or care decisions.

At one point Anne observed that Clare's mother had a tendency to focus on the details of the technological care but that Clare's father would tell her "not to sweat the small details." Although Anne recognized that Clare's parents had different coping styles, she also perceived that Clare's mother might be feeling powerlessness in the present situation. In addition, Anne recognized that a loss of control might threaten the self. Clare's mother may feel threatened and therefore make issues out of little things. Anne took an opportunity to discuss her perceptions with Clare's mother, who validated that she did not feel like a mother and claimed that she could do nothing for Clare as her mother because the nurses did everything.

Taken together, the concepts of interaction, perception, communication, transaction, self, role, stressors/stress, growth and development, time, and personal space constitute the Theory of Goal Attainment. Through communication and interaction, Clare's parents and Anne clarified their perceptions of reality and mutually established the goal of identifying aspects of care that they could provide within the constraints of Clare's physical condition and treatment. Anne's role was to teach and assist them to care for Clare safely. Within several days, Anne observed that Clare's mother independently initiated aspects of care and was becoming adept at performing them even within the confined space. As her confidence in herself increased, Clare's mother became less focused on minor changes in blood gas levels or ventilator settings and began to function in her role as parent. Clare's mother demonstrated growth and development in behavioral activities related to parenting in the environment and social system of the NICU. Anne observed that verbal and nonverbal manifestations of stress decreased for both parents.

The process of goal attainment occurs within the context of time, with one event leading to another. Discussion and clarification of perceptions leads to judgment, action, and reaction for both Clare's parents and Anne. These activities were followed by mutual establishment of goals during the process of interaction, which led to achievement of goals. Achievement of goals is transaction. Transactions lead to improved health—in this case, the ability to be parents to their infant.

At one point during Clare's hospitalization, her parents faced a major ethical dilemma. They had to make a decision to use an experimental treatment (nitric oxide) to try to save her life. Anne used the nursing process and King's transaction process model to help Clare's parents arrive at a decision (King, 1999).

Anne first assessed their perceptions of the situation. The fact that they had discussed organ donation indicated that Clare's parents understood that Clare might not survive. They were also concerned about any pain and suffering that Clare might be experiencing. In addition, they did not seem sure of the best outcome for their daughter. Anne knew that it was critical to communicate with Clare's parents and to interact with them.

Acknowledging that there is an ethical dilemma present in a situation is a very difficult step. Engaging in dialogue about it is even more difficult, considering the emotional roller coaster that Clare's parents have experienced. Anne is able to help them explore their values and beliefs regarding this situation. She provides them with specific information about the nitric oxide treatment and about the process of organ donation, should treatment be unsuccessful.

It is clear that Clare's parents are concerned about the issue of quality versus sanctity of life. They are not sure what impairments she may have as a result of this illness, and the uncertainty makes a decision less clear. Clare's parents appear to value the sanctity of life. They consider experimental treatment for their daughter because they want to try to save her life at all costs. The fact that they have a son who is developmentally delayed but still want Clare to have a chance to survive despite any later difficulties is testimony to their support for the sanctity of life. They also appear to value the quality of life. They waited 6 years to have another child so they could devote themselves to their son, maximize his opportunities to develop, and give their second child the care and attention she would need.

Once Clare's parents have had an opportunity to interact with the physicians and Anne, they decide on a plan of action. Clare's parents decide to give Clare the chance to survive by agreeing to the experimental treatment, which represents a transaction, according to King (1999). Despite the fact that Clare's condition deteriorated, the ultimate goal was achieved, and Clare survived. Clare's parents understand that it will be long time before they will be able to evaluate their decision. As they raise their daughter, they will reflect on whether any limitations she develops detract from her quality of life to the point that they wish they had made a different decision. Anne knows they will agonize over whether they have made the right decision. She continues to communicate and interact with Clare's parents to help them explore their perceptions and evaluate the outcome of their decision.

Over time, Clare's physical condition continues to improve to the point at which survival is likely, but the need for special care when she goes home remains high. This represents a critical time for parental participation in setting goals and developing plans to meet those goals so they are prepared to assume full-time parenting roles and skills when they get home. For example, infants who have been receiving ECMO are often slow to establish bottle-feeding. Anne will communicate this information to Clare's parents to decrease potential stress caused by unrealistic expectations and to coordinate a consultation with occupational therapy to teach Clare's parents feeding strategies that will promote adequate weight gain and growth.

The challenge to nurses working in the NICU is to look beyond the technological care they provide to the importance of interaction and transaction early in the hospitalization of a sick infant. Families expect technological care to be appropriate and competent. In addition, they need a caring relationship with nurses. As one mother put it when discussing her son's NICU experience, "The facts of his history will remain the same. How we perceive the experience may be changed. The memories are tempered by the relationships we formed. In partnership, you will make a permanent, positive difference in the life in an NICU family" (Busch, 1992, p. 8).

King's Theory of Goal Attainment (1981) provides direction for nursing practice in the NICU because it emphasizes the processes of communication, interaction, and transactions, which are the foundations for promoting and maintaining the health status of individuals and families (Norris & Hoyer, 1993). The relationships that nurses establish with parents based on mutual respect and trust also attain the goal of nursing, which is "to help individuals to maintain their health so that they can function in their roles" (King, 1981, pp. 4-5). Nurses who work with parents to mutually establish and attain goals will influence health outcomes of personal and interpersonal systems.

CRITICAL THINKING EXERCISES

1. Identify three nursing diagnoses you would expect to develop for Debbie. What is the relevant assessment data for each diagnosis? What are possible mutually derived goals for Debbie? What is the priority nursing diagnosis? Why did you choose this diagnosis?
2. Conduct a comprehensive assessment of Clare and her parents with respect to the ethical dilemma they face. What are the relevant concepts from each of King's systems (personal, interpersonal, and social) that organize Anne's thinking about the care of this family? What additional information does Anne need to complete her assessment? Why is this information important to your decision making?

3. Throughout the case discussion of Clare and her parents, several goals are identified. Were these goals attained? If so, explain why you think these goals were attained. If they were not attained, propose possible reasons why they were not attained. What other courses of action could be taken to achieve these goals? If you could not decide based on the case discussion, what evidence would you need to come to a conclusion?

4. Individuals are called personal systems in King's framework. The concept of self is relevant for understanding Anne as a human being and as a professional nurse. What attitudes and values appear to influence Anne's practice as a professional nurse? If you were the nurse caring for Clare, what would you do differently?

5. You are a senior in college and are sharing an apartment with two other students. Parents' weekend is 3 days away, and all of your parents will be visiting the apartment for the first time. It has not been cleaned or straightened up since the beginning of the semester 8 weeks ago. Two weeks ago, you all agreed that you wanted the apartment to look nice for your parents so they would be proud of you. Describe the personal, interpersonal, and social system factors that have contributed to everyone's share of this mess. How will you achieve your goal over the next 3 days?

References

Alligood, M. R. (1995). Theory of goal attainment: Application to adult orthopedic nursing. In M. A. Frey & C. L. Sieloff (Eds.), *Advancing King's systems framework and theory for nursing* (p. 212). Thousand Oaks, CA: Sage.

Busch, J. (1992). Partners in care: Parents and professionals in the NICU. *NANNews, 5*(5), 1, 6-8.

Carter, K. F. & Dufour, L. T. (1994). King's theory: A critique of the critiques. *Nursing Science Quarterly, 7*(3), 128-133.

Daubenmire, M. J. & King, I. M. (1973). Nursing process: A system approach. *Nursing Outlook, 21*(8), 512-517.

Doornbos, M. M. (1995). Using King's systems framework to explore family health in the families of the young chronically mentally ill. In M. A. Frey & C. L. Sieloff (Eds.), *Advancing King's systems framework and theory of nursing* (pp. 192-205). Thousand Oaks, CA: Sage.

Fawcett, J. (1989). *Analysis and evaluation of conceptual models.* Philadelphia: F. A. Davis.

Frey, M. A. (1996). King's systems framework for nursing. In J. Fitzpatrick & A. Whall (Eds.), *Conceptual models of nursing: Analysis and application* (3rd ed., pp. 225-242). Norwalk, CT: Appleton & Lange.

Frey, M. A. & Norris, D. (1997). King's systems framework and theory in nursing practice. In M. R. Alligood & A. Marriner-Tomey (Eds.), *Nursing theory: Utilization and application* (p. 75). St. Louis: Mosby.

Frey, M. A. & Sieloff, C. L. (1995). *Advancing King's systems framework and theory for nursing.* Thousand Oaks, CA: Sage.

Gonot, P. W. (1989). Imogene King's conceptual framework of nursing. In J. Fitzpatrick & A. Whall (Eds.), *Conceptual models of nursing: Analysis and application* (2nd ed., pp. 271-283). Norwalk, CT: Appleton & Lange.

Jersild, A. T. (1952). *In search of self.* New York: Teacher's College.

Kameoka, T. (1995). Analyzing nurse-client interaction in Japan. In M. A. Frey & C. L. Sieloff (Eds.), *Advancing King's framework and theory for nursing* (pp. 261-277). Thousand Oaks, CA: Sage.

King, I. M. (1968). A conceptual frame of reference. *Nursing Research, 17*(1), 27-31.

King, I. M. (1971). *Toward a theory for nursing.* New York: John Wiley.

King, I. M. (1981). *A theory for nursing: Systems, concepts, process.* Albany, NY: Delmar.

King, I. M. (1986). *Curriculum and instruction in nursing: Concepts and process.* Norwalk, CT: Appleton-Century-Crofts.

King, I. M. (1988). Concepts: Essential elements in theories. *Nursing Science Quarterly, 1*(1), 22-25.

King, I. M. (1990). Health as the goal for nursing. *Nursing Science Quarterly, 3*(3), 123-128.

King, I. M. (1991). Nursing theory 25 years later. *Nursing Science Quarterly, 4*(3), 94-95.

King, I. M. (1992). King's Theory of Goal Attainment. *Nursing Science Quarterly, 5*(1), 19-26.

King, I. M. (1993, June). *King's conceptual system and Theory of Goal Attainment.* Paper presented at the meeting of Sigma Theta Tau International Sixth International Nursing Research Congress, Madrid, Spain.

King, I. M. (1994). Quality of life and goal attainment. *Nursing Science Quarterly, 7*(1), 29-32.

King, I. M. (1995a). A systems framework for nursing. In M. A. Frey & C. L. Sieloff (Eds.), *Advancing King's systems framework and theory of nursing* (pp. 14-22). Thousand Oaks, CA: Sage.

King, I. M. (1995b). The Theory of Goal Attainment. In M. A. Frey & C. L. Sieloff (Eds.), *Advancing King's systems framework and theory of nursing* (pp. 23-32). Thousand Oaks, CA: Sage.

King, I. M. (1996). The Theory of Goal Attainment in research and practice. *Nursing Science Quarterly, 9*(2), 61-66.

King, I. M. (1997). King's Theory of Goal Attainment in practice. *Nursing Science Quarterly, 10*(4), 180-185.

King, I. M. (1999). A Theory of Goal Attainment: Philosophical and ethical implications. *Nursing Science Quarterly, 12*(4), 292-296.

King, I. M. (2000). World view: King's conceptual system and middle range Theory of Goal Attainment. In M. Parker (Ed.), *Nursing theories and nursing practice* (2nd ed.). Philadelphia: F. A. Davis.

King, I. M. Personal Communication, February 8, 2001.

Lazarus, R. S. & Folkman, S. (1984). *Stress, appraisal, and coping.* New York: Springer.

Magan, S. J. (1987). A critique of King's theory. In R. R. Parse. (Ed.), *Nursing science: Major paradigms, theories, and critiques* (pp. 115-133). Philadephia: W. B. Saunders.

Meleis, A. (1991). *Theoretical nursing: Development and progress* (2nd ed.). Philadelphia: J. B. Lippincott.

Meleis, A. (1997). *Theoretical nursing: Development and progress* (3rd ed.). Philadelphia: J. B. Lippincott.

Norris, D. M. & Hoyer, P. J. (1993). Dynamism in practice: Parenting within King's framework. *Nursing Science Quarterly, 6*(2), 79-85.

Rubenfeld, M. G. & Scheffer, B. K. (1999). *Critical thinking in nursing: An interactive approach* (2nd ed.). Philadelphia: Lippincott.

Sieloff, C. L., Frey, M., & Killeen, M. (2000). Application of King's work to practice. In M. Parker (Ed.), *Nursing theories and nursing practice* (2nd ed., pp. 228-313). Philadelphia: F. A. Davis.

Yura, H. & Walsh, M. (1983). *The nursing process.* Norwalk, CT: Appleton-Century-Crofts.

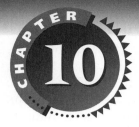

Levine's Conservation Model in Nursing Practice

Karen Moore Schaefer

"Nursing is a profession as well as an academic discipline, always practiced and studied in concert with all of the disciplines that together form the health sciences. . . . Scientific knowledge from many contributing disciplines is, in fact, connected to nursing, as an adjunct to the knowledge that nursing claims for its own." (From M. E. Levine, Nursing Science Quarterly 1[1], p. 16-21, copyright © 1988 by Sage Publications, Inc. Reprinted by permission of Sage Publications, Inc.)

HISTORY AND BACKGROUND

The conservation model was originally developed as an organizing framework for teaching undergraduate nursing students (Levine, 1973a). Levine's book *Introduction to Clinical Nursing* (1973a) made a significant contribution to the "why"s of nursing actions. Levine was intent on not simply teaching the skill of nursing but also on providing a rationale for the behaviors. She has shown a high regard for the integration of the adjunctive sciences to develop a theoretical basis of nursing, has been a clear voice for the development of the discipline, and has called attention to the rhetoric of nursing theory (Levine, 1988, 1989b, 1989c, 1994, 1995).

The universality of the conservation model is supported by its use with a variety of patients of varied ages in a wide range of settings. This model

---

This chapter is dedicated to the memory of Myra E. Levine.

has been successfully used in critical care (Brunner, 1985; Langer, 1990; Litrell & Schumann, 1989; Lynn-McHale & Smith, 1991; Taylor, 1989; Tribotti, 1990), acute care (Foreman, 1991; Molchany, 1992; Roberts, Brittin, Cook, & deClifford, 1994; Roberts, Brittin, & deClifford, 1995; Schaefer, 1991; Schaefer, Swavely, Rothenberger, Hess, & Willistin, 1996), and long-term care (Burd, Olson, Langemo, Hunter, Hanson, Osowki, & Sauvage, 1994; Clark, Fraaza, Schroeder, & Maddens, 1995; Cox, 1991). The conservation model has also been used with the neonate (Tribotti, 1990), infant (Newport, 1984; Savage & Culbert, 1989), young child (Dever, 1991), pregnant woman (Roberts, Fleming, & Yeates-Giese, 1991), young adult (Pasco & Halupa, 1991), woman with chronic illness (Schaefer, 1996) and elderly (Cox, 1991; Foreman, 1991; Happ, Williams, Strumpf, & Burger, 1996; Hirschfeld, 1976). It has been successfully used in the community (Dow & Mest, 1997; Pond, 1991), emergency room (Pond & Taney, 1991), extended care facility (Cox, 1991; personal communication, February 21, 1995), critical care unit (Brunner, 1985; Molchany, 1992), primary care clinic (Schaefer & Pond, 1994), and operating room (Crawford-Gamble, 1986). The model has been used as a framework for wound care and enterostomal therapy (Cooper, 1990; Neswick, 1997), care of intravenous sites (Dibble, Bostrom-Ezrati, & Ruzzuto, 1991), as a framework for management of patients on long-term ventilation (Higgins, 1998), and for patients undergoing treatment for cancer (O'Laughlin, 1986; Webb, 1993). Recently, the model has been used to assess and intervene on issues associated with staff nurse productivity, burnout, and satisfaction (Jost, 2000).

OVERVIEW OF LEVINE'S CONSERVATION MODEL

According to Levine (1973a), "nursing is human interaction" (p. 1). "The nurse enters into a partnership of human experience where sharing moments in time—some trivial, some dramatic— leaves its mark forever on each patient" (Levine, 1977, p. 845). As a human science, the profession of nursing integrates the adjunctive sciences (e.g., chemistry, biology, anatomy and physiology, psychology, sociology, anthropology, philosophy, medicine) to develop the practice of nursing.

There are three major concepts that form the basis of the model and its assumptions: conservation, adaptation, and wholeness. Conservation is natural law that is fundamental to many basic sciences.

Levine (1973a) explains that individuals continuously defend their wholeness. Conservation is the keeping together of the life system. To keep together means, on one hand, to maintain a proper balance between active nursing interventions coupled with patient participation and, on the other, the safe limits of the patient's ability to participate. Individuals defend that system in constant interaction with their environments and choose the most economical, frugal, energy-sparing options available to safeguard their integrity. Energy source cannot be directly observed, but the consequences (clinical manifestations) of its exchange are predictable, manageable, and recognizable (Levine, 1991). Conservation is about achieving a balance of energy supply and demand that is within the unique biological realities of the individual.

Adaptation is the ongoing process of change whereby individuals retain their integrity within the realities of their environments (Levine, 1989a). Change is the life process, and adaptation is the method of change. The achievement of adaptation is "the frugal, economic, contained, and controlled use of environmental resources by the individual in his or her best interest" (Levine, 1991, p. 5). Every individual possesses a range of adaptive responses that is unique to that individual. These ranges may vary as one ages or is challenged by illness. This trend is evidenced as the hypoxic drive provides the stimulus for breathing in individuals with chronic obstructive pulmonary disease.

History, specificity, and redundancy characterize adaptation. Adaptations are grounded in history and await the challenges to which they respond (Levine, 1995). The severity of individual responses and their adaptive patterns will vary based on the specific genetic structure and the influence of social, cultural, and experiential factors.

Redundancy represents the fail-safe anatomical, physiological, and psychological options available to the individual to ensure continued adaptation (Levine, 1991). Levine (1991) argues that "[a]chieving health is predicated on the deliberate selection of redundant options" (p. 6). Survival depends on these redundant options, which are challenged and often limited by illness, disease, and aging.

Wholeness exists when the interactions or constant adaptations to the environment permit the assurance of integrity (Levine, 1991). Nurses promote wholeness through the use of the conservation principles. Their recognition of an open, fluid, constantly changing interaction between the individual and the environment is the basis for holistic thought, which views the individual as whole. Wholeness is health; health is integrity. Health is a pattern of adaptive change, the goal of which is well-being.

The conservation model includes the metaparadigm concepts of person, nursing, health, and environment. Levine (1988) referred to these concepts as commonplaces of the discipline in that they are necessary for any description of nursing. The person is a holistic being who is sentient, thinking, future-oriented, and past-aware. The wholeness (integrity) of the individual demands that the "isolated aspects . . . can have meaning outside of the context within which the individual experiences his or her life" (Levine, 1973a, pp. 325-326). Persons are in constant interaction with the environment, responding to change in an orderly, sequential pattern. Thus they adapt to forces that shape and reshape the essence of the person. According to Levine (1973a), the person can be defined as an individual, an individual in a group (family), or an individual in a community (Pond, 1991).

The environment completes the wholeness of the person. Each individual is viewed as having his or her own internal and external environments. The internal environment combines the physiological and pathophysiological aspects of the patient. The internal environment is challenged constantly by changes in the external environment.

The external environment includes those factors that impinge on and challenge the individual. Acknowledging the complexity of the environment, Levine (1973a) adopted the three levels of environment identified by Bates (1967): perceptual, operational, and conceptual. The perceptual environment includes aspects of the world that individuals are able to intercept or interpret through the senses. The operational environment includes elements that may physically affect individuals but are not directly perceived by them (e.g., radiation and microorganisms). The conceptual environment includes the cultural patterns characterized by spiritual existence and mediated by symbols of language, thought, and history. This includes factors that affect behavior (e.g., values and beliefs).

Health and disease are patterns of adaptive change, the goals of which include well-being (Levine, 1971b). Health from a social perspective is defined by the question "Do I continue to function in a reasonably normal fashion?" (Levine, 1984). Health (wholeness) is implied to be the unity and integrity of the individual, which is the goal of nursing.

Illness is described as adaptation to noxious environmental forces. Levine (1971a) argues that "[d]isease represents the individual's effort to protect self-integrity, such as the inflammatory system's response to injury" (p. 257). Disease is unregulated and undisciplined change that must be stopped to prevent death (Levine, 1973a).

Nursing involves engaging in "human interaction" (Levine, 1973a, p. 1). Individuals seek nursing care when they are no longer able to adapt. The goal of nursing is to promote adaptation and maintain wholeness. This goal is accomplished through the conservation of energy and structural, personal, and social integrity.

Energy conservation depends on free energy exchange with the environment so that living systems can constantly replenish their energy supplies (Levine, 1991). Conservation of energy is integral to the individual's range of adaptive responses. The conservation of structural integrity depends on an intact defense system that supports repair and healing and that is responsive to the challenges from the internal and external environments.

The conservation of personal integrity recognizes the individual who establishes his or her wholeness in response to the environment. It acknowledges that individuals strive for recognition, respect, self-awareness, human-ness, holiness, independence, freedom, selfhood, and self-determination.

Conservation of social integrity recognizes that individuals function in a society that helps to establish the boundaries of the self. Social integrity is created by family and friends, workplace and school, religion, personal choices, and cultural and ethnic heritage (Levine, 1996). With its political and economic controls, the healthcare system is part of the social system to which the individual belongs. Levine (1991) contends that "[c]onservation of integrity is essential to assuring wholeness and providing the strength needed to confront illness and disability" (p. 3).

Levine (1973a) makes explicit the importance of understanding the medical plan of care and the results of diagnostic studies to an accurate understanding of patient problems. To this understanding the nurse brings knowledge of nursing science, a careful history of the patient's illness, the patient's perception of the current predicament, information gained from family and friends, and acute observation of the patient and his or her interactions with others (Levine, 1966a). This integrated approach to patient-centered care provides the basis for collaborative care and the establishment of partnerships in the delivery of comprehensive care. Treatment focuses on the management of the organismic responses to the illness.

Organismic responses include flight/fight, inflammatory/immune system, stress, and perceptual awareness responses. The flight/fight response is the most primitive. The inflammatory/immune system response provides for structural continuity and promotion of healing. The stress response is recorded over time and is influenced by the accumulated experience of the individual. Prolonged stress can lead to damage to the systems. The perceptual awareness response involves the gathering of information from the environment and converting it to a meaningful experience. These four responses work together to protect the individual's integrity and are essential components of the individual's whole response.

The goal of nursing care is to promote adaptation and well-being. Because adaptation is predicated on redundant options and is rooted in history and specificity, therapeutic interventions will vary, depending on the unique nature of each person's response.

THEORIES FOR PRACTICE

The model provides the basis for three theories for practice: the Theory of Conservation, the Theory of Therapeutic Intention, and the Theory of

Redundancy. Alligood (1997) made the Theory of Conservation explicit. The Theory of Conservation is rooted in the universal principle of conservation, which provides the foundation for the model. The purpose of conservation is to "keep together." According to Levine (1973a), "To keep together means to maintain a proper balance between active nursing interventions coupled with patient participation on the one hand and the safe limits of the patient's abilities to participate on the other" (p. 13). The patient interacts with the environment in a singular but integrated fashion. The person represents a system that is more than the sum of its parts and that reacts as a whole being. As part of the patient's environment, the nurse, supports the patient's responses. All nursing acts of conservation are devoted to restoring symmetry of response with the goal of maintaining wholeness (Levine, 1969).

In developing the Theory of Therapeutic Intention, Levine (in Fawcett, 1995) was "seeking a way of organizing nursing interventions out of the biological realities which the nurse had to confront" (p. 198). Therapeutic regimens should support the following goals (Fawcett, 1995):

- Facilitate integrated healing and optimal restoration of structure and function through natural response to disease
- Provide support for a failing autoregulatory portion of the integrated system (medical/surgical treatments)
- Restore individual integrity and well-being
- Provide supportive measures to ensure comfort and promote human concern when therapeutic measures are not possible
- Balance a toxic risk against the threat of disease
- Manipulate diet and activity to correct metabolic imbalances and to stimulate physiological processes
- Reinforce or antagonize usual response to create a therapeutic change

Levine (in Fawcett, 1995) proposed that the Theory of Redundancy, seemingly grounded in adaptation, "redefines almost everything that has to do with human life" (p. 199). Redundancy seems to be predicated on the ability of the individual to "monitor its own behavior by conserving the use of resources required to define its unique identity" (Levine, 1991, p. 4). Inherent in this ability to select from the environment is the availability of options from which choices can be made.

There are currently no studies that test the application of the three theories. Anecdotal reports, although stated simply here, suggest that the theories are consistent with practice observations. For example, a patient with diabetes who follows a diet and exercise program is more likely to control his or her blood sugar levels (therapeutic intention) than one who does not follow the same program. The patient with emphysema who spaces activity to conserve energy will be more satisfied with daily life than the patient who does not space activities (conservation). The patient with a chronic illness will manage his or her life better if he or she has options from which to select for treatment than the patient who is not provided with options (redundancy). According to Levine (1991), failure of redundant options (loss of hearing in one ear) helps to explain aging. The Theory of Redundancy might explain the process of aging because as one ages, organ function declines, in some cases as a part of the aging process. If a kidney fails, the Theory of Redundancy no longer operates because only one kidney remains. The same happens if one can only hear out of one ear; the option to hear out of one or the other no longer exists. Of course, if a hearing aid helps to restore hearing in the ear that has less than optimal function, then the Theory of Redundancy is supported through the use of technology and all the nursing that accompanies the use of an assistive aid.

CRITICAL THINKING IN NURSING PRACTICE WITH LEVINE'S MODEL

Levine (1973a, 1973b) proposes that nurses use their scientific and creative abilities to provide nursing care to the patient. The nursing process incorporates these abilities, enhancing the nurse's ability to think critically about the patient. See Table 10-1 for Levine's nursing process using critical thinking.

CASE HISTORY OF DEBBIE

Debbie is a 29-year-old woman who was recently admitted to the oncology nursing unit for evaluation after sensing pelvic "fullness" and noticing a watery, foul-smelling vaginal discharge. A Papanicolaou smear revealed class V cervical cancer. She was found to have a stage II squamous cell carcinoma of the cervix and underwent a radical hysterectomy with bilateral salpingoooophorectomy.

Her past health history revealed that physical examinations had been infrequent. She also reported that she had not performed breast self-examination. She is 5 feet, 4 inches tall and weights 89 pounds. Her usual weight is about 110 pounds. She has smoked approximately two packs of cigarettes a day for the past 16 years. She is gravida 2, para 2. Her first pregnancy was at age 16, and her second was at age 18. Since that time, she has taken oral contraceptives on a regular basis.

Debbie completed the eighth grade. She is married and lives with her husband and her two children in her mother's home, which she describes as less than sanitary. Her husband is unemployed. She describes him as emotionally distant and abusive at times.

She has done well following surgery except for being unable to completely empty her urinary bladder. She is having continued postoperative pain and nausea. It will be necessary for her to perform intermittent self-catheterization

TABLE 10-1 Levine's Nursing Process Using Critical Thinking

Process	Decision Making
ASSESSMENT	
Collection of provocative facts through interview and observation of challenges to environments, with consideration of conservation principles	The nurse observes the patient for organismic responses to illness, reads medical reports, evaluates results of diagnostic studies, and talks with the patient about his or her needs for assistance. The nurse assesses for challenges to both internal and external environments of the patient. Guided by conservation principles, the nurse assesses for additional challenges in environments. The nurse assesses for challenges that interfere with:*
1. Energy conservation	1. Balance of energy supply and demand.
2. Structural integrity	2. Body's defense system.
3. Personal integrity	3. Person's sense of self-worth and personhood.
4. Social integrity	4. Person's ability to participate in social system. These data are provocative facts.
JUDGMENT—TROPHICOGNOSIS†	
Nursing diagnosis—gives the provocative facts meaning	Provocative facts are arranged in a way that they provide meaning to the patient's predicament. A judgment is made about the patient's needs for assistance. This judgment is the trophicognosis.†
HYPOTHESES	
Direct the nursing interventions with the goal of maintaining wholeness and promoting adaptation	Based on his or her judgment, the nurse seeks validation with the patient about the problem. The nurse then proposes hypotheses about the problem and its solution. This becomes the plan of care.
INTERVENTIONS	
Tests hypothesis	The nurse uses the hypothesis to direct care. In essence, the nurse tests proposed hypotheses. Interventions are designed based on conservation principles: conservation of energy, structural integrity, personal integrity, and social integrity. The expectation is that this approach will maintain wholeness and promote adaptation.
EVALUATION	
Observation of organismic response to interventions	The outcome of hypothesis testing is evaluated by assessing for organismic response that means the hypothesis was supported or not supported. Consequences of care are either therapeutic or supportive: therapeutic consequences improve one's sense of well-being; supportive consequences provide comfort when the downward course of illness cannot be influenced. If hypothesis is not supported, the plan is revised and a new hypothesis is proposed.

*Although use of the conservation principles to guide the assessment of challenges in the environments was not part of the original model, it helps the novice nurse, in particular, to organize the provocative facts in a manner that directs the hypotheses. For the experienced nurse, this is integrated into the assessment of the environments as in nursing care of Alice. (see text).

†*Trophicognosis* is a nursing care judgment arrived at through the use of the scientific process (Levine, 1966b). The scientific process is used to make observations and select relevant data to form hypothetical statements about the patient's predicaments (Schaefer, 1991).

at home. Her medications are (1) an antibiotic, (2) an analgesic as needed for pain, and (3) an antiemetic as needed for nausea. In addition, she will be receiving radiation therapy on an outpatient basis.

Debbie is extremely tearful. She expresses great concern over her future and the future of her two children. She believes that this illness is a punishment for her past life.

NURSING CARE OF DEBBIE WITH LEVINE'S MODEL

Debbie is very concerned about her future and the future of her children. She requires nursing care because of the environmental challenges that have threatened her integrity and interfered with her ability to adapt. The nurse assesses for the challenges to her internal and external environments.

Challenges to Debbie's Internal Environment

Challenges that reduce Debbie's energy resources include her 20 pound weight loss and smoking. She has had radical surgery, which challenges her structural integrity. The resulting loss of reproductive ability poses a challenge to her personal integrity. After the surgery, she is having difficulty completely emptying her bladder. She smokes and has taken oral contraceptives on a regular basis. The results of diagnostic studies and vital signs would provide additional indices about the challenges to her internal environment.

Challenges to Debbie's External Environment

Debbie's husband is emotionally distant and at times abusive. Considering these facts, the nurse would investigate available patient records for any indication (bruises, burns, broken bones, chronic pain) that the abuse has precipitated other healthcare visits.

She is living in a home that she describes as "less than sanitary." She is concerned about her future and the future of her two children.

Assessment

Energy conservation. Challenges that result in an energy drain on Debbie's resources include recent weight loss, nausea, pain, and smoking. She has pain despite the pain medication. She is concerned about the care of her two children.

Structural integrity. Debbie's structural integrity is threatened by a surgical procedure with the potential for skin breakdown and infection. She is currently receiving an antibiotic prophylactically to prevent infection of the surgical wound. In addition, she is having difficulty emptying her bladder. Risk assessment includes oral contraceptive administration, smoking, early childbirth, and her recent diagnosis of cancer. On discharge, she will undergo radiation therapy. Radiation therapy poses additional challenges of skin breakdown, destruction of normal cells, pain, potential nausea, and hair loss in the irradiated area.

Personal integrity. Debbie feels as though her illness is a punishment for past behaviors. The surgery and the consequences of the surgical technique may further jeopardize her sense of self-worth. Debbie is only 29 years old, and she could have had more children were it not for this surgery. The impact of not being able to give birth to more children could be devastating. Further, the impact of this situation on the family must be considered. Debbie identifies her husband as being emotionally distant and acknowledges that he may not be capable of providing her with emotional support.

Social integrity. Debbie will experience premature menopause and all the emotional and physical effects of that experience. Many young women her age have infants and menstrual cycles; she will not. Her own and her children's concern about whether she will live to raise them may cause considerable anxiety and fear about the future. Debbie's relationship with her husband may experience added strain. Both the emotional impact of the surgery on him and his potential for abuse must be evaluated.

Judgments
The following trophicognoses (diagnoses) are identified for Debbie:
1. Inadequate nutritional status
2. Pain
3. Engaging in risky behavior
4. Potential for wound and bladder infection
5. Need to learn self-catheterization
6. Preparation for radiation therapy
7. Decreased self-worth, feelings of guilt
8. Potential for abuse
9. Premature menopause
10. Concern for her children's future

Hypotheses
Using the conservation model, the nurse proposes hypotheses about Debbie's needs to develop a plan of care with her. Some of the hypotheses might include the following:
1. Providing Debbie with a nutritional consultation will assist her to find foods that she can tolerate and that will provide her with the energy she needs for strength and healing.

2. Careful use of food and medicine for nausea will improve her tolerance for food.
3. Adequate teaching and return demonstration of urinary self-catheterization will reduce the potential for infection.
4. Observation and cleansing of the surgical wound will reduce the chance for infection.
5. Preparation for radiation treatment, by discussing expected effects and ways to reduce the effects will promote structural integrity (maintain skin integrity) and personal integrity (provide the patient with control if she desires some control).
6. Encouraging Debbie to talk about her concerns and fears about what having a hysterectomy means to her will help her resolve fears, defuse myths associated with loss of femininity, and prepare her for some of the emotional/physical effects, including premature menopause.
7. Arranging a visiting nurse follow-up visit (post-discharge visit) for Debbie will provide her with emotional (sharing) and physical support (self-catheterization reinforcement).
8. Teaching Debbie about her discharge medications will maximize their effect (pain relief) and reduce the risk of potential side effects.
9. Teaching alternate approaches for pain management (relaxation) will enhance the effects of the pain medication.
10. Providing information about risky behaviors and including ways to reduce those behaviors will give Debbie control over her health and reduce or control her risky behaviors.
11. Providing Debbie with time to talk about why she thinks her diagnosis is punishment for past behavior will help her understand that she did not cause her illness and subsequently will improve her sense of self-worth.

Nursing Interventions

When providing care to Debbie, the nurse uses the conservation principles to maintain wholeness and promote adaptation.

Energy conservation. A nutritional consultation will assist Debbie in identifying foods that will reduce nausea, improve caloric intake, and maintain the required intake for her size. If nausea continues, careful administration of the medication before eating may help to reduce associated nausea. The frequency and intensity of the pain can be controlled by identifying those activities that aggravate the pain and by offering the medication or other pain management interventions to reduce the pain. Because patients commonly experience fatigue after a total hysterectomy and the radiation treatment, Debbie will be prepared to expect normal fatigue and to balance her activity and rest periods. Rest will become very important while her body heals.

Structural integrity. Debbie's wound will be assessed for signs of healing. The antibiotic will be administered as ordered, and she will be given instructions on how to take it at home. The nurse will stress the importance of completing the prescriptions as ordered.

Debbie will learn self-catheterization. Return demonstrations will improve her confidence in performing the task.

Before discharge, Debbie will be prepared for outpatient radiation treatments. The following points should be stressed:

1. The importance of laboratory work to monitor the body's response to the therapy
2. The importance of skin protection to reduce skin irritation associated with the radiation
3. The avoidance of situations that support infection (e.g., a child with a cold) because of the body's decreased ability to fight infection

Personal integrity. Debbie will be encouraged to talk about having her uterus removed because of cancer. If she chooses not to discuss how she feels, the nurse will respect her privacy.

Because Debbie feels that her illness is punishment for her past behavior, Debbie needs to be reassured. If appropriate, a referral to a mental health clinical nurse specialist should be made.

Social integrity. The nurse will also assess the potential for abuse from Debbie's husband and family needs for support. The nurse will explore resources available in the community (e.g., church, support groups, shelters) that may be sources of support to Debbie and her family.

Organismic Responses

In response to the interventions, the nurse would observe for the following possible organismic responses:

1. Abdominal wound healing
2. Clean urinary self-catheterization
3. Dialogue about how Debbie feels about the hysterectomy and cancer
4. Improved appetite and weight gain
5. Recognition that her past behavior did not cause the disease
6. Restful sleep and increased energy level
7. Controlled pain
8. Husband and children are providing assistance within their capabilities

CASE HISTORY OF ALICE

Alice was diagnosed with fibromyalgia (FM) in 1988. At the time of the assessment, she was 44 years old, married, and childless. She worked as a secretary for temporary services that required computer skills. She had quit her full-time job because of the extreme stress of the environment and the overtime hours it required. The nurse met her when she had inquired about a study to examine the health patterns of women with FM. She described herself as desperate for anything that would help her. The nurse clarified for her that the study was not meant to help her but to describe the patterns of health in women with the disorder.

At the time of assessment, Alice had been missing a lot of work because of the amount of pain and fatigue she was experiencing when she woke in the morning. Her pain was severe enough that she was unable to lift a cup of coffee. At times she had difficulty cleaning herself after bowel movements because of the pain in her arm when she extended it backward. Sometimes her pain and fatigue were so severe that she had to cancel social engagements. This situation often resulted in feelings of self-pity and bouts of crying. Severe headaches were of particular concern for her. She reported that her libido was significantly decreased. She said her husband told her that she has a split personality—when she was not tired, she was fine; when she was getting tired, she was mean and verbally abusive. Her husband tried to understand, but his patience was wearing thin.

She was under the care of a physician who had prescribed an antidepressant. She chose not to take any medication except an antiinflammatory medication for menstrual cramps. She was particularly adverse to taking the antidepressant because of the stigma associated with depression. Her physician had ruled out all other possible sources of pain through his diagnostic workup and through that of a consulting neurologist. She was searching for help and had thought about going to support group meetings but had not done so at the time of assessment. She was continuously trying to determine what she did or ate that might cause her pain and fatigue so she could change patterns even during a single day. She had learned that pacing herself when she had a lot to do helped to reduce the intensity of the pain. Massage sometimes temporarily reduced the achiness and pain. She observed that damp, rainy weather made her feel worse. She agreed to keep a daily diary to help identify her patterns of health and illness. The nurse hoped that this would provide her with information about her predicament and give her some control over her health.

NURSING CARE OF ALICE WITH LEVINE'S MODEL

Fibromyalgia (FM) is a chronic painful muscle disorder that is most commonly first diagnosed in women between the ages of 20 and 45 years (Rothchild, 1991). The individuals feel terrible, yet most diagnostic studies are normal. The symptoms generally mimic the flu and include muscle aches and pains, stiffness, nausea, and fatigue (Boissevain & McCain, 1991).

According to Levine (1971a), the focus of nursing care is the maintenance of wholeness (integrity, oneness) and the promotion of adaptation. Alice was very open to discussion about what she might be able to do for herself. She was desperate and frustrated with the notion that nothing seemed to be helping her.

Continuous pain and fatigue were getting her down. She continued to visit her physician, who ordered additional testing to ensure that nothing new was causing the pain. In the interim, she was seeking some relief. Levine's conservation model directs the nurse to involve the patients in decisions about their care.

As the nurse entered into a relationship with Alice, she encouraged her to explain her predicament. Attention to the environmental factors and the integrities help nurses to ensure that the patient's sense of oneness is maintained, even during an initial encounter. Patients often doubt their integrity and feel, like Alice, that they no longer have control over their lives, that they are not taken seriously, and that their concerns are not perceived as valid (Schaefer, 1995).

Challenges to Alice's Internal Environment

Assessment revealed that Alice had "been treating pains for years." All the diagnostic tests were normal. She reported a history of difficult menstrual periods, premenstrual syndrome (PMS), and migraine headaches. All the physiological and pathophysiological aspects of her internal environment were found to be normal.

Challenges to Alice's External Environment

Alice noticed that she experienced migraine headaches after she ate Italian food and concluded that she might be allergic to the sauce. She claimed she felt better since she had begun being more careful. This finding supported Levine's notion that a person seeks, selects, and tests information from the environment in the context of his or her definition of self, thus defending his or her safety, identity, and purpose (1991).

Adaptation to the conceptual environment is sometimes threatened by a response that implies that the complaints associated with the illness are not valid. Alice was fortunate that her physicians acknowledged her pain; however, family members had a difficult time believing that something really was wrong. Socially, she felt as though people thought she was malingering, and she felt sorry for herself when she could not keep her social engagements.

Judgment (Trophicognosis)

Alice was diagnosed with FM, a chronic illness about which little is known. The major problems are fatigue and pain, which have threatened her ability to adapt and maintain wholeness. Considering the conservation principles, the nurse tried to help her adapt in a positive manner and to return to a level of perceived wholeness.

Hypotheses

1. Encouraging the combined use of pharmacological and nonpharmacological sleep interventions (relaxation, hot showers) will improve the subjective quality of Alice's sleep and improve her energy level.
2. Losing weight will help reduce Alice's aches and pains.
3. Encouraging Alice to keep a diary of her symptoms and the internal and external environmental challenges to her integrity will improve Alice's understanding of her unique patterns of FM.
4. Adequate teaching about the medications Alice can take for FM will help her decide about the use of pharmacological interventions.
5. Encouraging Alice to communicate openly and honestly will help reduce her anger.
6. When Alice feels physically better, she will feel better about herself and will be able to engage in social activities.

Nursing Interventions

Energy conservation. Both emotional stress and managing multiple responsibilities at work and home drained Alice's energy. She elected to work part-time rather than stay in an environment that seemed unhealthy for her.

Alice reported in her diary that she frequently had difficulty getting a good night's sleep. She believed that the more restless her night, the more pain she experienced in the morning. Her diary supported this claim. Sleep improved slightly when she used her relaxation tapes to fall asleep. The nurse suggested that her sleep may be improved by taking a warm bath before bedtime, drinking warm milk at bedtime, and avoiding heavy foods 3 to 4 hours before bedtime. She was encouraged to establish a bedtime routine that she practiced on a daily basis. The notion of routine is critical to these interventions.

When discussing possible ways to improve Alice's sleep, the nurse reviewed the drugs Alice was taking and their possible effects. It was at this time that Alice indicated that she had a prescription for an antidepressant but chose not to take it. The nurse informed Alice that the drug is frequently helpful in reducing the severity and frequency of pain, but that it may take up to 3 weeks for the benefits to be noticed. She also told her that women have stopped taking the drug because of the inability to tolerate the side-effects. She reviewed the effects of dry mouth, fast pulse, and constipation and noted that eating a diet with grains and vegetables and drinking 10 glasses of water a day reduces these side-effects. Alice tried taking the medicine but did so only sporadically. She found that if she took the drug every night she felt much better and had more energy. She subsequently was able to plan social outings without the constant fear that she would have to cancel her plans because of the pain and fatigue.

Alice had identified the importance of pacing activities when she had a lot to do. Planning for additional sleep needs was an extension of her established pattern of behavior. During times of stress (e.g., deadlines at work, illness, menstrual periods), she would plan to get extra sleep at night or find a time when she could nap in the afternoon. If sleep is not possible, rest accompanied by relaxation, such as slow rhythmic breathing and imagery, has the potential to replenish energy needs.

Alice was about 10 pounds overweight. She agreed to try to slowly lose some of the weight. Her physician believed that the weight reduction would reduce the strain on her back and help control her aches and pains.

Alice noted that she thought foods such as tomatoes or spices precipitated her headaches. She was encouraged to keep a record of the food she ate and the pattern of symptoms she experienced.

A review of her diary, her reported experiences, and the results of cross-correlation analysis revealed that weather changes lagged the pain and fatigue by up to 2 days. This helped her to realize that some of the pain and fatigue was temporary and would decrease once the weather changed. This recognition helped her deal with the discomfort in a more positive way, if only to simply get more rest when challenged by external environmental factors.

Structural integrity. Alice understood that, because of the uncertainty about the symptoms, other illness must be ruled out to ensure that appropriate interventions were ordered. Because Alice was taking antidepressants, she needed to know about the possibility of weight gain, dry membranes, and constipation. Eating complex carbohydrates can help reduce the hunger associated with the increased serotonin levels. Drinking more water and eating a balanced diet may help reduce the dryness and constipation. Heart rate changes are associated with some antidepressants and should be reported to the physician or nurse practitioner. She was also reassured that alternative medications are available if she is unable to tolerate the prescribed drug. Because she expressed an interest in homeopathy, she was warned that herbs and other over-the-counter remedies can be equally harmful and that she should not take any of these homeopathic treatments without supervision.

Alice was encouraged to continue taking hot showers in the morning and listening to her tapes at night. Because she admitted to having a few alcoholic drinks before bed, she was encouraged to not drink more than two drinks a day and to avoid drinking for 3 hours before bedtime.

Personal integrity. Regaining a sense of selfhood for Alice meant being able to do things around the house and to enjoy social events with her husband and her family. She expressed satisfaction with the fact that she "seemed to be getting better" and could do most of the things she hoped to be able to do.

Social integrity. Alice was encouraged to attend a support group. Alice said that the support groups made her feel excited, that she finally found people who have the same problem, that she has learned a lot about her illness, that she likes interacting with the other members, and that she feels good when she attends the meetings. Alice is a very outgoing person, and with her pain under control, she was able to reach out to other people at the support groups.

It is important to encourage the patient to communicate openly and honestly. Alice felt that her husband did not really understand her illness; he simply tolerated it. Although this made her angry, it also gave her cause for concern that their marriage was suffering. After Alice attended the support groups and shared her positive experience with her husband, she had her first "emotional feeling" talk with him in years. She felt extremely good about this.

Organismic Responses

Success of the interventions is measured through the observation of organismic responses. Responses observed in Alice included the following:

- Reduction in reported pain or need for pain control
- Reported improved quality of sleep
- Reported improved ability to anticipate and plan for exacerbations
- Better understanding of illness
- Comfort in sharing of stories

- Reduction in stress
- Reported improved quality of life
- Better communication with her husband
- Increased energy
- Satisfaction because she was feeling better

CRITICAL THINKING EXERCISES

1. Select and read a pathography (autobiography or biography involving a story about illness) of interest to you in your area of clinical practice (e.g., *The Alchemy of Illness;* Duff, 1993). Use Levine's conservation model to evaluate the health and healthcare of the individual in the story. Consider the medical plan of care, environmental challenges, and organismic responses. Evaluate the use of the model relative to the identification of the nursing care needs of the patient and the potential use of the model in promoting adaptation and maintaining wholeness. Explore how the patient defines adaptation and wholeness. What questions would be asked to gather the information found in the book? Compare these questions to the questions that would be asked if you were using Levine's conservation model. Make a judgment about the value of the model with attention to its strengths and weaknesses.

2. Write a story about when you were ill or when a family member or friend was ill. Given the nature of the illness, what was needed for you or the friend/family member to feel well? How would you help them get to that point? What were the actual outcomes, and how would the use of the conservation model change or support those outcomes?

3. List the assumptions on which Levine's conservation model is based. Determine whether the assumptions are or are not consistent with your beliefs. Identify the knowledge that supports these assumptions. Determine how you could support or refute their validity (truthfulness).

4. Consider and write about a nursing situation that you have recently encountered. Use this situation to determine the kind of knowledge needed to provide nursing care. Distinguish between that which is nursing knowledge and that which is knowledge from the adjunctive disciplines. Determine how adjunctive knowledge becomes nursing knowledge in this situation. What knowledge is missing? What other information is needed?

References

Alligood, M. R. (1997). Models and theories: Critical thinking structures. In M. R. Alligood & A. Marriner-Tomey (Eds.), *Nursing theory: Utilization and application* (pp. 31-45). St. Louis: Mosby.

Bates, M. (1967). A naturalist at large. *Natural History, 76*(6), 8-16.

Boissevain, M. D. & McCain, G. A. (1991). Toward an integrated understanding of fibromyalgia syndrome: II. Psychological and phenomenological aspects. *Pain, 45,* 239-248.

Brunner, M. (1985). A conceptual approach to critical care nursing using Levine's model. *Focus on Critical Care, 12*(2), 39-44.

Burd, C., Olson, B., Langemo, D., Hunter, S., Hanson, D., Osowki, K. F., & Sauvage, T. (1994). Skin care strategies in a skilled nursing home. *Journal of Gerontological Nursing, 20*(11), 28-34.

Clark, L. R., Fraaza, V., Schroeder, S., & Maddens, M. E. (1995). Alternative nursing environments: Do they affect hospital outcomes? *Journal of Gerontological Nursing, 21*(11), 32-38.

Cooper, D. H. (1990). Optimizing wound healing: A practice within nursing domains. *Nursing Clinics of North America, 25*(1), 165-180.

Cox, R. A., Sr. (1991). A tradition of caring: Use of Levine's model in long-term care. In K. M. Schaefer & J. B. Pond (Eds.), *The conservation model: A framework for nursing practice* (pp. 179-197). Philadelphia: F. A. Davis.

Cox, R. A. Personal Communication, February 21, 1995.

Crawford-Gamble, P. E. (1986). An application of Levine's conceptual model. *Perioperative Nursing Quarterly, 2*(1), 64-70.

Dever, M. (1991). Care of children. In K. M. Schaefer & J. B. Pond (Eds.), *The conservation model: A framework for nursing practice* (pp. 71-82). Philadelphia: F. A. Davis.

Dibble, S. L., Bostrom-Ezrati, J., & Ruzzuto, C. (1991). Clinical predictors of intravenous site symptoms. *Research in Nursing and Health, 14*, 413-420.

Dow, J. S. & Mest, C. G. (1997). Psychosocial interventions for patients with chronic obstructive pulmonary disease. *Home-Healthcare-Nurse, 15*(6), 414-420.

Duff, K. (1993). *The alchemy of illness.* New York: Pantheon Books.

Fawcett, J. (1995). *Conceptual models of nursing* (3rd ed.). Philadelphia: F. A. Davis.

Foreman, M. D. (1991). Conserving cognitive integrity of the hospitalized elderly. In K. M. Schaefer & J. B. Pond (Eds.), *The conservation model: A framework for nursing practice* (pp. 133-150). Philadelphia: F. A. Davis.

Happ, M., Williams, C. C., Strumpf, N. E., & Burger, S. G. (1996). Individualized care for frail elderly: Theory and practice. *Journal of Gerontological Nursing, 22*(3), 7-14.

Higgins, P. A. (1998). Patients' perception of fatigue while undergoing long-term mechanical ventilation: Incidence and associated factors. *Heart and Lung: Journal of Acute and Critical Care, 27*(3), 177-183.

Hirschfeld, M. H. (1976). The cognitively impaired older adult. *American Journal of Nursing, 76*, 1981-1984.

Jost, S. (2000). An assessment and intervention strategy for managing staff needs during change. *Journal of Nursing Administration, 30*(1), 34-40.

Langer, V. S. (1990). Minimal handling protocol for the intensive care nursery. *Neonatal Network, 9*(3), 23-27.

Levine, M. E. (1966a). Adaptation and assessment: A rationale for nursing intervention. *American Journal of Nursing, 66*, 2450-2453.

Levine, M. E. (1966b). Trophicognosis: An alternative to nursing diagnosis. In *American Nurses' Association Regional Clinical Conference, Volume 2.* (pp. 55-70). New York: American Nurses Association.

Levine, M. E. (1969). The pursuit of wholeness. *American Journal of Nursing, 69*, 93-98.

Levine, M. E. (1971a). Holistic nursing. *Nursing Clinics of North America, 6*(2), 253-263.

Levine, M. E. (1971b). *Renewal for nursing.* Philadelphia: F. A. Davis.

Levine, M. E. (1973a). *Introduction to clinical nursing* (2nd ed.). Philadelphia: F. A. Davis.

Levine, M. E. (1973b). On creativity in nursing. *Image, 3*(3), 15-19.

Levine, M. E. (1977). Nursing ethics and the ethical nurse. *American Journal of Nursing, 77*(5), 845-849.

Levine, M. E. (1984, August). *Myra Levine.* Paper presented at the Nurse Theorist Conference, Edmonton, Alberta, Canada. (Cassette recording).

Levine, M. E. (1988). Antecedents from adjunctive disciplines: Creation of nursing theory. *Nursing Science Quarterly, 1*(1), 16-21.

Levine, M. E. (1989a). The conservation model: Twenty years later. In J. P. Riehl-Sisca (Ed.), *Conceptual models for nursing practice* (pp. 325-337). Norwalk, CT: Appleton & Lange.

Levine, M. E. (1989b). Ration or rescue: The elderly in critical care. *Critical Care Nursing, 12*(1), 82-89.

Levine, M. E. (1989c). The ethics of nursing rhetoric. *Image, 21*(1), 4-5.

Levine, M. E. (1991). The conservation model: A model for health. In K. M. Schaefer & J. B. Pond (Eds.), *The conservation model: A framework for nursing practice* (pp. 1-11). Philadelphia: F. A. Davis.

Levine, M. E. (1994). Some further thoughts on nursing rhetoric. In J. F. Kikuchi & H. Simmons (Eds.), *Developing a philosophy of nursing* (pp. 104-109). Thousand Oaks, CA: Sage.

Levine, M. E. (1995). The rhetoric of nursing theory. *Image, 27*(1), 11-14.

Levine, M. E. (1996). The conservation principles: A retrospective. *Nursing Science Quarterly, 9*(1), 38-41.

Litrell, K. & Schumann, L. (1989). Promoting sleep for the patient with a myocardial infarction. *Critical Care Nurse, 9*(3), 44-49.

Lynn-McHale, D. J. & Smith, A. (1991). Comprehensive assessment of families of the critically ill. In J. S. Leske (Ed.), *AACN clinical issues in critical care Nursing* (pp. 195-209). Philadelphia: J. B. Lippincott.

Molchany, C. A. (1992). Ventricular septal and free wall rupture complicating acute MI. *Journal of Cardiovascular Nursing, 6*(4), 38-45.

Neswick, R. S. (1997). Myra E. Levine: A theoretical basis for ET nursing. *Professional Practice, 24*(1), 6-9.

Newport, M. A. (1984). Conserving thermal energy and social integrity in the newborn. *Western Journal of Nursing Research, 6*(2), 175-197.

O'Laughlin, K. M. (1986). Changes in bladder function in the woman undergoing radical hysterectomy for cervical cancer. *Journal of Obstetric, Gynecologic, and Neonatal Nursing, 15*(5), 380-385.

Pasco, A. & Halupa, D. (1991). Chronic pain management. In K. M. Schaefer & J. B. Pond (Eds.), *The conservation model: A framework for practice* (pp. 101-117). Philadelphia: F. A. Davis.

Pond, J. B. (1991). Ambulatory care of the homeless. In K. M. Schaefer & J. B. Pond (Eds.), *The conservation model: A framework for practice* (pp. 167-178). Philadelphia: F. A. Davis.

Pond, J. B. & Taney, S. G. (1991). Emergency care in a large university emergency department. In K. M. Schaefer & J. B. Pond (Eds.), *The conservation model: A framework for practice* (pp. 151-166). Philadelphia: F. A. Davis.

Roberts, J. E., Fleming, N., & Yeates-Giese, D. (1991). Perineal integrity. In K. M. Schaefer & J. B. Pond (Eds.), *The conservation model: A framework for practice* (pp. 61-70). Philadelphia: F. A. Davis.

Roberts, K. L., Brittin, M., Cook, M., & deClifford, J. (1994). Boomerang pillows and respiratory capacity. *Clinical Nursing Research, 3*(2), 157-165.

Roberts, K. L., Brittin, M., & deClifford, J. (1995). Boomerang pillows and respiratory capacity in frail elderly women. *Clinical Nursing Research, 4*(4), 465-471.

Rothchild, B. M. (1991). Fibromyalgia: An explanation for the aches and pains of the nineties. *Comprehensive Therapy, 17*(6), 9-14.

Savage, T. A. & Culbert, C. (1989). Early intervention: The unique role of nursing. *Journal of Pediatric Nursing, 4*(5), 339-345.

Schaefer, K. (1991). Care of the patient with congestive heart failure. In K. M. Schaefer & J. B. Pond (Eds.), *The conservation model: A framework for practice* (pp. 119-132). Philadelphia: F. A. Davis.

Schaefer, K. M. (1995). Struggling to maintain balance: A study of women with fibromyalgia. *Journal of Advanced Nursing, 21*, 95-102.

Schaefer, K. M. (1996). Levine's conservation model: Caring for women with chronic illness. In P. H. Hinton & B. Neuman (Eds.), *Blueprint for use of nursing models: Education, research, practice, and administration* (pp. 187-227). New York: NLN Press.

Schaefer, K. M. & Pond, J. B. (1994). Levine's conservation model as a guide to nursing practice. *Nursing Science Quarterly, 7*(2), 53-54.

Schaefer, K. M., Swavely, D., Rothenberger, C., Hess, S., & Willistin, D. (1996). Sleep disturbances post–coronary artery bypass surgery. *Progress in Cardiovascular Nursing, 11*(1), 5-14.

Taylor, J. W. (1989). Levine's conservation principles. Using the model for nursing diagnosis in a neurological setting. In J. P. Riehl-Sisca (Ed.), *Conceptual models for nursing practice* (3rd ed., pp. 349-358). Norwalk, CT: Appleton & Lange.

Tribotti, S. (1990). Admission to the neonatal intensive care unit: Reducing the risks. *Neonatal Network, 8*(4), 17-22.

Webb, H. (1993). Holistic care following a palliative Hartmann's procedure. *British Journal of Nursing, 2*(2), 128-132.

Neuman's Systems Model in Nursing Practice

Raphella Sohier

"Wholism, implicit in the Neuman Systems Model, is both a philosophical and a biological concept, implying relationships and processes arising from wholeness, dynamic freedom, and creativity in adjusting to stressors in the internal and external environments. Using a wholistic systems approach to both protect and promote client welfare, nursing action must be skillfully related to the meaningful and dynamic organization of the various parts and subparts of the whole affecting the client. The various interrelationships of the parts and subparts must be appropriately identified and analyzed before relevant nursing action can be taken." (From Neuman, B. [1995]. The Neuman Systems Model *[3rd ed.]. Norwalk, CT: Appleton & Lange. Reprinted by permission of Pearson Education, Inc. Upper Saddle River, NJ 07458.)*

HISTORY AND BACKGROUND

Neuman first designed her systems model in the early 1970s as a teaching tool to assist psychiatric/mental health nursing students in their early encounters with clients in community mental health centers. Neuman conceptualizes the "client system" or focus of nursing practice as a person, dyad, family unit, group, population stratum, entire community, or society (Neuman & Koertvelyessey, 1986; Neuman & Young, 1972; Neuman, 1974, 1980, 1982, 1989a, 1989b, 1990, 1995). Literature addressing the application of the Neuman Systems Model in practice with each of these foci can be found in the major works of Neuman (1990, 1995). The model has been extensively applied in practice and in educational and management settings and has been a focus for research. In the final section of the most recent edition of her book, Neuman (1995) discusses the trajectory from the past, into the present, and on into the future, detailing the uses of the model in various settings (pp. 669-703).

Nursing has embarked on the twenty-first century with Neuman's Systems Model as relevant now as when it was first developed in the early 1970s. Recent literature utilizes the model in research and clinical work related to advanced practice nursing (Hassell, 1996; Martin, 1996), nursing education (McHolm & Geib, 1998), instrument development (Flannery, 1995), spiritual care (Carrigg & Weber, 1997; Martsolf & Mickley, 1998), crosscultural research (Hanson, 1999; Neuman, 1996; Taggart & Mattson, 1996), psychiatric nursing (Barker, Robinson, & Brautigan, 1999), women's health (Gigliotti, 1999; Lowry, Saeger, & Barnett, 1997), and in chronic illness care of dialysis patients (Breckenridge, 1997), cancer patients (Molassiotis, 1997; Sabo & Michael, 1996), patients with chronic obstructive pulmonary disease (COPD) (Narsavage, 1997), and patients with human immunodeficiency virus (HIV) (Mill, 1997).

In Neuman's model, each client system, whether it is an individual or an aggregate, is visualized as an open system that experiences stressors developing from internal or external environments. Neuman (1995) explains that a systems perspective was chosen for her model because it permits "the precise comprehensive analysis of the relations in space and time on which they [the clients] largely depend" (p. 10).

Systems models have two equally important features: structure and process. All systems consist of subsystems. Each system and each subsystem is complete in itself. The sum of the subsystems or parts that make up the system is said to be greater than the sum of its parts (von Bertalanffy, 1968). As open systems, human systems accept input from outside the system, process the input in a phase called *throughput,* and export it in a phase called *output.* Equilibrium (a stable state) is the goal of the system. Change (e.g., input, throughput, output) is a feature of the process, and the end product (output) is necessarily different from what is entered into the system (input). Neuman describes people as open systems in constant interaction with their internal and external environments.

The Neuman Systems Model is health-oriented. Neuman (1995) describes health as a continuum from wellness to illness and speaks of an "optimal state of wellness" as "the best possible state of health for a client system at any given point in time" (p. 32). Equilibrium is the healthy state of the system, and disequilibrium is the unhealthy or diseased state of the system. Neuman offers a general proposition that the healthier the system, the lower the reaction to stress. Additionally, the greater the control over disequilibrium is proportionately greater, and a return to stability can be achieved that much more quickly. Prevention of disequilibrium or illness is a central focus and goal; thus Newman (1995) describes her model as a wellness model.

OVERVIEW OF NEUMAN'S SYSTEMS MODEL

Neuman (1995) claims that "[t]he intent of the Neuman Systems Model or conceptual framework is to set forth a structure that depicts the parts and subparts and their interrelationship for the whole of the client as a complete system" (p. 15). Neuman depicts the client system as a person or persons constantly bombarded by environmental stressors (Selye, 1950). Whereas the client system is exposed to stressors from within and outside the system, the client system as visualized by Neuman is also protected by a series of concentric buffers that minimize the impact of stressors and act as safety zones between environments and the central core. The greater the quality of the client system's health, the greater the protection provided by the buffers or safety zones. The central core consists of functions basic or essential to human life. When the client system is in equilibrium (i.e., well), all the protective circles are in place. Figure 11-1 provides a visual depiction of Neuman's model.

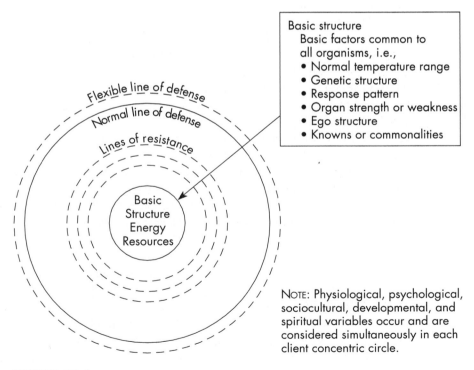

Basic structure
Basic factors common to
all organisms, i.e.,
• Normal temperature range
• Genetic structure
• Response pattern
• Organ strength or weakness
• Ego structure
• Knowns or commonalities

Flexible line of defense
Normal line of defense
Lines of resistance

Basic
Structure
Energy
Resources

NOTE: Physiological, psychological, sociocultural, developmental, and spiritual variables occur and are considered simultaneously in each client concentric circle.

FIGURE 11-1

The client system. (From Neuman, B. [1995]. *The Neuman Systems Model.* [3rd ed.]. Norwalk, CT: Appleton & Lange.)

At the outside of the circle is the flexible line of defense (FLD). This protective mechanism has a great deal of flexibility and an accordian-like effect in the healthy client system. If the client takes appropriate health measures (e.g., eats a healthy diet, gets adequate rest), the client system can tolerate normal life stress and even extraordinary stress for a time. When the system is healthy, the FLD is extended far away from the next buffer, which is called the normal line of defense (NLD). As long as stressors are not extreme and the organism continues to live healthily, the flexibility of this buffer will permit a measure of give-and-take. For example, a busy student who has a part-time job, a full-time school schedule, and shared responsibility for home and children will survive as long as he or she eats properly, exercises, rests appropriately, and gets some recreation. However, if this person ignores body language (tiredness) or body needs (hunger), resistance is weakened; susceptibility to stressors is increased; and he or she soon becomes vulnerable to a common infection such as a cold virus. The FLD is breached, and the NLD is threatened. In the same fashion, without appropriate action to care for the system, a common cold may become bronchitis or even pneumonia. At that point the NLD has also been breached, and the internal buffer—the lines of resistance (LOR), or the life-protecting buffer—is threatened. In that case, if the pneumonia state becomes acute, a life-threatening situation can arise.

When the client system is well, stable, and in equilibrium, the protective mechanisms are all in place. As these mechanisms are breached, the client enters a state of disequilibrium during which nursing interventions are needed. To intervene using the Neuman model, the nurse must understand that stressors threatening the integrity of the system may be intrapersonal, interpersonal, or extrapersonal. For example, if the client system is a person with a medical condition, that condition constitutes an intrapersonal stressor. If the client system is a family in disequilibrium, the stressor is interpersonal in nature. If the client system is a community that has experienced an external threat, the stressor is an extrapersonal stressor. Stressors of all three types are often at work simultaneously in clients' lives.

To determine the nature of the stressors affecting clients and to provide direction for the nursing process, the nurse carries out a thorough and "wholistic assessment" (Neuman, 1995, p. 10). The client system is assessed from five perspectives: physiological, psychological, developmental, sociocultural, and spiritual. On first contact with the client, the nurse carries out a very detailed assessment. Later it may be sufficient to update the original accessment.

Addressing the variables one by one provides the detailed essentials for an accurate diagnosis and differential diagnoses. To maintain the wholistic focus central to Neuman's model, the assessment data relating to the five variables are reintegrated to form a wholistic picture of the client system. Neuman focuses on the client's perspective, which is obtained by asking him or her several questions regarding the problem that brings him or her to the care provider. The objective results from the nursing assessment are repeated to the client to ensure that the nurse has understood the problem from the client's perspective (Sohier, 1995). A primary diagnosis and differential diagnoses emerge through analysis of the data and are congruent with this subjective-objective comparison. A plan of care is constituted based on these data.

The nurse categorizes the data in terms of stressors and their nature (intrapersonal, interpersonal, or extrapersonal). The data are shared with the client system; individual or aggregate feedback is considered and incorporated in the data; and the client is encouraged to express all of his or her opinions regarding the accuracy of the conclusion at this step and throughout the nursing process. When the nurse and client have agreed on appropriate nursing interventions, the client is encouraged to comment on whether he or she believes the goals can be achieved by a proposed method. Sometimes it may be appropriate to contract with the client about how goals are to be achieved and to share responsibility for meeting them between the client and the provider. This feature of caregiver-client cooperation in the application of the Neuman model also facilitates crosscultural care (Sohier, 1995). Permitting the client to clarify his or her comprehension of the problem, propose acceptable ways to address the problem, and accept a measure of responsibility for achieving goals places the responsibility in a shared context and allows a culture-centered view to emerge. This shared responsibility continues throughout the caregiver-client contact and is included in the exit interview and evaluation of outcomes. Unique to the Neuman nursing process format is that both client and caregiver perceptions are considered for relevant goal setting (Neuman, 1995).

Client strengths are often reflected in response to the question "Have you had a similar problem before, and if so, how did you deal with it?" (Neuman, 1990, p. 61). Evaluation of client strengths and weaknesses in the face of stressors assists the nurse in developing a client-centered plan of care. The initial question "What do you see as your greatest problem at this moment?" occasionally produces surprising responses. The reason for the client's referral or the obvious need observed by the caregiver may not form the focus of the client's need. This type of occurrence challenges the nurse to recognize the client's perspective in order to facilitate achievement of long-term goals (Neuman, 1995).

Because wellness provides a central focus in the Neuman model, nursing interventions are conceptualized as preventions, and the actions of the nurse are conceptualized as reconstitutions. Neuman identifies three types of nursing intervention and labels all as preventions: (1) *primary prevention*—when a threat to health exists but no stressor invasion reaction has occurred; (2) *secondary prevention*—when stressor invasion has occurred and action is taken to prevent the state of disequilibrium from progressing to the point at which basic structures become threatened; and (3) *tertiary prevention*—aimed at reconstituting a system seriously impacted by stressors to restore the system to equilibrium, optimal wellness, or its stable state (Neuman, 1995). Interventions at more than one level of prevention may take place concomitantly. For example, the nurse may offer assistance at the tertiary level in terms of reconstitution of a health state while applying primary or secondary teaching interventions in an attempt to prevent a recurrence of the response in the future. Because optimal client stability is the goal of nursing intervention in the Neuman model, it is to be expected that interventions will consist of more than one type of prevention. The prevention-as-intervention approach—primary, secondary, and tertiary—is illustrated in the case studies described later in the chapter.

CRITICAL THINKING IN NURSING PRACTICE WITH NEUMAN'S MODEL

Nursing in the Neuman model facilitates and requires critical thinking on the part of the nurse. A thorough assessment following Neuman's guidelines is essential to support the development of a diagnostic statement, determine the appropriate interventions, and evaluate outcomes. Using the Neuman systems, the nurse is concerned with acquiring significant and comprehensive client data to determine the actual or possible impact of environmental stressors on the defined client system. This process fully explains the client condition and provides the logic or rationale for subsequent nursing action. That is, it provides the basis for a broad, comprehensive, umbrella-like diagnostic statement that concerns the entire client condition. Logically defensible goals are easily and accurately derived from such a statement (Neuman, 1995).

Neuman and Martin (1998) offered a new perspective on the linkage of the Neuman Systems Model with the Omaha System to describe, measure, and evaluate practice. The Neuman Systems Model is viewed as the "wide umbrella," or general theoretical framework, whereas the more specific Omaha System terms and codes offer a method of describing the detailed level of problem identification, interventions, and outcome measures. Neuman and Martin further suggest that these two systems used together provide practitioners with an organizing framework and a set of tools that facilitate working in partnership with clients and providing evidence-based quality care.

The nursing process based on Neuman's model is an interactive process between the client and the nurse that requires critical thought on the nurse's part. Following Neuman's guidelines and assessment phase provides objective, client-centered information. The task of the nurse is to synthesize these elements, interpret them according to the model, develop a comprehensive diagnostic statement, develop goals in interaction with the client, provide care in terms of the three preventions, and evaluate the outcomes. Evaluation of progress and renegotiation of goals based on the client experience are important elements in the Neuman approach to the nursing process. Table 11-1 illustrates the interaction of the nurse with the client in the nursing process as guided by Neuman's model. Nursing based on Neuman's model requires critical analytical thought and interaction between the nurse and the client before relevant nursing action can take place.

CASE HISTORY OF DEBBIE

Debbie is a 29-year-old woman who was recently admitted to the oncology nursing unit for evaluation after sensing pelvic "fullness" and noticing a watery, foul-smelling vaginal discharge. A Papanicolaou smear revealed class V cervical cancer. She was found to have a stage II squamous cell carcinoma of the cervix and underwent a radical hysterectomy with bilateral salpingooophorectomy.

Her past health history revealed that physical examinations had been infrequent. She also reported that she had not performed breast self-examination. She is 5 feet, 4 inches tall and weights 89 pounds. Her usual weight is about 110 pounds. She has smoked approximately two packs of cigarettes a day for the past 16 years. She is gravida 2, para 2. Her first pregnancy was at age 16, and her second was at age 18. Since that time, she has taken oral contraceptives on a regular basis.

Debbie completed the eighth grade. She is married and lives with her husband and her two children in her mother's home, which she describes as less than sanitary. Her husband is unemployed. She describes him as emotionally distant and abusive at times.

She has done well following surgery except for being unable to completely empty her urinary bladder. She is having continued postoperative pain and nausea. It will be necessary for her to perform intermittent self-catheterization at home. Her medications are (1) an antibiotic, (2) an analgesic as needed for pain, and (3) an antiemetic as needed for nausea. In addition, she will be receiving radiation therapy on an outpatient basis.

Debbie is extremely tearful. She expresses great concern over her future and the future of her two children. She believes that this illness is a punishment for her past life.

TABLE 11-1   Critical Thinking and the Neuman Nursing Process

Nurse	Client
1. Approach client, introduce self, make some small talk (weather, etc.).	Allow client opportunities to respond and relax.
2. As verbal and nonverbal contact proceeds, nurse asks, "What do you think is your greatest problem right now?"	Allow client to explain problem in own terms.
3. Question: "Have you ever had to deal with this problem in the past?"	Allow time for response.
4. If response is "yes," nurse asks, "How did you deal with it then?"	Allow time for response. Note strengths indicated by response.
5. Nurse then explains to client that he/she will carry out complete examination and history to detect all problems.	Assist client to prepare for examination.
6. Carry out complete assessment and history in the five variables: physiological, psychological, sociocultural, developmental, and spiritual.	Consider the client's needs (e.g., modesty, disability, culture). Maintain a caring attitude.
7. While client dresses, collate data and reach tentative comprehensive diagnosis. Share diagnosis with client and ask for feedback.	Ask client what he/she thinks would help alleviate problem. Client clarifies perspective on problem.
*8. Use nursing judgment about need for immediate action or new appointment with client at earliest possible time. Provide telephone number where you can be reached. Reassure client. Respond to any questions from client.	Client and nurse mutually agree on plan.
*9. Collate all data and determine nature of stressors facing client (intrapersonal, interpersonal, or extrapersonal).	
*10. Consider client strengths.	
*11. Develop problem list. Prioritize needs. Develop long-term and short-term goals.	Client clarifies priority needs and agrees to goals.
12. Meet with client and discuss findings. Propose plan of care. Listen to feedback, and adjust plan of care if necessary. Contract with client ways to achieve goals, and identify the role that the nurse will play as well as expectations for client. Make any referrals or arrangements necessary for client to proceed with management plan. Reinforce identified strengths. Make future appointment.	Client provides feedback on plan. Client considers making contract with nurse to achieve mutual goals.
13. Meet with client, evaluate status, discuss progress, praise achievement or improvement, discuss reasons for failures, and renegotiate as necessary, listening carefully to client's position. Propose new plan as necessary. Make future appointment.	

*Steps 8, 9, 10, and 11 take place out of the client's presence.

NURSING CARE OF DEBBIE WITH NEUMAN'S MODEL
Assessment Data

The case history is considered in the Neuman model according to the five client variables.

Physiological. These variables describe class V cervical cancer—stage II squamous cell carcinoma followed by radical hysterectomy/salpingo-oophorectomy, serious weight loss (21 pounds), urinary retention, need for catheterization, and upcoming radiation treatment.

Psychological. These variables paint a picture of a very frightened young woman expressing concerns about her future and about the future of her children, with little support from her husband.

Sociocultural. Debbie has minimal education and became pregnant at age 16. She is a guest in her mother's home, where she lives with her two children and her unsupportive, "emotionally distant and abusive at times" husband. She has smoked continually and excessively since age 13. The home is described as "unsanitary."

Developmental. The Neuman assessment would evaluate Debbie as a 29-year-old woman and mother of two who has a life-threatening illness. A Neuman assessment requires consideration of the adult developmental tasks appropriate to a 29-year-old woman, wife, and mother. It is also important to ask whether her psychological development is such that she will be able to assess problems and tasks that face her in an accurate manner and tackle them when she feels better.

Spiritual. Debbie is tearful and fearful and "believes her illness is a punishment for her past life."

Organization of Data

The next step in a Neuman nursing process is the organization of data in relation to the five variables assessed, identifying the nature of each stressor described by the client and/or observed by the nurse. Several areas in this case study require additional data. For example, it would be useful to know more about Debbie's mother and the quality of their relationship and about Debbie's children and the quality of their shared lives. It would be useful to know whether Debbie is a spiritual person and whether she is or has been affiliated with a church. To avoid duplication of work, it would be important to know whether a social work consultation took place before her discharge from the acute-care setting. It would also be valuable to know whether Debbie's husband is looking for work and whether he is discouraged or even depressed. These factors are important in the assessment because the Neuman model is a systems model. Systems models always propose that whatever occurs at the system boundaries (e.g., between Debbie and her husband) can cause disequilibrium in the total family system. To clarify Debbie's problems and her needs, it is useful to plot the information in a chart like the one in Table 11-2.

TABLE 11-2	Debbie's Stressors		
Stressors	**Intrapersonal**	**Interpersonal**	**Extrapersonal**
Physiological	Cancer: radiation therapy planned Nausea Pain Catheter care— danger of infection Weight loss Smokes	Catheter care	
Psychological	Fear about future	Fear about future of children Lack of support from husband Mother (no data)	
Sociocultural	Basic education Fear of effects of smoking	Unsupportive, sometimes abusive husband Responsible for two children	Limited income Husband unable to obtain employment
Developmental	Has two children First pregnancy at 16 years of age	Mother of one teenager: 13 Mother of one preteen: 11	
Spiritual	Spiritual distress related to past life and present state		Concern over past behavior related to societal norms

This organization of stressors reported in Debbie's case history permits the nurse to establish an initial understanding of Debbie's needs and to develop a tentative priority list. This list, however, must be discussed with Debbie to be certain that she agrees with this assessment of her problems. A comprehensive diagnostic statement and mutual goals then can be chosen. It is also useful to create a prioritized list of the problems from the nurse's objective perspective and again from Debbie's subjective perspective. The client does not always agree with the nurse. For example, the nurse might place Debbie's physiological needs at the top of the list; Debbie, on the other hand, might place psychological and sociocultural stressors regarding the future of her children before concern for self. These discrepancies must be respected, discussed, balanced, and fit into a care plan that meets the client's satisfaction. The nurse who fails to approach the situation in this way is less likely to achieve the goals essential to the client's obtaining optimal wellness. Neuman describes optimal wellness as the best possible state of health the client can attain at any point in time.

Neuman's philosophical view is wholistic. The idea of a client composed of subsystems that together form a system greater than the sum of its parts forms the foundation for examining the five client variables and then restructuring the data to form a whole. According to Neuman (1995), "The various interrelationships of the parts and subparts must be appropriately identified and analyzed before relevant nursing action can be taken" (p. 11).

Problem List

When the nurse considers the stressors listed in Table 11-2, he or she develops a problem list like the one that follows. This list would be shared with Debbie to verify that these are her problems as she sees them.
1. Pain, nausea, serious weight loss; understanding of catheter care; unsanitary conditions
2. Fear—lack of family support, concern about children
3. Spiritual distress—fear of possible eternal punishment

The nurse might approach Debbie in the following way to clarify the problems and her priorities:

Nurse: Debbie, I want to help you to be as comfortable as you can be now that you are home. What would you like me to help you with first? What do you see as your biggest problem?

Debbie: Well, my life just seems to be one big problem now; I am weak and tired, and sometimes I hurt and feel nauseated. My mother has to work so she can't help me, and my husband seems more distant than ever since I got sick. And then I'm so scared about what will happen to my kids. I don't want them to be like me. I want them to stay in school and I don't want them to smoke because I know that cancer and smoking are related. And look at this place—it's such a mess! I just turn to the wall and cry. I don't know what to do! I think I'm to blame for all of this. I ran around a lot and got pregnant when I was 16.

Nurse: Debbie, have you ever felt this way before?

Debbie: Well, sometimes when my husband was abusive and so on, but that wasn't the same.

Nurse: What helped you then?

Debbie: (crying) Well, you know, I went to work then so I could get away from it. And my kids and I used to have fun, and I'd get them to help me clean up the place. But I've lost so much weight and been so sick, they stay away a lot at their friends' houses, and I don't want them to smoke!

Nurse: What would help?

Debbie: (sobbing) I don't believe I know, but if the place were cleaned up and my kids stayed home some more, that might help.

Reflection on Data

When the nurse compares these two sets of data, it becomes clear that her priorities are different from Debbie's. Of course, it is important for the nurse to determine whether Debbie understands the medications, is taking them as ordered, and finds them effective. In addition, the nurse should evaluate the state of the catheter, whether Debbie has been taught and understands good sterile technique, and Debbie's personal state of cleanliness. However, these concerns obviously are not foremost for Debbie.

Debbie is frightened about her life and the future of her children, and she has a need from a developmental perspective as a mother to have the home clean so she can experience some close time with her children. It also seems as if she wants teach her children to understand the dangers of smoking and the importance of education.

Synthesis and Analysis of Data

Applying the Neuman model, the nurse considers all the data and the available resources and decides that she will propose cleaning services for Debbie if she agrees. Because Debbie said her children has helped her around the home in the past, the nurse considers some way to involve the children with the housecleaner so they can help in some way with Debbie's care. She also plans to request Meals-on-Wheels for Debbie, who is often alone during the day when her husband leaves her without food. The nurse wonders whether he can be taught to accept more responsibility to help. She makes a note to meet with Debbie's husband.

Although it is not clear to the nurse what Debbie thinks caused her illness, it is clear that she is spiritually distressed. It is important to try to find out who might help Debbie with her spiritual distress. The nurse thinks of a female pastor at the hospital who is very empathetic. With Debbie's permission she decides to ask the pastor to start visiting Debbie.

Having clarified the nature and strength of the stressors, the nurse asks how interventions can be structured so they reduce the actual stressors, improve the client's strengths, and prevent the same stressors from causing disequilibrium in the future.

The three preventions are used to develop interventions for this purpose. In Debbie's case, all three types of prevention are needed. Secondary and tertiary preventions can restore her to optimal wellness; tertiary preventions can reconstruct the family; and primary preventions can teach Debbie about self-catheterization and teach her children about smoking and cancer, their mother's needs, and how to take care of their own needs. In addition, primary preventions are necessary to teach the husband about his wife's illness and needs. Secondary preventions could assist in repairing the husband's self-esteem, and tertiary preventions may be necessary if he is diagnosed with depression. The whole family is affected by Debbie's illness and needs to be considered in the health plan. On each visit, the nurse will reassess the situation, evaluate the health of the protective mechanisms, and intervene as necessary.

CASE HISTORY OF HOMELESS WOMEN

The client targeted in this application of the Neuman approach to the nursing process (nursing assessment, diagnoses, and intervention) is a group of 16 homeless women who are clients of a 22-bed shelter in urban Boston. The shelter has religious affiliations and is supported by state, local, and private funding. The philosophical stance at this shelter is to assist women to move out of homelessness by increasing their self-esteem and by building skills that will allow them to become self-supporting, thereby increasing the likelihood of their success when job and housing opportunities arise. The 22 beds are full most of the time. Only three or four clients are long-term residents; the others are transitory, often returning after failed attempts to resolve their situations on their own.

The assessment of this client required patience and time, because the same women were not always present. The Neuman approach provides ways for the nurse to focus on aggregate clients such as a group or a system, and it facilitates the evaluation of a changing structure as easily as a stable one. This assessment reflects the perspectives of a changing group with certain common features that identify them as one system over time.

An individual Neuman physical assessment of the 16 women was carried out over a 3-month period. Because the identified client is the group of women, these physiological data were pooled at the end of the assessment phase to provide an accurate and objective picture of the health of the group. This objective assessment was then related to the psychological, sociocultural, developmental, and spiritual assessment also carried out in group context.

NURSING CARE OF HOMELESS WOMEN WITH NEUMAN'S MODEL

This case illustrates a situation in which the Neuman model is applied to the nursing care of the aggregate client. A group of homeless women using an urban shelter forms the focus of the application.

Assessment Data

Physiological. As expected, the general physiological status of the group was very poor. All individuals showed signs of malnutrition, poor hygiene, and skin conditions. Most of the women smoked, and many reported substance abuse. Tests provided evidence of infectious diseases, including tuberculosis, HIV, and AIDS. Some women had seriously elevated blood pressure, and several had diabetes.

Psychological. The psychological assessment provided information about lifetime patterns of abuse, including early sexual abuse, rape, incest, self-abuse, and self-mutilation. Generalized or episodic depression was reported together with a corresponding mistrust of society in general and of the people with whom they had contact in particular.

Sociocultural. The group was predominately Caucasian and from low socioeconomic families. Some were Hispanic, and a few were African-American. Educational status was generally low. Most had dropped out of school, but a few were college graduates. It was evident from observing the group that they felt little trust for each other and distrusted most authority figures. Some had made attempts to become established outside the shelter but had not succeeded, and they blamed their lack of success on the absence of support systems. Some spoke excitedly about ways they could succeed (e.g., job and training opportunities) and identified greater support networks as missing links. Others expressed helplessness in the face of societal stresses. Because they felt little trust for each other, community bonds were not developed. Despite their common experience, they were not a cohesive group.

Developmental. The youngest person was in her late twenties, and the oldest was in her sixties. Many had never learned to trust, and others were very manipulative in their attempts to manage the system. The general physiological development of the women appeared normal.

Spiritual. All of the group members exhibited high-intensity spiritual beliefs and evidence of religiosity or superstition. They said that certain good behaviors would be rewarded by a "greater force" that "looked out for them."

Neuman's Assessment Questions

When asked what they saw as their greatest problem, the women agreed that it was "having no permanent place to live" (Neuman, 1990, pp. 56-63). Many said it was "being without a job" (Neuman, 1990, pp. 56-63). A few spoke of the lack of "safe spaces" and "the gentrification of the city's North End" that had reduced the number of available low-income dwelling spaces (Neuman, 1990, pp. 56-63). Several complained about their inability to stay clean, about "dirt," and about "bingeing" whenever food or drink was available (Neuman, 1990, pp. 56-63).

Homelessness confronts nurses with what appear to be insurmountable problems. Applying Neuman's model helps the nurse obtain a clearer picture of the mountain to be tackled and guides the nurse to develop a clearer comprehension of where to begin to overcome the problems.

Organization of Data

While assisting at the shelter, the nurse realized that although the ultimate objective of the staff and the clients is to assist the women with finding jobs and making the transition from the shelter into permanent housing, other problems interfere with this long-term goal. Many of these problems require nursing action. Organizing the data according to the Neuman model helps prioritize those problems according to the client's needs and identify shorter-term goals to help them solve their problems.

Table 11-3 presents the stressors of these women according to their intrapersonal, interpersonal, and extrapersonal nature.

The comprehensive diagnosis is disenfranchisement from society, as expressed by homelessness.

Problem List

1. Individual physical problems
2. Generalized low self-esteem and lack of trust
3. Depression, fear
4. Residual mental health problems related to history of abuse
5. Lack of education and job skills
6. Lack of job training opportunities

Reflection on Data

Long-term goals

1. Rehabilitate and house all those who can be rehabilitated
2. Find jobs for those who can work
3. Find resolution in a permanent sheltered situation for those who cannot work

TABLE 11-3   Stressors of Aggregate Client of Homeless Women

Stressors	Intrapersonal	Interpersonal	Extrapersonal

Physiological	Malnutrition
	High blood
	  pressure
	HIV, TB, STDs, AIDS,
	  diabetes
	Hygiene, skin
	  problems
		HIV, TB, AIDS, STDs
		Hygiene
			Malnutrition
			TB

Psychological	Abuse (residual and actual) Fear Depression Lack of trust Low self-esteem	Abuse Depression Lack of trust Fear of people	Lack of trust Fear of society

Sociocultural	Lack of trust
	Lack of skills
		Lack of support
		Inability to trust those
		  who try to help
			Lack of support
			  sytems
			Society's cruelty
			Lack of job training
			  and opportunities
			  to develop skills
			No money

Developmental	Lack of trust
	Absence of self-
	  esteem
	Lack of responsibility
		Lack of trust
		Absence of self-
		  esteem
			Lack of trust in
			  homeless
			Absence of self-
			  esteem
			Failure in society

Spiritual	Fear of life and
	  society
		Common belief in
		  "something"
		Superstitious
			Inability to profit
			  from religion
			  because of lack
			  of trust of society

TB, tuberculosis; *STDs,* sexually transmitted disease.

The long-term goals for the group were identified by the nurse after synthesizing and analyzing the data. When these goals were presented to the women, they agreed that the long-term goals would meet their needs and were listed in the correct order of importance. As in all nursing process approaches, Neuman suggests breaking long-term goals into shorter-term objectives that facilitate the achievement of the end goal and should incorporate the nursing process, utilizing nursing diagnosis, nursing goals, and nursing outcomes (Neuman, 1990).

Those who work with the urban homeless are acutely aware of the low measure of success their clients generally experience. Many of the problems are virtually intractable, and few respond to short-term intervention. Nevertheless, short-term goals provide a measure of hope for achieving success. The following short-term goals were formulated for this group of urban homeless women:

Short-term goals
1. Improve the physical health of each woman
2. Increase self-esteem in all clients
3. Reduce fear
4. Increase skills
5. Assist in the job search
6. Provide long-term mental health counseling
7. Find training for clients

Working with this particular client group provides a clear example of the necessity of approaching the task from a wholistic perspective. For example, without a reasonable measure of physical well-being, interventions will not help the women increase their self-esteem or reduce their fear of vulnerability. Likewise, unless they are reasonably well, there is little chance that they will be able to learn new skills or take up the challenge of a job search. Unless long-term mental health counseling is available, the women who are short on self-confidence will have difficulty believing in success or believing that anyone will give them a new opportunity to learn and succeed. The disenfranchisement from society experienced by this group of women and the odds they face require simple, open approaches.

Sharing the initial assessment material with this group required an educative posture. First, the women needed assistance to understand the following facts about the process of rehabilitation: (1) it is slow; (2) it demands work on some aspects of self and society to accomplish the long-term goals; (3) the shelter staff and volunteers want to help in the process; and (4) they also must participate in the process.

The women were asked whether they agreed with the problem list and whether they could see that their first priority might require a short-term goal of increased physical and psychological strength. A general consensus was reached, and the discussion proceeded to short-term goals. The details for a contract were drawn up. In order to achieve these short-term goals with and for the client, the nurse must intervene by applying all three levels of prevention.

The improvement of each woman's physical health stabilizes the core by using tertiary prevention. As physical health improves, secondary prevention is brought to bear on the psychological and sociocultural deficits, which improves the women's chances of getting off the street. New types of skills and education for jobs and survival success in the real world (primary prevention) are eventually added, and constant tertiary and secondary interventions based on ongoing reassessment are tailored according to individual need.

Recognition that the women are buffeted by intrapersonal, interpersonal, and extrapersonal stressors that create total vulnerability, leads to interventions that contribute to an occasional success story. Some of the women increase their trust levels sufficiently to the point that they believe in the good intentions of the people who assist them and in the shared experience of their peers.

Synthesis and Analysis of Data

When the short-term goals and interventions are clear, the client is asked how and in what way she would contract to work on self with assistance from the nurse. The plan of care is a "working with the client" plan; therefore if the client has reasonable ideas of other ways to meet goals, the plan is renegotiated until the client can commit herself to a plan or to part of it (Table 11-4). Owning the plan helps the client achieve the short-term goals.

TABLE 11-4 Plan of Care for Homeless Urban Women Applying the Neuman Approach	
Nurse	**Women**
1. Make appointments for doctor's care for each person.	Support each other in keeping appointments.
2. Arrange for beautician for hair care and hand care.	Keep appointments. Support each other in doing so.
3. Conduct group therapy directed at increasing self-esteem.	Attend group. Acknowledge each other's successes.
4. Provide foot care (nurse and students).	Request foot care.
5. Obtain women's commitment to stay drug- and alcohol-free while in shelter.	Provide support for these efforts.
6. Provide education on communicable diseases.	Attend classes.
7. Investigate skills training and/or job training or schooling possibilities for client.	Accept opportunities as possible.
8. Assist in job finding and house search.	Believe in possibility of success.
9. Provide (with staff) opportunities for fun.	Participate.
10. Commit self as long-term care provider at the shelter.	Acknowledge commitment.
11. Lobby for needed programs and opportunities.	Participate if possible.

Each intervention is evaluated for effectiveness at each contact. If the elements of the plan are failing, they need to be discussed and renegotiated until a working plan is constructed.

Actual proof of the effectiveness of the plan and intervention is reaching the long-term goal—in this case, permanent housing and job placement for the client. Needless to say, rehabilitation of homeless women with such complex histories and problems requires long-term effort and commitment. Some of the women will succeed; some will succeed and relapse; some will need permanent shelter in mental health facilities; and some will choose to live permanently on the streets, returning to the shelter for respite from time to time.

There is no question that the flexible and comprehensive nature of the Neuman model assists in visualizing, organizing, planning, and delivering the complex care needs of the client. The assessment of the five client variables and organization of the data as intrapersonal, interpersonal, or extrapersonal stressors offer a clear picture of the challenges facing the homeless women at the shelter and provide the information to develop a plan of care to reconstitute their personal health and strengthen their protective mechanisms.

CRITICAL THINKING EXERCISES

1. Conduct a Neuman assessment on a friend by using the five variables, and determine the stressors. Use observational, clinical, and cognitive skills. Evaluate client experiential background and strengths.
2. Organize the data into a meaningful, wholistic picture, and generate a stressor list, identifying the nature of each stressor.
3. Develop a primary diagnosis and a differential or alternative diagnosis, and discuss it with your friend.
4. Take the nursing care plan and from a patient for whom you have previously cared. Sort the data from the plan according to the five client variables of Neuman's model; classify the stressors as intrapersonal, interpersonal, or extrapersonal; and develop a comprehensive diagnosis.
5. Using the case history of Debbie and the Neuman Systems Model, identify and classify the stressors for her children and her husband.
6. Think back to the last time you became ill. Develop an assessment of yourself at that time according to the five client variables. Sort the stressors as intrapersonal, interpersonal, and extrapersonal to explore how your stressors may have contributed to lowered resistance.

References

Barker, E., Robinson, D., & Brautigan, R. (1999). The effect of psychiatric home nurse follow-up on readmission rates of patients with depression. *Journal of the American Psychiatric Nurses Association, 5,* 111-116.

Breckenridge, D. M. (1997). Decisions regarding dialysis treatment modality: A holistic perspective. *Holistic Nursing Practice, 12,* 54-61.

Carrigg, K. C. & Weber, R. (1997). Development of the Spiritual Care Scale. *Image, 29,* 293.

Flannery, J. (1995). Cognitive assessment in the acute care setting: Reliability and validity of the Levels of Cognitive Functioning Assessment Scale (LOCFAS). *Journal of Nursing Measurement, 3,* 43-58.

Gigliotti, E. (1999). Women's multiple role stress: Testing Neuman's flexible line of defense. *Nursing Science Quarterly, 12,* 36-44.

Hanson, M. J. (1999). Crosscultural study of beliefs about smoking among teenaged females. *Western Journal of Nursing Research, 21,* 635-651.

Hassell, J. S. (1996). Improved management of depression through nursing model application and critical thinking. *Journal of the American Academy of Nurse Practitioners, 8,* 161-166.

Lowry, L. W., Saeger, J., & Barnett, S. (1997). Client satisfaction with prenatal care and pregnancy outcomes. *Outcomes Management for Nursing Practice, 1,* 29-35.

Martin, S. A. (1996). Applying nursing theory to the practice of nurse anesthesia. *ANNA Journal, 64,* 369-372.

Martsolf, D. S. & Mickley, J. R. (1998). The concept of spirituality in nursing theories: Differing worldviews and extent of focus. *Journal of Advanced Nursing, 27,* 294-303.

McHolm, F. A. & Geib, K. M. (1998). Application of the Neuman Systems Model to teaching health assessment and nursing process. *Nursing Diagnosis, 9,* 23-33.

Mill, J. E. (1997). The Neuman Systems Model: Application in a Canadian HIV setting. *British Journal of Nursing, 6,* 163-166.

Molassiotis, A. (1997). A conceptual model of adaptation to illness and quality of life for cancer patients treated with bone marrow transplants. *Journal of Advanced Nursing, 26,* 572-579.

Narsavage, G. L. (1997). Promoting function in clients with chronic lung disease by increasing their perception of control. *Holistic Nursing Practice, 12,* 17-26.

Neuman, B. (1974). The Betty Neuman health-care systems model: A total person approach to patient problems. In J. P. Riehl & C. Roy (Eds.), *Conceptual models for nursing practice* (pp. 99-114). Norwalk, CT: Appleton-Century-Crofts.

Neuman, B. (1980). The Betty Neuman health-care systems model: A total person approach to patient problems. In J. P. Riehl & C. Roy (Eds.), *Conceptual models for nursing practice* (2nd ed., pp. 119-134). Norwalk, CT: Appleton-Century-Crofts.

Neuman, B. (1982). *The Neuman Systems Model: Application to nursing education and practice.* Norwalk, CT: Appleton-Century-Crofts.

Neuman, B. (1989a). *The Neuman Systems Model.* Norwalk, CT: Appleton & Lange.

Neuman, B. (1989b). The Neuman nursing process format: Family. In J. Riehl-Sisca (Ed.), *Conceptual models for nursing practice* (3rd ed., pp. 49-62). Norwalk, CT: Appleton & Lange.

Neuman, B. (1990). Health on a continuum based on the Neuman Systems Model. *Nursing Science Quarterly, 3*(3), 129-135.

Neuman, B. (1995). *The Neuman Systems Model* (3rd ed.). Norwalk, CT: Appleton & Lange.

Neuman, B. (1996). The Neuman Systems Model in research and practice. *Nursing Science Quarterly, 9,* 67-70.

Neuman, B. & Koertvelyessey, A. (1986). *The Neuman Systems Model and nursing research.* Paper presented at Nursing Theory Congress, Ryerson School of Nursing, Toronto, Ontario, Canada.

Neuman, B. M. & Martin, K. S. (1998). Neuman Systems Model and the Omaha System. *Image, 30,* 8.

Neuman, B. & Young, R. J. (1972). A model for teaching a total person approach to viewing patient problems. *Nursing Research, 21*(3), 264-269.

Sabo, C. E. & Michael, S. R. (1996). The influence of personal message with music on anxiety and side effects associated with chemotherapy. *Cancer Nursing, 19,* 283-289.

Selye, H. (1950). The physiology and pathology of exposure to stress. *ACTA,* 12-13.

Sohier, R. (1995). Nursing care for the people of a small planet. In B. Neuman (Ed.), *The Neuman Systems Model* (pp. 101-117). Norwalk, CT: Appleton & Lange.

Taggart, L. & Mattson, S. (1996). Delay in prenatal care as a result of battering in pregnancy: Crosscultural implications. *Health Care for Women International, 17,* 25-34.

von Bertalanffy, L. (1968). *General system theory.* New York: Braziller.

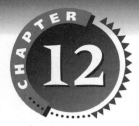

Orem's Self-Care Deficit Nursing Theory in Practice

Violeta A. Berbiglia

"Nurses work in life situations with others to bring about conditions that are beneficial to persons nursed. Nursing demands the exercise of both the speculative and practical intelligence of nurses. In nursing practice situations, nurses must have accurate information and be knowing about existent conditions and circumstances of patients and about emerging changes in them. This knowledge is the concrete base for nurses' development of creative practical insights about what can be done to bring about beneficial relationships or conditions that do not presently exist. Asking and answering the questions 'what is?' and 'what can be?' are nurses' points of departure in nursing practice situations." (Orem, 1995)

HISTORY AND BACKGROUND

The Self-Care Deficit Nursing Theory (SCDNT) is one of the nursing theories most commonly used in practice. Orem's dedication to the concept of self-care resulted in a nursing theory appropriate for present and future healthcare scenes. The earliest development of the theory occurred in 1956 (Orem, 1985). Orem's purpose was to define the following: (1) nursing's concern—"man's need for self-care action and the provision and management of it on a continuous basis in order to sustain life and health, recover from disease or injury, and cope with their

The author wishes to thank Irma Lopez, B.S.N., R.N., who assisted with data collection and nursing system design for the case of Ms. Davila.

effects" (Orem, 1959, p. 3) and (2) nursing's goal—"overcoming human limitations" (Orem, 1959, p. 4).

The concept of self-care evolved into a theory as Orem and colleagues discussed and formulated the concept into a working description of nursing. Orem's model supports nursing through the following three central theories:

1. Nursing is required because of the inability to perform self-care as the result of limitations (Theory of Self-Care Deficit).
2. Maturing or mature adults deliberately learn and perform actions to direct their survival, quality of life, and well-being (Theory of Self-Care).
3. The product of nursing is nursing system(s) by which nurses use the nursing process to help individuals meet their self-care requisites and build their self-care or dependent-care capabilities (Theory of Nursing Systems).

The significance of the utilization of Orem's model in practice has been explicit since the publication of the first edition of *Nursing: Concepts of Practice* (Orem, 1971). Early use of the theory in practice began with the work of the Nursing Development Conference Group (NDCG) (1973). The group initiated their adventure into theory-based practice by integrating the developing concepts of the model into their clinical teaching of students. As the conceptualizations evolved, they were incorporated into nursing care.

The reality of nursing was further addressed by NDCG members who were in positions in which they could assert control on nursing systems (Allison, 1973; Backscheider, 1971). Members of the NDCG valued their work in practice settings for supporting their conceptualizations and revealing the importance of the broad conceptualizations to structure practice. The Center for Experimentation and Development in Nursing at Johns Hopkins Hospital was one of the early sites for the development of the theory through practice. Later, in 1976, Allison (1989) implemented SCDNT-based practice in the Mississippi Methodist Hospital and Rehabilitation Center.

Gradually, theory development in the practice arena began to filter into a variety of practice settings. Selected practice strategies are shown in Table 12-1. Patient education was addressed by Goodwin's programmed instruction for self-care in postsurgical patients (1979). Graduate students at the University of Texas ventured out to implement the SCDNT in extended-care services and found that the self-care concept was growth-producing for the nurses and the patients and showed the potential for cost-effectiveness (Anna, Christensen, Hohon, Ord, & Wells, 1978). Underwood (1980) brought the concept of self-care into the area of psychiatric nursing.

TABLE 12-1   Utilization of Orem's Model in Selected Practice Settings

Author	Practice Setting	Conceptual Focus
Allison, 1973	Diabetic clinic	Nurse action
Allison, 1989	Rehabilitation hospital	Self-care agency
		Dependent-care agency
		Therapeutic self-care demand
Anna, Christensen, Hohon, Ord, & Wells, 1978	Administration	Self-care
Backscheider, 1971	Ambulatory care	Nursing system
Buckwalter & Kerfoot, 1982	Psychiatry	Self-care
Crumbley, Ice, & Cassidy, 1999	Nurse-managed wound clinic	Nursing system
Furlong, 1996	Inpatient cardiac unit	Self-care
Hildebrandt, 1996	Public health	Self-care
		Nursing system
Intarasombat, 1995	Hospital	Dependent-care
Marz, 1989	Public health	Nursing situation
Norris, 1991	Transplant outpatient service	Nursing system
Taylor & McLaughlin, 1991	Community	Multiperson situations
Taylor & Renpenning, 1995	Community	Multiperson situations
Taylor & Robinson Purdy, 1989	Hospital discharge protocol	Self-care
		Dependent-care
Underwood, 1980	Psychiatric unit	Self-care
Walborn, 1980	Hospice	Nursing system
Walker, 1986	Nursing administration	Nursing system
Weis, 1988	Cooperative care unit	Self-care
		Dependent-care
Whitener, Cox, & Maglich, 1998	Public school	Foundational capabilities

The literature of the 1980s reveals numerous efforts that further established the SCDNT in practice. This was a time when the theory was being explicated for use with specific nursing situations and in varying types of practice settings. The efforts that focused on nursing situations often centered on how patients managed illness through self-care (Dodd, 1982, 1983; Kubricht, 1984; Whelan, 1984). SCDNT-guided practice began to thrive in many settings, including the following:

- *Hospice*—implementation of primary-care and self-care nursing (Walborn, 1980)
- *Public health departments*—administration and delivery of care (Walker, 1986; Marz, 1989)
- *Rehabilitation center*—evaluation of patient outcome (Allison, 1989)
- *Cooperative care unit*—fostering of maximum self-care in acute-care patients (Weis, 1988)

SCDNT-guided practice continues to abound in a variety of settings and situations. Discharge protocols for self-care and dependent-care (Taylor & Robinson Purdy, 1989) and for specific populations such as the elderly (Kennedy, 1990) have been designed. Steel and Sterling (1992) recommended helping method-specific interventions that are conducive to discharge readiness. Prescriptions for specialized practice—such as transplant nursing (Norris, 1991) and for the provision of culturally-sensitive care (Howard & Berbiglia, 1997)—are appearing. The trend toward community-based practice has been supported by further explication of the SCDNT for use with multiperson units (i.e., community and family) (Taylor & McLaughlin, 1991), interdisciplinary care systems (Taylor & Renpenning, 1995), and community-based case management (Holzemer, 1992). More recent reports on utilization of SCDNT reveal an emphasis on practice and model/theory development.

Several practice-focused articles portrayed the value of SCDNT-based practice. Furlong's phenomenological perspective (1996) of the rationales for adopting and applying the self-care philosophy in an inpatient unit indicated that the approach evolved through patient need. The practice of self-care on the unit seemed to center around four patient themes: patient control, involvement, dignity, and coping. Hart's assessment of self-care in pregnancy revealed that strengthening self-care agency through prenatal care produced more positive outcomes in infant birth weight and maternal hemoglobin levels (1996). Renker (1999) studied the effects of physical abuse, social support, and self-care on pregnancy outcomes of older adolescents. The SCDNT-related predictors of infant birth weight were self-care agency, self-care practice, and two basic conditioning factors. Freston, Young, Calhoun, Fredericksen, Salinger, Malchodi, and Egan (1997) assessed the knowledge base of healthy preterm pregnant women concerning appropriate actions to take for symptoms of preterm labor and stated nursing implications for helping women to increase their knowledge base.

Recent intervention studies centered on cancer care. An informative videotape was developed to prepare women for receiving chemotherapy for breast cancer by assisting them in the development of anticipatory coping and self-care behaviors (McDaniel & Rhodes, 1998). Another study assessed subjects by using the Exercise of Self-Care (ESCA) Scale. Findings showed that subjects with higher ESCA scores used more self-care measures to alleviate side effects of chemotherapy, whereas the intervention (multiple phone calls and oral and written messages) did not increase the use or effectiveness of self-care measures (Craddock, Adams, Usui, & Mitchell, 1999). Another study measured the effect of a structured intervention for applying the self-care model to ambulatory cancer patients receiving chemotherapy or radiation therapy (Benor, Delbar, & Krulik, 1998). Results suggested that the self-care approach was effective in improving quality of life of unstable cancer patients through the reduction of suffering and increase in controlling capabilities.

A nurse-managed ambulatory clinic successfully applied nurse case management in caring for chronic and complex wounds by combining the process of case management with the philosophy of self-care (Crumbley, Ice, & Cassidy, 1999). Nursing case management was viewed on a continuum with the goal of bringing patients to self-care and healing wounds.

Reports of model/theory development feature the combining of the SCDNT with other models/theories as well as theory explication and verification studies. One example is the blending of cognitive development theories with selected foundational capabilities and dispositions from the SCDNT to isolate five concrete factors for design and delivery of health messages for children (Whitener, Cox, & Maglich, 1998). Another example is the SCDNT combined with the Self-Regulation Theory to provide the vehicle for assessing hospice patients' and nurses' perceptions of self-care deficits based on symptom experience. Ulbrich (1999) developed a theory of exercise through triangulation of the SCDNT, the transtheoretical model of exercise behavior, and characteristics of a population at risk for cardiovascular disease.

Orem's theory was tested with Mexican-Americans for the purpose of verifying the use of the SCDNT with diverse populations (Villarruel, 1997). Hartweg's study (1995) of African-American and Caucasian subjects was conducted to explicate the concept of health promotion self-care requisites. Subsequently, Hartweg and Berbiglia (1996) piloted the Health Promotion Self-Care Interview Guide to assess cultural sensitivity of the instrument in the Mexican-American population.

Lipson and Steiger (1996) published an informative book, *Self-Care Nursing in a Multicultural Context*. A reviewer of the text characterized the publication as "a successful attempt to examine and present the interface of two main components of nursing self-care and culturally competent care. A refreshing feature of the book is that it provides an integrative perspective based upon a wide-ranging analysis of self-care in relation to clinical practice in different settings" (Rassool, 1997, p. 859). In their 1999 book *Nursing Administration in the 21st Century: A Self-Care Theory Approach*, Allison and McLaughlin-Renpenning examined the changing nature of healthcare systems and implications for nursing. The authors discussed models of administration, population descriptions, administrative processes, nursing system designs, clinical documentation, and other adminstration-related factors.

The International Orem Society for Scholarship and Nursing Science (IOS) provides a continuing forum for the exchange of SCDNT practice models (Isenberg, 1993). A sampling of the practice models presented at the IOS's Fourth International Self-Care Deficit Nursing Theory

Conference revealed the structure that the SCDNT provides in innovative practices. In Germany, nurses are becoming proactive in their practices and are anticipating that the theory will assist in the transformation of nursing practice (Berbiglia & Bekel, 1995). In Thailand, family participation in patient care of the elderly is stimulated by the self-care framework (Intarasombat, 1995). In the United States, a clinic for homeless men uses Orem's five methods of helping to guide nursing practice (Martin, 1995). In some healthcare institutions, innovative computer programming has facilitated a blending of theory-based practice and information systems (Bliss-Holtz & Sayer, 1995; Riggs, 1995).

The Fifth International Self-Care Deficit Nursing Theory Conference featured the use of the SCDNT in practice, research, and education. Themes addressed in the sessions included the following: self-care and culture; developing nursing agency; teaching self-care nursing science; self-care and well-being; self-care of children and home health services; self-care agency of the elderly; self-care and pregnancy, childbearing; self-care and cancer; diabetes; self-care and cardiovascular disease; self-care and renal failure, chronic lung disease; self-care and family; integration of SCDNT in practice and management; instrumentation research; middle-range theories; and concept clarification (Fifth International Self-Care Deficit Nursing Theory Conference Abstracts, 1997). A keynote address presented a systems theory model of collaboration and the role of the philosophical beliefs of the SCDNT in achieving connections in the healthcare paradigm of the new millennium (Sullivan, 1997). Isenberg and Evers described an "ongoing program of international collaborative research designed to advance nursing science derived from Self-Care Deficit Nursing Theory" (1997, p. 24).

The Sixth International Self-Care Deficit Nursing Theory Conference provided opportunities for exploring research, education, and practice from an SCDNT perspective as well as an assessment of the progress made through international collaboration (Sixth International Self-Care Deficit Nursing Theory Conference Abstracts, 2000). Thai representatives summarized their research accomplishments and the research agenda for the future (Hanucharurnkul, 2000) and presented the World Health Organization South-East Asia Regional Office goal for *Health for All and Self-Care* (Sungkalobol, 2000). Organizing themes for presentations were the following: measurement of self-care agency/meaning of self-care; education; outcomes; older adults/basic conditioning factors; HIV/AIDS; respiratory/cardiovascular; practice model development; culture; interventions; oncology; self-care/self-management; caregiver issues; child/adolescent; fatigue; action research; and self-care behaviors/diabetes mellitus (Sixth International Self-Care Deficit Nursing Theory Conference Abstracts, 2000).

This review of the role the SCDNT plays in practice demonstrates its versatility. A product of the post–World War II period, the theory continues into the new millennium as a guidepost for the profession. The timelessness of Orem's theory, its practical approach, and the utility of the theory in decision making are essential to practice.

OVERVIEW OF OREM'S SELF-CARE DEFICIT NURSING THEORY

Nursing practice oriented by the SCDNT represents a caring approach that uses experiential and specialized knowledge (science) to design and produce nursing care (art). The body of knowledge that guides the art and science incorporates empirical and antecedent knowledge (Orem, 1995). Empirical knowledge is rooted in experience and addresses specific events and related conditions that have relevance for health and well-being. It is empirical knowledge that supports observations, interpretations of the meaning of those observations, and correlations of the meaning with potential courses of action. Antecedent knowledge includes previously mastered knowledge and identified fields of knowledge, conditions, and situations.

Orem (1995) identified eight fields of knowledge essential for understanding nursing practice. Seven of those emanate from previously developed fields of knowledge found in the sciences and other disciplines, including sociology, profession/occupation, jurisprudence, history, ethics, economics, and administration. The eighth, nursing science, is knowledge about nursing practice created by nurses through scientific investigations that yield an understanding of the field of nursing and provide foundations for nursing practice. The practical science establishes essential content for courses focused on nursing practice. Personal knowledge of self and the other provides a screen through which input about the other is objectified. Insights gained facilitate a reality orientation to self and the other and contribute to the "giving" characteristics of nursing: care, responsibility, and respect.

Practice knowledge is systematized, validated, and conducive to dynamic processes. Dynamic knowledge leads the user to acceptance and owning of the theory (Orem, 1988). Allison (1988) noted the dynamic quality of the theory and commented that the SCDNT always keeps the nurse in an action mode. Orem (1988) emphasized that today's nurses must be scholars within the developing theory. In doing so, nurses are committed to an awareness of the relationship between what they know and what they do. From this awareness comes a healthy sense of professionalism.

Awareness is heightened by access to and ascription to nursing knowledge. Orem (1995) referred to two categories of knowledge in practical science: speculatively practical knowledge and practically practical knowledge. She indicated that the theories and conceptual elements of the SCDNT are in the speculative category, whereas the practically practical knowledge is more particularized. It is knowledge that prepares one to practice. Practically practical knowledge framed within the SCDNT prepares one to practice by organizing knowledge necessary for practice in accordance with actions and outcome.

CRITICAL THINKING IN NURSING PRACTICE WITH OREM'S THEORY

SCDNT-based critical thinking emanates from four structured cognitive operations: diagnostic, prescriptive, regulatory, and control. Each operation fulfills a distinct phase in the use of the theory. Sequencing of the phases may vary throughout the process in order to reassess and continue to prescribe and regulate the nursing system for the best interest of self-care. The operations are intended to be collaborative and to provide the self-care agent or dependent-care agent input into the decision making. Examples of the four cognitive operations are found in this chapter's discussion of the nursing care for two clients. Table 12-2 outlines the critical thinking requirements for SCDNT-based decision making. Critical thinking exercises are featured at the end of this chapter.

Diagnostic Operations

The first phase, diagnostic operations (see Table 12-2), begins with establishing the nurse-client relationship and proceeds to contracting to work toward identifying and discussing current and potential therapeutic self-care demands. Basic conditioning factors are noted and considered in relationship to a thorough review of universal, developmental, and health deviation self-care requisites and related self-care actions. The projected value of requisites is estimated. An analysis of the assessment data results in a diagnosis concerning the type of self-care demands. Self-care agency is addressed through an assessment of self-care practices and the effects of related limitations and abilities. Personal characteristics such as intellect, skill performance, and willingness are evaluated. From these data, inferences about the adequacy and potential of self-care agency are made, validated, and treated as diagnostic of self-care agency. Finally, self-care deficits are diagnosed by reflecting on the adequacy of agency to meet specific requisites. In instances in which self-care agency is inadequate, a self-care deficit is stated.

Prescriptive Operations

In the prescriptive phase, ideal therapeutic self-care requisites for each self-care requisite are determined by reviewing possible helping methods, considering related basic conditioning factors, and identifying the most

TABLE 12-2   Critical Thinking with Orem

DIAGNOSTIC OPERATIONS

Establish therapeutic relationship	Enter into and maintain relationship
	Contract to collaborate in identifying and analyzing existing/potential therapeutic self-care demands
	Assess for basic conditioning factors
	Review existing/projected universal, developmental, and health deviation requisites
	Estimate value and expected changes in value of each requisite
	Consider interaction between basic conditioning factors and requisites
	Identify and describe self-care practices
	State specific limitations and abilities related to practices
	Make inferences about effect of limitations and abilities on engaging in self-care
	Validate inferences through continued observation
	Determine adequacy of knowledge, skills, and willingness to meet therapeutic self-care demands
	Estimate potential for development of self-care agency
Diagnose self-care deficits (existing or projected)	Make judgments about degree of ability to provide self-care
	Inform client of presence or absence of self-care deficit

PRESCRIPTIVE OPERATIONS

Calculate ideal therapeutic self-care demand	Review possible helping methods
	Consider validity and reliability of each method in relationship to basic conditioning factors
	Identify most appropriate methods
	Review identified methods with client/family
	Explain to client/family the sets and sequences of actions required for selected methods
Design therapeutic self-care demands	Consider time-specific relationships between requisites, economy of time and effort, and compatibility with personal and family life
	Plan for adjustment in design as requisites change or new requisites emerge
Prioritize therapeutic self-care demands	Prioritize in this order:
	First: Those essential for life processes
	Second: Those that prevent personal harm/injury or health deterioration
	Third: Those that maintain or promote health
	Fourth: Those that contribute to well-being
Prescribe client role and nurse role	Identify what client should do, should not do, and is willing to do
	Determine potential for continued development of self-care agency

Continued

TABLE 12-2   Critical Thinking with Orem—cont'd

REGULATORY OPERATIONS

Design regulatory nursing system for prescribed therapeutic self-care demands	Take into consideration the basic conditioning factors of age, developmental state, health state, and healthcare system
	Provide for effective regulation of health and developmental state by setting forth relationships among components of therapeutic self-care demands
	Specify timing, amount of nurse-client contact, and reasons for contact
	Identify actions of nurse, client, and others
	Take into consideration positive or negative cooperation
Plan for regulatory operations	Set forth the organization and timing of essential tasks/roles responsibilities
	Specify time, place, environmental conditions, equipment/supplies, and type and number of personnel necessary
Production of regulatory care	Perform and regulate self-care tasks or assist client in performing self-care tasks
	Coordinate self-care task performance
	Bring about accomplishment of self-care that is satisfying to client
	Guide, direct, and support client in exercise of self-care agency
	Stimulate client interest in self-care
	Support and guide client learning
	Support and guide client through experiences in meeting ongoing self-care requisites
	Monitor and assist client to monitor self in self-care measures

CONTROL OPERATIONS

Observe and appraise regulatory operations	Make judgments about quantity and quality of self-care, development of self-care agency, and nursing assistance
	Judge effect of measures on well-being of client
	Make or recommend adjustments in nursing care system
	Determine whether:
	Regulatory operations are performed according to nursing system design
	Operations are in accord with client condition and environment for which they were prescribed
	Operations are still valid
	Regulation of client functioning has been achieved
	Developmental change is in progress and is adequate
	Client is adjusting to any decline in self-care ability

appropriate helping methods. Actions required to meet the therapeutic self-care demands are discussed with the client and are designed for maximum efficiency and compatibility. Priority is given to those therapeutic self-care demands that are the most essential to physiological processes. Client and nurse expectations are formalized and recognized as supportive of continued development of self-care agency.

Regulatory Operations

The prescriptions that evolve are used in the regulatory phase to design, plan, and produce the regulatory nursing system. Factors entering into decisions about design include basic conditioning factors, effective regulation of health and developmental state, timing, assignment of actions, and degree of cooperation. Further planning specifies conditions for the regulatory operations such as frequency, equipment/supplies, and personnel needed. Throughout the production of regulatory care, there is a strong emphasis on development of self-care agency by using helping methods that encourage learning, increase feelings of well-being, and stimulate interest in self-care.

Control Operations

Evaluation occurs in the control phase. The effectiveness of regulatory operations and client outcome is estimated. Regulatory operations are evaluated for correctness and appropriateness. Client outcome is appraised for regulation of functioning, developmental change, and adjustments to varying levels of self-care ability.

CASE HISTORY OF DEBBIE

Debbie is a 29-year-old woman who was recently admitted to the oncology nursing unit for evaluation after sensing pelvic "fullness" and noticing a watery, foul-smelling vaginal discharge. A Papanicolaou smear revealed class V cervical cancer. She was found to have a stage II squamous cell carcinoma of the cervix and underwent a radical hysterectomy with bilateral salpingooophorectomy.

Her past health history revealed that physical examinations had been infrequent. She also reported that she had not performed breast self-examination. She is 5 feet, 4 inches tall and weights 89 pounds. Her usual weight is about 110 pounds. She has smoked approximately two packs of cigarettes a day for the past 16 years. She is gravida 2, para 2. Her first pregnancy was at age 16, and her second was at age 18. Since that time, she has taken oral contraceptives on a regular basis.

Debbie completed the eighth grade. She is married and lives with her husband and her two children in her mother's home, which she describes as less than sanitary. Her husband is unemployed. She describes him as emotionally distant and abusive at times.

> She has done well following surgery except for being unable to completely empty her urinary bladder. She is having continued postoperative pain and nausea. It will be necessary for her to perform intermittent self-catheterization at home. Her medications are (1) an antibiotic, (2) an analgesic as needed for pain, and (3) an antiemetic as needed for nausea. In addition, she will be receiving radiation therapy on an outpatient basis.
>
> Debbie is extremely tearful. She expresses great concern over her future and the future of her two children. She believes that this illness is a punishment for her past life.

NURSING CARE OF DEBBIE WITH OREM'S THEORY
Goal for Theoretical Guidance

The goal for the application of the SCDNT to the care of Debbie is to prescribe the type of nursing system appropriate to meet Debbie's self-care requisites. The system designed should provide the optimum effect in the achievement of regulation of Debbie's self-care agency and meeting of her therapeutic self-care demands. A revised version of Laschinger's data collection and nursing system design tool (1990) is used for data analysis and critical thinking.

Diagnostic and Prescriptive Operations

Table 12-3 places the data from Debbie's case into the SCDNT framework. A review of Debbie's basic conditioning factors, shown in section A of Table 12-3, reveals a young woman caught up in what Sheehy (1976) calls "Age 30 passage," a time to claim full adult status in society (p. 175). However, Debbie is lacking the characteristics necessary for the transition. The effects of early sociocultural factors (limited education, teenage pregnancies) are compounded by adult experiences: an insecure, intergenerational family system of limited resources living in the the unacceptable environment of Debbie's mother's home. Debbie's past history and her present illness represent negative influences that impinge on her universal, developmental, and health deviation requisites. Essential universal self-care requisites (air, prevention of hazards, and prevention of harm), shown in section B of Table 12-3, have been threatened by a history of smoking, inadequate relationships, and psychological dependency. Her advanced stage of cancer and recent surgery have taken their toll, both physiologically and psychologically. In section C of Table 12-3, it is clear that Debbie's failure to meet developmental self-care requisites places her at risk. The health deviation self-care requisites reflected in section D of Table 12-3 represent requisites influenced by Debbie's basic

TABLE 12-3 Data Collection for Debbie

A. Basic Conditioning Factors

Age (years)	Gender	Developmental State	Health State	Sociocultural Orientation	Healthcare System	Family System	Patterns of Living	Environment	Resources
29	Female	Early adult-hood 30s transition	Acute phase of chronic illness	8th grade education Teenage pregnancies No work	Diagnosis Surgery Treatment Plan	Married Children at home (2)	Lives at mother's home	Unclean	Extremely limited Husband out of work

B. Universal Self-Care Requisites

Air	Water	Food	Elimination
730 pack/year smoking history	No restrictions	No restrictions Weight: 89 lb Weight loss (19%) Nauseated Phenergan (25 mg per rectum prn nausea)	Urinary retention Intermittent self-catheterization

Activity/Rest	Solitude/Social Interaction	Prevention of Hazards	Promotion of Normalcy
Pain, nausea Percocet (1-2 tabs qd)	Tearful Expresses concerns	Husband abusive Keflex (500 mg po qid)	Dissatisfied with home environment Dependent on mother Radiation therapy

Continued

TABLE 12-3   Data Collection for Debbie—cont'd

C. Developmental Self-Care Requisities

Maintenance of Developmental Environment	Prevention/Management of Conditions Threatening Normal Development
Teenage pregnancies (2)	No breast self-examinations
Oral contraceptives for 10 years	Infrequent physical examinations
Dependent on mother	No hormone replacement therapy
Husband emotionally distant	Educational deprivation
	Poor health
	Oppressive living conditions

D. Health Deviation Self-Care Requisites

Seeking Medical Assistance When Health Status Altered	Awareness/Management of Disease Process
Seeks medical attention infrequently for overt symptoms	Aware of disease
	No evidence of ability to understand/manage effects

Adherence to Medical Regimen	Awareness of Potential Problems Associated with Regimen
Will perform intermittent self-catheterization	No awareness of need for hormone replacement therapy
Will receive radiation therapy	No awareness of radiation side effects

Modification of Self-Image to Incorporate Changes in Health Status	Adjustment of Lifestyle to Accommodate Changes in Health Status and Medical Regimen
Views illness as punishment for past life	Concerned for future of self and children

conditioning factors and developmental self-care requisites. Limited resources, developmental threats, and weak self-care agency surface in Debbie's own awareness/perception of her health deviation self-care requisites. She is expected to perform self-care and undergo extensive treatment although she lacks the knowledge, skills, and psychological security to do so.

The nurse encounters Debbie 1 day before discharge and is plagued by the weak self-care agency shown in Debbie's healthcare history: early sexual activity, a 704 pack/year smoking habit, and a relative deficit in managing developmental self-care requisites. The goal is to make a difference in Debbie's self-care agency. Using sections B, C, and D of Table 12-3, the nurse quickly identified the therapeutic self-care demands and stated these demands in the nursing system design (Table 12-4) for discharge. There are four priority diagnoses that are indicated with asterisks (see Table 12-4) and are discussed here. First priority is given to the therapeutic self-care demands related to the following: (1) elimination (provide care for eliminative process), and (2) adherence to medical regimen (ensure adherence) because elimination is essential for life processes. Prevention of spousal abuse takes second priority in that it will prevent harm/injury. Lowest priority goes to the therapeutic self-care demand for modifying self-image. Although self-image is important, low priority is assigned to self-image–related therapeutic self-care demands because they involve only contributing to well-being.

Regulatory and Control Operations

The supportive-educative nursing system design was intended to return control to Debbie and ultimately to strengthen her self-care agency. The design was supportive-educative because the prescribed helping methods were designed to support—not compensate for—Debbie's self-care ability, primarily through teaching and guiding. The regulatory operations assisted Debbie to perform her self-care within a unified system of care. The support and guidance promoted her interest in self-care and brought her unexpected satisfaction with attainment of specific universal and health deviation self-care requisites. There was a possibility that a partly compensatory system would evolve if Debbie were unsuccessful in learning and performing intermittent self-catheterization and the nurse had to assume that action. However, control operations revealed effective regulations. For example, regulatory operations for intermittent self-catheterization provided for a self-catheterization every 8 hours until Debbie had less than 60 ml postvoid residual. A routine urinalysis revealed no evidence of urinary tract infection subsequent to the self-care actions.

TABLE 12-4   Nursing System Design for Debbie: Supportive-Educative

| Therapeutic Self-Care Demand | Diagnostic Operations | | Prescriptive Operations |
	Adequacy of Self-Care Agency	Nursing Diagnosis	Methods of Helping
AIR Maintain effective respiration	Inadequate	Potential for impaired respiratory status related to smoking	Guiding and directing
WATER At present, no problem	Adequate	Potential for fluid imbalance related to nausea	Teaching
FOOD Maintain sufficient food intake	Inadequate	Actual nutritional deficit related to nausea and cachexia of cancer	Providing physical support
ELIMINATION Provide care for eliminative process	Inadequate	Actual eliminative disturbance related to postoperative urinary retention*	Teaching
ACTIVITY/REST Maintain balance	Inadequate	Actual activity/rest imbalance related to pain and nausea	Providing physical and psychological support
SOLITUDE/SOCIAL INTERACTION Maintain balance	Inadequate	Potential for social isolation related to emotional distress and husband's distancing	Providing and maintaining environment that supports personal development
PREVENTION OF HAZARDS Prevent spouse abuse	Inadequate	Potential for personal injury related to abusive husband*	Guiding and directing
PROMOTION OF NORMALCY Improve living environment and lifestyle	Inadequate	Actual deficits in environment related to shared housing	Guiding and directing
MAINTAIN DEVELOPMENTAL ENVIRONMENT Support increased normalcy in environment	Inadequate	Actual delay in normal human development related to early parenthood dependence on mother, and level of education	Guiding and directing Providing psychological support
PREVENT/MANAGE DEVELOPMENTAL THREATS Manage/decrease threats by receiving appropriate therapy	Inadequate	Actual developmental deficit related to lifestyle and surgical loss of reproductive organs	Providing physical and psychological support

MAINTENANCE OF HEALTH STATUS Promote health	Inadequate	Potential for continued alterations in health status related to inadequate health-seeking behaviors, financial status, and knowledge deficits	Teaching Guiding and directing
AWARENESS/MANAGEMENT OF DISEASE PROCESS Develop understanding of disease effects and management	Inadequate	Potential for urinary tract infection related to intermittent self-catheterizations	Teaching Guiding and directing
ADHERENCE TO MEDICAL REGIMEN Ensure adherence	Inadequate	Potential for decreased adherence in self-catheterization and outpatient radiation therapy related to no apparent patient teaching*	Teaching
AWARENESS OF POTENTIAL PROBLEMS Understand treatment plan	Inadequate	Actual deficit in awareness of advisability of hormone replacement and management of radiation side effects related to no discharge planning	Teaching
MODIFY SELF-IMAGE TO INCORPORATE CHANGED HEALTH STATUS Adjust to loss of reproductive ability and develop healthy view of etiology of illness	Inadequate	Actual threats to self-image related to disease, treatment, and guilt feelings*	Providing psychological support
ADJUST LIFESTYLE TO ACCOMMODATE HEALTH STATUS CHANGES AND MEDICAL REGIMEN Plan for future	Inadequate	Actual self-deficit to planning for future needs related to resources	Guiding and directing

*Priority diagnosis.

CASE HISTORY OF MS. DAVILA

Ms. Davila, age 64, is under the care of a home health agency. Because of rheumatoid arthritis, she has been mostly homebound for 6 years. The home healthcare was begun at the time of her diagnosis with type II diabetes mellitus 3 years ago. She is pleased to report that she has never been hospitalized—even for the birth of her two children. Since age 50, she has had her share of health problems, including osteoporosis, intense arthritic pain and impaired mobility, diabetes, anemia, and a weight problem. Recent laboratory reports showed triglyceride 250 mg/dl, LDH 290, Hb_{A1} 15, and RBC 3.65. Her blood sugar tests are usually somewhat elevated, but her diabetes continues to be managed by diet alone. She is 5 feet tall and weighs 180 pounds. Weight has never been viewed as a liability in her Hispanic upbringing. Good times are always associated with eating.

Ms. Davila dropped out of school midway through high school to get married. Now, as a widow, she provides a home in the country for her son. Her daughter and grandchildren live in the nearby city. Although her husband left her a small retirement fund, she relies mostly on Social Security income and receives healthcare through Medicare.

Home care has met her needs well and has minimized expenses. Her largest bill each month is to the pharmacy for Darvocet N-100, calcium, and monthly vitamin B12 injections. She looks forward to the home health aide's assistance twice a day and to the weekly visit of the registered nurse. These visits are a source of social contact, which she rarely has anymore. (See Table 12-5).

NURSING CARE OF MS. DAVILA WITH OREM'S THEORY

A complete data collection compiled from Ms. Davila's agency records and a home visit is shown in Table 12-5. Section A of Table 12-5 reveals that Ms. Davila has limited resources, has changed her lifestyle to accommodate chronic health problems, and receives home healthcare. In Section B of Table 12-5, there are concerns for the universal self-care requisites of food (abnormal laboratory findings and nonadherence to diet) and activity/rest (pain and impaired mobility). Ms. Davila has become somewhat developmentally dependent (section C of Table 12-5). She requires assistance in food preparation, hygiene, and toileting. The relationship of her universal and developmental self-care requisites to her health deviation self-care requisites emerges clearly in section D of Table 12-5. Ms. Davila is nonadherent to her diet, has not modified her self-image to include dietary precautions, and seems to deny any diet-associated difficulties.

TABLE 12-5 Data Collection for Ms. Davila

A. Basic Conditioning Factors

Age (years)	Gender	Developmental State	Health State	Sociocultural Orientation	Healthcare System	Family System	Patterns of Living	Environment	Resources
64	Female	Ego integrity vs. despair	Disability due to health conditioning	10th grade education Hispanic	Home healthcare	Widow 1 son, 1 daughter, several grandchildren	Lives at home Son lives with her Leaves home only for physician appointments	Rural Items needed for ADLs in easy reach: shower chair and safety bars in bathroom, wheelchair ramp	Social Security income Medicare Son makes small contributions Refrigerator and pantry well supplied

B. Universal Self-Care Requisites

Air	Water	Food	Elimination
Breathes without difficulty Skin warm, dry Normal color for client	Fluid intake sufficient No edema Skin turgor normal for age	Triglyceride 250 mg/dl LDH 290 RBC 3.65 Hb_{A1} 15 2000-calorie ADA diet Does not adhere to diet Weight: 180 lb Height: 60 inches Calcium (1500 mg po qd) Vitamin B_{12} (IM q Monday) Blood sugar tests bid (usually between 90 and 120)	Voids without difficulty Last BM 4/20, normal

ADLs, activities of daily living; *LDH,* lactate dehydrogenase; *RBC,* red blood count; *ADA,* American Diabetes Association.

Continued

TABLE 12-5   Data Collection for Ms. Davila—cont'd

Activity/Rest	Solitude/Social Interaction	Prevention of Hazards	Promotion of Normalcy
Requires frequent rest periods due to pain with ambulation	Isolated—homebound and decreased mobility related to pain	Requires reminders	Has good relationship with son and daughter
Uses wheelchair at home	Communicates with daughter by phone frequently	Needs instructions on foot care	
Nalfon for joint pain (especially hands)	Home health aide present 2 ×/day	Prefers to walk barefooted	
Careless scheduling pain medication	Nurse visits once a week		
Pain not completely relieved			

C. Developmental Self-Care Requisites

Maintenance of Developmental Environment	Prevention/Management of Conditions Threatening Normal Development
Able to feed self once meals are prepared for her	Discusses condition and medical regimen with home health nurse and aide and family
Needs assistance bathing, grooming, toileting	

D. Health Deviation Self-Care Requisites

Reports to home health nurse any changes in conditions:	Aware of disease processes
blood glucose, pain, prescribed medications	Not compliant with diet or prevention of hazards

Adherence to Medical Regimen	Awareness of Potential Problems Associated with Regimen
Cooperates with medications	Aware of side effects of medications
Aware of medications and side effects	Appears to deny problems associated with nonadherence to diet
Aware of medical regimen	
Does not follow ADA diet well	

Modification of Self-Image to Incorporate Changes in Health Status	Adjustment of Lifestyle to Accommodate Changes in Health Status and Medical Regimen
Accepting of general health condition	Has adapted well to home healthcare services
Has adapted to limitations in mobility	
Has not been able to include healthy eating habits and weight loss in her self-image	

Diagnostic and Prescriptive Operations

Table 12-6 presents the nursing system design. All three priority diagnoses (denoted by asterisks) are classified as second priority because the therapeutic self-care demands are related to preventing health deterioration. In Ms. Davila's case, the SCDNT proposes a supportive-educative nursing system (with a partly compensatory component) that is designed to individualize her care. The individualization of the nursing system was accomplished through the overlay of basic conditioning factors and developmental self-care requisites (in sections A and C of Table 12-5) on the therapeutic self-care demands. The expected outcome is health status maintenance, health promotion, and prevention of further health deviations through strengthening self-care agency. The helping methods shown in Table 12-6 foster self-care. As noted earlier, the nursing system design would benefit from the addition of a partly compensatory component to supplement patient agency related to food intake. For example, supervised, restricted eating times, although they would seem developmentally appropriate, would produce increased adherence to the American Diabetes Association (ADA) diet. If Ms. Davila becomes extremely nonadherent to her diet, the nursing system design will change to partly or fully compensatory in an effort to promote physiological functioning and prevent health deterioration.

Regulatory and Control Operations

The SCDNT has been found to be especially useful in cases in which multiple chronic illnesses and medically-prescribed interventions existed, such as the case of Ms. Davila. The theory guided the operations away from disease to the strengths/weaknesses of the self-care agent. In section C of Table 12-5, it is evident that Ms. Davila does seek to prevent/manage conditions threatening her development, yet she requires assistance in this area. The most significant self-care deficits are related to food. Section D of Table 12-5 shows that just under one half of the health deviation self-care requisites involved food in some way.

The theory also guided the nurse to analyze the self-care agency from the perspective of the basic conditioning factors. Culturally, we know it is common and socially acceptable for a Hispanic woman to be overweight, center her needs on caring for her family, and become more sedentary and gain weight at this age. Thus although the nurse-developed supportive-educative system may appear to be a successful way to intervene, a closer look at the adequacy of the self-care agent and the potential for Ms. Davila to actually become motivated to alter her food-related habits should be taken. Are there motivators that will strengthen her agency? Is it possible to alter sociocultural views at this late time in her life?

TABLE 12-6 Nursing System Design for Ms. Davila: Supportive-Educative			
	Diagnostic Operations		Prescriptive Operations
Therapeutic Self-Care Demand	Adequacy of Self-Care Agency	Nursing Diagnosis	Methods of Helping
AIR			
WATER			
FOOD			
Increase adherence to ADA diet	Adequate Adequate Inadequate	Potential for becoming insulin-dependent related to failure to control diet and weight*	Teaching Guiding and directing Providing psychological support
ELIMINATION	Adequate		
ACTIVITY/REST	Inadequate	Ineffective pain control related to no real schedule for analgesic	Teaching Guiding and directing
Cope with/manage pain on ambulation			
SOLITUDE/SOCIAL INTERACTION	Adequate	Potential for social isolation related to solitary living arrangements	Providing psychological support
Continue to maintain family, social, and home care contacts			
PREVENTION OF HAZARDS	Inadequate	Potential for diabetic foot problems related to carelessness in using shoes	Teaching Guiding and directing Providing physical support
Maintain safe ambulation		Potential for falls and fractures related to rheumatoid arthritis, osteoporosis, and obesity	
PROMOTION OF NORMALCY	Adequate		
MAINTAIN DEVELOPMENTAL ENVIRONMENT	Inadequate	Potential for deterioration of health status related to any future discontinuing of home health service*	Guiding and directing Providing psychological support
Continue to receive home healthcare assistance			
PREVENT/MANAGE DEVELOPMENTAL THREATS	Adequate	Potential for misunderstandings related to mixed messages	Providing/maintaining environment that supports personal development
Keep communication lines open and clear with providers			

MAINTENANCE OF HEALTH STATUS	Adequate		
AWARENESS/MANAGEMENT OF DISEASE PROCESS Increase understanding of interrelationships of disease processes, diet, and hazards	Inadequate	Potential for diabetic complications, falls, and decreased mobility related to 3 chronic health problems*	Teaching Guiding and directing Providing physical support Providing/maintaining environment that supports personal development
ADHERENCE TO MEDICAL REGIMEN Increase adherence to ADA diet Regulate administration of analgesic Continue routine medications	Inadequate	Nonadherence to ADA diet related to lifestyle, motivation, and knowledge deficits Inadequate pain relief related to timing of analgesic Self-care deficit related to inability to inject medications	Teaching Guiding and directing Providing psychological support Acting for or doing for another
AWARENESS OF POTENTIAL PROBLEMS Gain better understanding of cause/prevention of problems	Inadequate	Potential for exacerbations and increased disability related to knowledge deficits concerning problems	Teaching Guiding and directing
MODIFY SELF-IMAGE TO INCORPORATE CHANGED HEALTH STATUS Attain ideal body weight	Inadequate	Inability to maintain ideal body weight related to lifestyle, motivation, and knowledge deficits	Providing psychological support Teaching
ADJUST LIFESTYLE TO ACCOMMODATE HEALTH STATUS CHANGES AND MEDICAL REGIMEN Adjust eating habits	Inadequate	Inability to maintain ideal body weight related to cultural attitudes toward eating and weight gain and meal preparation by aide	Guiding and directing Providing/maintaining environment that supports personal development

ADA, American Diabetes Association.
*Priority diagnosis.

The theory guidance provides an ample framework and fosters maintenance through the nursing system. However, it is evident that much of the responsibility for prevention and health promotion rests in Ms. Davila's hands. Thus in retrospect, it becomes imperative to further analyze her developmental self-care requisites (section C of Table 12-5), prescribe and regulate helping methods that center on the maintenance of the appropriate developmental environment, and—at the same time—prescribe a system that is partly compensatory in the area of food requirements.

The extensive diagnostic operations in this case led to an important recognition: do not expect one type of nursing system design to fit all therapeutic self-care demands. Plan at the beginning to supplement patient agency when the patient is faced with overbearing basic conditioning factors and/or problematic developmental self-care demands. This insight prevents wasted time, energy, and expense; is more reality-based; and places more responsibility on the nurse agency.

CRITICAL THINKING EXERCISES

1. The hospital where you are assistant nurse manager for the inpatient medical unit is revising the patient information booklet. Your responsibility is to develop a succinct statement of the nursing framework (SCDNT) that guides overall care at the hospital. Develop this statement using the outline provided by the vice-president for nursing. Remember, this statement is for *lay persons.*
   Outline
   I. Overall goal of nursing
   II. Five premises concerning the self-evident characteristics of human beings being served
   III. Three subtheories (self-care, self-care deficit, and nursing systems)
   IV. Nursing: Helping methods
   V. Attainment of therapeutic self-care requisites

2. Nurses in your unit perceived you as a resource person on the use of the SCDNT and have included in the annual inservice program schedule a program on the theory to be presented by you. The title they suggest is "Inherent Values in Utilizing the Self-Care Deficit Nursing Theory in Inpatient Settings." As you develop the inservice program outline, what are the six values you list?

3. Looking back at the case study of Debbie, reconsider the basic conditioning factors. Which one do you think influenced her current health status the most? If that one factor could have been changed early in her life, what predictable changes in Debbie's self-care agency would have been possible? Project the ways that altered self-care agency would have prevented/limited the health deviations Debbie is experiencing now.

4. Mr. and Mrs. Cowan, parents of a 27-year-old man who is receiving inpatient rehabilitation for extensive burns incurred in an offshore oil rig fire, have an appointment scheduled with you to discuss their son's nursing care. Their major complaint is "We are paying over $1000 a day for his rehabilitation! Why don't the nurses do more for him? He is so unfortunate and needs all the help he can get here." With the five-point outline presented above, you use your understanding of the SCDNT to reply.

5. James, an 8-year-old boy, faces a lengthy hospitalization as the result of recent injuries in a private plane crash. Both of his parents died in the crash. He has multiple fractures but luckily no neurological deficits. Identify three health deviation therapeutic self-care demands for James. Plan for these in a way that methods of helping will assist him to meet his developmental self-care requisites.

6. As you design the nursing system for James, do you perceive the nurse to be providing dependent-care? If so, what factors in the nursing system indicate this?

7. Recently you were appointed to the cost-effectiveness department of a home health agency that is facing nursing fee reorganization. Explain to the department leaders the validity/reliability of designing a fee structure that utilizes the SCDNT framework. Explain how the fee structure can vary by nursing system design and specific helping methods.

8. Your high school class reunion will occur this summer. The reunion organizer has requested that each graduate develop a brief personal history to share with the class. Which of your basic conditioning factors are you most likely to keep secret? What universal self-care requisites do you think they would find interesting? Which developmental self-care requisite do you especially want to explain to the class? Have a great class reunion!

References

Allison, S. E. (1973). A framework for nursing action in a nurse-conducted diabetic management clinic. *Journal of Nursing Administration, 3*(4), 53-60.

Allison, S. E. (1988). *Making theory-based practice work: An administrator's view.* Paper presented at the meeting of the Self-Care Deficit Theory Institute, Vancouver, British Columbia.

Allison, S. E. (1989). Patient outcomes identified through theory-based practice. In *Clinical and cultural dimensions around the world* (pp. 147-156). Columbia, MO: Curators of the University of Missouri.

Allison, S. E. & McLaughlin-Renpenning, K. (1999). *Nursing administration in the 21st century: A self-care theory approach.* Thousand Oaks, CA: Sage.

Anna, D. J., Christensen, D. G., Hohon, S. A., Ord, L., & Wells, S. R. (1978). Implementing Orem's conceptual framework. *Journal of Nursing Administration, 4*, 8-11.

Backscheider, J. E. (1971). The use of self as the essence of clinical supervision in ambulatory patient care. *Nursing Clinics of North America, 6*, 53-60.

Benor, D. E., Delbar, V., & Krulik, T. (1998). Measuring impact of nursing intervention on cancer patients' ability to control symptoms. *Cancer Nursing, 21*(5), 320-334.

Berbiglia, V. A. & Bekel, G. (1995, February). *The changing face of nursing in Germany: How can Self-Care Deficit Nursing Theory assist in the transformation?* Paper presented at the meeting of the Fourth International Self-Care Deficit Nursing Theory Conference, San Antonio, TX.

Bliss-Holtz, J. & Sayer, P. (1995, February). *ISAAC: A theory-based information system.* Paper presented at the meeting of the Fourth International Self-Care Deficit Nursing Theory Conference, San Antonio, TX.

Buckwalter, K. & Kerfoot, K. (1982). Teaching patients self-care. *Journal of Psychiatric Nursing and Mental Health Services, 20*(5), 15-20.

Craddock, R. B., Adams, P. F., Usui, W. M., & Mitchell, L. (1999). An intervention to increase use and effectiveness of self-care measures for breast cancer chemotherapy patients. *Cancer Nursing, 22*(4), 312-319.

Crumbley, D. R., Ice, R. C., & Cassidy, R. (1999). Nurse-managed wound clinic: A case study in success. *Nursing Case Management, 4*(4), 168+.

Dodd, M. J. (1982). Assessing patient self-care for side-effects of cancer chemotherapy—Part I. *Cancer Nursing, 5,* 447-451.

Dodd, M. J. (1983). Self-care for side-effects in cancer chemotherapy: An assessment of nursing interventions—Part II. *Cancer Nursing, 6,* 63-67.

Fifth International Self-Care Deficit Nursing Theory Conference Abstracts. (1997). Leuven, Belgium: Catholic University.

Freston, M. S., Young, S., Calhoun, S., Fredericksen, T., Salinger, L., Malchodi, C., & Egan, J. F. X. (1997). Responses of pregnant women to potential preterm labor symptoms. *Journal of Obstetric, Gynecologic, and Neonatal Nursing, 26*(1), 35-41.

Furlong, S. (1996). Self-care: The application of a ward philosophy. *Journal of Clinical Nursing, 5*(2), 85-90.

Goodwin, J. O. (1979). Programmed instruction for self-care following pulmonary surgery. *International Journal of Nursing, 16*(1), 29-38.

Hanucharurnkul, S. (2000). Ten years of self-care research: What we have accomplished and where we should go. *Sixth International Self-Care Deficit Nursing Theory Conference Abstracts.*

Hart, M. A. (1996). Nursing implications of self-care in pregnancy. *The American Journal of Maternal/Child Nursing, 21*(3), 137-143.

Hartweg, D. (1993). Self-care actions of healthy middle-aged women to promote well-being. *Nursing Research, 42*(4), 221-227.

Hartweg, D. & Berbiglia, V. (1996). Determining the adequacy of a health promotion self-care interview guide with healthy, middle-aged, Mexican-American women: A pilot study. *Healthcare for Women International, 17*(1), 57-68.

Hildebrandt, E. (1996). Building community participation in healthcare: A model and example from South Africa. *Image, 28*(2), 155-159.

Holzemer, W. L. (1992). Linking primary healthcare and self-care through case management. *International Nursing Review, 39*(3), 83-89.

Howard, J. & Berbiglia, V. (1997, November/December). Caring for childbearing Korean women. *Journal of Obstetric, Gynecologic, and Neonatal Nursing, 26*(6), 665-671.

Intarasombat, P. (1995, February). *Promoting family participation in healthcare for the hospitalized elderly.* Poster session presented at the meeting of the Fourth International Self-Care Deficit Nursing Theory Conference, San Antonio, TX.

Isenberg, M. (1993). From the president. *The International Orem Society Newsletter, 1*(1).

Isenberg, M. & Evers, G. (1997). An international collaborative model for advancing self-care nursing science. *Fifth International Self-Care Deficit Nursing Theory Conference Abstracts.*

Kennedy, L. M. (1990). The effectiveness of self-care medication education protocol on the home medication behaviors of recently hospitalized elderly. Unpublished doctoral dissertation, University of Texas—Austin; Austin, Texas.

Kubricht, D. W. (1984). Therapeutic self-care demands expressed by outpatients receiving external radiation therapy. *Cancer Nursing, 7,* 43-51.

Laschinger, H. S. (1990). Helping students apply a nursing conceptual framework in a clinical setting. *Nurse Educator, 5*(3), 20-24.

Lipson, J. G. & Steiger, N. J. (1996). *Self-care nursing in a multicultural context.* Thousand Oaks, CA: Sage.

Martin, B. (1995, February). *Promoting self-care behaviors with clients who are homeless.* Paper presented at the meeting of the Fourth International Self-Care Deficit Nursing Theory Conference, San Antonio, TX.

Marz, C. E. (1989). New York referral intake and disposition: An application of Orem's classification of nursing situations. In *Clinical and cultural dimensions around the world* (pp. 107-126). Columbia, MO: Curators of the University of Missouri.

McDaniel, R. W. & Rhodes, V. A. (1998). Development of a preparatory sensory information videotape for women receiving chemotherapy for breast cancer. *Cancer Nursing, 21*(2), 143-148.

Meleis, A. I. (1997). *Theoretical nursing development and progress.* New York: J. B. Lippincott.

Norris, N. G. (1991). Applying Orem's theory to long-term care of adolescent transplant recipients. *American Nephrology Nurses Association Journal, 18*(1), 45-47.

Nursing Development Conference Group. (1973). *Concept formalization in nursing: Process and product.* Boston: Little, Brown.

Orem, D. E. (1959). *Guides for developing curriculum for the education of practical nurses.* Washington, DC: U.S. Government Printing Office.

Orem, D. E. (1971). *Nursing: Concepts of practice* (1st ed.). New York: McGraw-Hill.

Orem, D. E. (1985). *Nursing: Concepts of practice* (3rd ed.). New York: McGraw-Hill.

Orem, D. E. (1988, June). *Changes in the nursing profession associated with nurses' use of the Self-Care Deficit Nursing Theory.* Paper presented at the meeting of the Self-Care Deficit Theory Institute, Vancouver, British Columbia, Canada.

Orem, D. E. (1995). *Nursing: Concepts of practice* (5th ed.). St. Louis: Mosby.

Rassool, G. H. (1997). Self-care nursing in a multicultural context (book review). *Journal of Advanced Nursing, 25*(4), 859-860.

Renker, P. R. (1999). Physical abuse, social support, self-care, and pregnancy outcomes in older adolescents. *Journal of Obstetric, Gynecologic, & Neonatal Nursing, 28*(4), 377-388.

Riggs, J. (1995, February). *Blending theory-based practice and computerization: The planning phase.* Poster session presented at the meeting of the Fourth International Self-Care Deficit Nursing Theory Conference, San Antonio, TX.

Sheehy, G. (1976). *Passages.* New York: E. P. Dutton.

Sixth International Self-Care Deficit Nursing Theory Conference Abstracts. (2000). Bangkok, Thailand: University of Missouri—Columbia; Columbia, MO.

Steel, N. F. & Sterling, Y. M. (1992). Application of the case study design: Nursing interventions for discharge readiness. *Clinical Nurse Specialist, 6*(2), 79-84.

Sullivan, T. (1997). Self-Care Deficit Nursing Theory: Building bridges in an era of connections. *Sixth International Self-Care Deficit Nursing Theory Conference Abstracts.*

Sungkalobol, D. (2000). Health for all and self-care. *Sixth International Self-Care Deficit Nursing Theory Conference Abstracts.*

Taylor, S. G. & McLaughlin, K. E. (1991). Orem's general theory and community nursing. *Nursing Science Quarterly, 4,* 153-160.

Taylor, S. G. & Renpenning, K. (1995). The practice of nursing in multiperson situations, family and community. In D. E. Orem (Ed.), *Nursing: Concepts of practice* (5th ed., pp. 348-380). St. Louis: Mosby.

Taylor, S. G. & Robinson Purdy, A. U. (1989). Assessing self-management and dependent care capabilities of hospitalized adults and caregivers in preparation for discharge. In *Clinical and cultural dimensions around the world* (pp. 4-16). Columbia, MO: Curators of the University of Missouri.

Ulbrich, S. L. (1999). Nursing practice theory of exercise as self-care. *Image, 31*(1), 65-70.

Underwood, P. (1980). Facilitating self-care. In P. Pothier (Ed.), *Psychiatric nursing: A basic text* (pp. 115-144). Boston: Little, Brown.

Villarruel, A. M. (1997). Testing Orem's theory with Mexican-Americans. *Image, 29*(3), 283-288.

Walborn, K. A. (1980). A nursing model for hospice: Primary and self-care nursing. *Nursing Clinics of North America, 15*(1), 205-217.

Walker, D. M. (1986). A nursing administration perspective on the use of Orem's Self-Care Deficit Nursing Theory. In M. E. Parker (Ed.), *Patterns of nursing theories in practice* (pp. 252-263). New York: National League for Nursing.

Weis, A. (1988). Cooperative care: An application of Orem's self-care theory. *Patient Education and Counseling, 11,* 141-146.

Whelan, E. G. (1984). Analysis and application of Dorothea Orem's self-care practice model. *Journal of Nursing Education, 23*(8), 342-345.

Whitener, L. M., Cox, K. R., & Maglich, S. A. (1998). Use of theory to guide nurses in the design of health messages for children. *Advances in Nursing Science, 20*(3), 21-35.

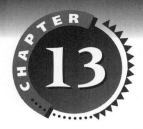

Rogers' Science of Unitary Human Beings in Nursing Practice

Kaye Bultemeier

"Nursing is both a science and an art. The uniqueness of nursing, like that of any other science, lies in the phenomenon central to its focus. Nurses' long-established concern with people and the world they live in is a natural forerunner of an organized abstract system encompassing people and their environments. The irreducible nature of individuals is different from the sum of the parts. The integralness of people and environment that coordinate with a multidimensional [later changed to pandimensional] universe of open systems points to a new paradigm: the identity of nursing as a science. The purpose of nurses is to promote health and well-being for all persons wherever they are. The art of nursing is the creative use of the science of nursing for human betterment." (From Barrett [Ed.], Visions of Rogers' Science-Based Nursing, *1990: National League for Nursing, New York, NY/Jones and Bartlett Publishers, Sudbury, MA WWW.jbpub.com. Reprinted with permission.)*

HISTORY AND BACKGROUND

The Rogerian model is an abstract system of ideas from which to approach the nursing care of the unitary human being. Rogers first introduced this model in 1970. The central concern of the model is the nursing of unitary human beings. Within this model, human beings are conceptualized as dynamic, constantly evolving energy fields rather than as homeostatic beings. Variation is expected and embraced within this homeodynamic perspective. Rogers' model, abstract in nature, becomes the basis for theory development that addresses the specific nature of nursing in caring for the unitary human being.

Nursing is considered an art and a science. The science of nursing is "a body of abstract knowledge emerging from scientific research and logical analysis" (Rogers, 1970, p. 86). The emergent knowledge is translated into nursing practice. From the Rogerian framework, nursing is a science, and the term *nursing* signifies a body of knowledge. Within Rogers' model, several assumptions regarding the nature of nursing are evident. First, nursing science is an organized body of abstract scientific knowledge that develops from research and analysis. This science of nursing helps to explain the human experience (Rogers, 1970). Second, Rogers contends that nursing is a learned profession and therefore must be based on solid scientific information. Third, Rogers' model is theoretical, and it is the predictive qualities of the model that provide the foundation for outlining practice. Theoretical structures that subsequently guide practice and research are formulated. Fourth, formulated knowledge is to be used creatively for human betterment (Rogers, 1970). Nursing knowledge provides the tools for the emergent artistic application for nursing care of the unitary human being (Rogers, 1970). Nurses use this scientific knowledge to care for and improve the lived experience of the unitary human being. Nursing is the creative use of nursing knowledge in caring for the unitary human being.

Rogers' model contends that the human being and the environment are energy fields that are irreducible and equal to more than the sum of their parts. Within the Rogerian model, the unitary human being and the environment are integral and therefore are viewed as a whole (Barnum, 1994; Malinski, 1986b). This wholistic perspective differentiates nursing from other sciences and identifies nursing's focus (Malinski, 1986a). Nursing's focus is the care of people and the life process of human beings. Its purpose is to identify and examine the phenomenon, the unitary human being, that is central to its concern and to make predictions regarding human field evolution (Malinski, 1986c). Nursing aims to accompany people while they achieve their maximum health potential. Maintenance and promotion of health, prevention of disease, nursing diagnosis, intervention, and rehabilitation encompass the scope of nursing (Rogers, 1970). According to Rogers (1970), "Professional practice in nursing seeks to promote symphonic interaction between human and environmental fields, to strengthen the integrity of the human field, and to direct and redirect patterning of the human and environment fields for realization of maximum health potential" (p. 122).

The life process of the unitary human being is one of wholeness, continuity, and dynamic and creative change. Within the Rogerian model, the concepts of health and illness are viewed as pattern manifestations. Health for the unitary human being signifies an irreducible human field pattern manifestation (Rogers, 1986). The manifestation of health emerges from the mutual, simultaneous pattern process of the human and environmental fields. This manifestation is an expression of the process of life as defined by individuals and their cultures (Rogers, 1970). Therefore what we know as health and illness are continuous expressions of the life process. The practice of nursing is accompanying unitary human beings in movement toward maximum health patterning. Clients define what health is for themselves, and nurses assist them in their movement toward that goal.

OVERVIEW OF ROGERS' SCIENCE OF UNITARY HUMAN BEINGS

Rogers' conceptual model is an abstraction that provides a way of viewing the unitary human being. Humans are viewed as integral with the universe. The unitary human being and the environment are one, not dichotomous. Nursing within Rogers' model focuses on people and the manifestations that emerge from the mutual human/environmental field process. A change in pattern and organization of the human field and the environmental field is propagated by waves. The manifestations of field patterning that emerge are observable events (Rogers, 1992). The identification of patterns that characterize a phenomenon provide knowledge and understanding of the human experience (Rogers, 1970). The following basic characteristics that describe the life process in humans are proposed: energy field, openness, pattern, and pandimensionality. Other concepts that provide clarity to the basic precepts of the Rogerian model include the unitary human being, environment, and homeodynamic principles.

Energy Field

The energy field is the conceptual boundary of all that is. The energy field is the fundamental unit of both the living and the nonliving. This energy field "provides a way to perceive people and their environment as irreducible wholes" (Rogers, 1986, p. 4). The energy field continuously varies in intensity, density, and extent.

Openness

The human field and the environmental field are constantly exchanging energy. There are no boundaries or barriers to inhibit energy flow between fields (Rogers, 1970).

Pattern

Pattern is defined as the distinguishing characteristic of an energy field perceived as a single wave. Rogers (1986) calls it "an abstraction" that "gives identity to the field" (p. 5).

Pandimensionality

Pandimensionality is defined as "a nonlinear domain without spatial or temporal attributes" (Rogers, 1990, p. 7). The parameters in language that human beings use to describe events are arbitrary. The present is relative; there is no temporal ordering of lives.

Unitary Human Being

A unitary human being is "an irreducible, indivisible, pandimensional energy field identified by pattern and manifesting characteristics that are specific to the whole and which cannot be predicted from knowledge of the parts" (Rogers, 1992, p. 27) and "a unified whole having its own distinctive characteristics which cannot be perceived by looking at, describing, or summarizing the parts" (Rogers, 1992, p. 27).

Environment

The environment is "an irreducible, pandimensional energy field identified by pattern and integral with the human field" (Rogers, 1992, p. 27). Figure 13-1 illustrates the coexistence of the fields without limits and boundaries. The fields coexist and are integral. Manifestations emerge from this field and are perceived.

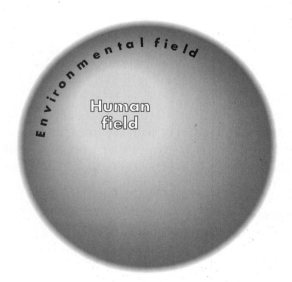

FIGURE 13-1

Conceptualization of human/environmental energy field. (From Bultemeier, K. [1993]. *Photographic inquiry of the phenomenon premenstrual syndrome within the Rogerian-derived Theory of Perceived Dissonance.* Unpublished doctoral dissertation, University of Tennessee—Knoxville; Knoxville, Tennessee.)

Homeodynamic Principles

Rogers' principles of homeodynamics provide a way of describing, explaining, and predicting a wide range of perceivable events (Malinski, 1986c). Because the fundamental unit of the living system is an energy field, three principles of homeodynamics are proposed by Rogers: (1) resonancy, (2) helicy, and (3) integrality. These principles describe the nature of the person/environment process. The principle of resonancy embraces the continuous variability of the human energy field as it evolves. Rogers defines it as "an ordered arrangement of rhythms characterizing both the human field and the environmental field that undergoes continuous dynamic metamorphosis in the human-environment process" (Rogers, 1970, p. 101). Helicy describes the unpredictable but continuous, nonlinear evolution of energy fields as evidenced by nonrepeating rhythmicities. The life process evolves in sequential stages along a curve that has the same general shape. Rhythmicities portend probabilistic predictions. Rogers (1970) states, "The principle of helicy postulates an ordering of the human's evolutionary emergence" (p. 100). Integrality embraces the mutual, continuous relationship of the human energy field and the environmental energy field (Rogers, 1990). Change can be understood to occur by the continuous repatterning of human and environmental fields by resonating waves (Rogers, 1970). The fields are one and integrated yet unique. The principles of homeodynamics postulate a way of perceiving unitary human beings. The homeodynamic principles have been refined and clarified since they were first introduced in Rogers' earlier works (Daily, Maupin, Satterly, Schnell, &Wallace, 1989).

THEORIES FOR PRACTICE

The Rogerian model provides the abstract philosophical framework from which to view the unitary human being and the environmental field. Within the Rogerian framework, nursing is based on theoretical knowledge that guides nursing practice. Historically, nursing commonly equated practice with the practical and theory with the impractical. More appropriately, theory and practice are two related components in a unified nursing practice. Alligood (1994) articulates how theory and practice direct and guide each other as they expand and increase nursing knowledge. Emerging from Rogers' model are theories that explain human phenomena and direct nursing practice. The Rogerian model, with its implicit assumptions, provides broad principles that conceptually direct theory development (Figure 13-2). Theory can and does emerge from each of the principles. Two theories derived from Rogers' model are used in this chapter: Bultemeier's Theory of Perceived Dissonance (1993) and Barrett's Theory of Power as Knowing Participation in Change (1986).

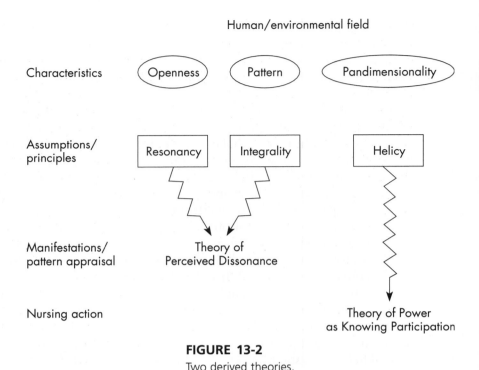

FIGURE 13-2

Two derived theories.

Theory of Perceived Dissonance

The Theory of Perceived Dissonance derived by Bultemeier (1993) from the Rogerian model provides a theoretical perspective for exploring situations of varying resonancy as manifest in healthcare concerns currently labeled *abnormal processes*. This theory emerges from the principles of resonancy and integrality. The theory provides a modality for pattern appraisal of manifestations of the human/environmental field during times labeled *illness*. The theory proposes that resonancy is altered periodically and rhythmically during the evolution of energy fields. The perception of dissonance during the rhythmical evolution of the human and environmental field is proposed. The theory of perceived dissonance articulates a human/environmental field process that is defined as illness within the healthcare system. The theory embellishes and embraces the evolution of natural rhythmicities and manifestations associated with this evolution.

Persons are viewed as energy fields manifesting in their environmental energy fields (see Figure 13-1). It is proposed that resonancy varies rhythmically during the evolution of natural rhythmicities. The inherent rhythmicity of fields can evolve into rhythms that vary and may manifest as discordant. During episodes of varying resonancy, the human and environmental field manifestations may be perceived as nonharmonic and as uncomfortable or unsettling to the person; thus the person views himself or herself as out of harmony, or ill. Likewise, others perceive the person in the same way. Personal feeling manifestations that are associated with episodes of discordant resonancy are identified.

Personal awareness of the emerging pattern manifestation is defined as being sentient to the evolutionary change of one's human energy field (Parker, 1989). A centered, receptive awareness is characteristic of integrality (a principle of homeodynamics) and is the means by which the person experiences varied resonancy, which may be perceived as dissonance (or illness). Alligood (1991) proposed that feeling attributes are a manifestation of the integrality of the human and environmental field pattern. Manifestations and feelings emerge with discordant rhythms that are associated with perceived dissonance.

The Theory of Perceived Dissonance adds clarity to how the nurse can draw on perceptions by the client and have his or her own perceptions to direct nursing care. The pattern manifestations that emerge during times of variability can be labeled *illness*. This is crucial to the practice of providing a wholistic assessment of the unitary human being.

Theory of Power as Knowing Participation in Change

The theory proposed by Barrett (1986)—power as knowing participation in change—emerges from the principle of helicy within the Rogerian model. This theory provides direction for the nurse participating in the care of the unitary human being. Within this theory, it is proposed that as knowledge increases, so does the capacity to participate knowingly. The theory proposes the capacity of human beings to pattern their human and environmental fields. This patterning manifests via nurse and client patterning process.

Barrett (1986) describes power as being aware of what one is choosing to do, feeling free to do it, and doing it. She calls power "a relative state characterized by the momentary continuously changing pattern; power is also a relative trait characterized by the more consistent organization of the human and environmental field pattern" (p. 174). She specifies that the person must be knowledgeable of his or her pattern manifestations for meaningful participation in the patterning process to occur.

Within the Rogerian framework, the nature of nursing is based on theoretical knowledge that guides nursing practice (Rogers, 1970). The theories previously outlined by Bultemeier and Barrett, which are derived from the Rogerian model, provide the descriptive, explanatory, and predictive principles that conceptually direct nursing practice. These conceptual features have relevance to understanding manifestation for practice.

CRITICAL THINKING IN NURSING PRACTICE WITH ROGERS' MODEL

Critical thinking is a process of conceptualizing, applying, analyzing, synthesizing, or evaluating information gathered from or generated by observation, experience, reflection, reasoning, or communication as a guide to belief and action. Within Rogers' model, the critical thinking process can be divided into three components: pattern appraisal, mutual patterning, and evaluation. This chapter presents a synthesis of the two theories previously discussed and builds on the guidelines for clinical practice proposed by Malinski (1986c). In addition, Cowling's work (1990) assists in outlining the critical thinking process for nurses working within the Rogers model.

Pattern Appraisal

The critical thinking process, which is outlined in Table 13-1, begins with a comprehensive pattern appraisal. The life process possesses its own unity and is inseparable from the environment. This appraisal requires the identification of patterns that reflect the whole. Pattern appraisal is a comprehensive assessment that incorporates cognitive input, sensory input, intuition, and language. The nurse gains additional knowledge during the interview process. Intuitive knowledge is gained from both the client and the nurse. The client has self-knowledge to share. The nurse accompanies the client in focusing on personal patterns and rhythms. Using emerging pattern manifestations during the appraisal allows for a departure from the linear cause-and-effect view. The nurse gains awareness of rhythmical fluctuations and their associated manifestations and perceptions. Patterning activities are based on probabilistic outcomes as they emerge from the appraisal of pattern evolution. Emergent human environmental rhythms and patterns are manifestations of the whole. Ongoing pattern appraisal with multiple manifestations can lead to prediction, patterning, and further pattern identification. The emergent rhythms are manifestations of the mutual process of human beings with their environments.

The client is encouraged to center and reflect on his or her personal pattern and on the pattern of those with whom he or she shares common experiences. Bultemeier (1997) introduced the use of photographs and written narrative to assist in pattern identification. Pattern appraisal

TABLE 13-1 Critical Thinking in Rogers' Model	
Nurse	**Client**
PATTERN APPRAISAL	**SELF-REFLECTION**
Comprehensive assessment of:	Nutrition
1. Human field patterns of	Work/leisure activities
communication, exchange,	Exercise
rhythms, dissonance, harmony	Sleep/wake cycles
2. Environmental field patterns	Relationships
of communication, rhythms,	Discomfort/pain
dissonance, harmony	Fears/hopes
Intuitive reflection	Dreams
Validate appraisal:	
1. With self	
2. With client	
3. With others	
MUTUAL PATTERNING OF HUMAN AND ENVIRONMENTAL FIELD	**PATTERNING ACTIVITIES**
	Meditation
Sharing knowledge	Imagery
Offering choices	Journaling
Empowering client	Modifying surroundings:
Fostering patterning	color, temperature, sounds,
	touch, music, art, humor
EVALUATION	**PERSONAL APPRAISAL**
Repeat pattern appraisal	Areas of dissonance
Identify dissonance/harmony	Areas of harmony
Validate appraisal with client	Patterning activities

includes multiple lifestyle rhythms, such as nutrition, work, exercise, pain, anger, depression, sleep/wake cycles, and safety. Another way to categorize rhythmicities is by utilizing the criteria developed by Kim and Moritz (1982). These rhythms include the following: (1) exchanging (eating, elimination, breathing, giving, and receiving), (2) communication (verbal and nonverbal), and (3) relating (spacing, touching, eye contact, belonging, and referencing). During the appraisal, special attention is given to rhythms of pain and discomfort or to areas about which the client is uncomfortable or concerned (Cowling, 1990). Another wholistic pattern appraisal method, the pattern portrait, is introduced by Butcher (1998).

The nurse uses the feeling or sensing level of knowing, which is often described as intuitive or instinctual. The intuitive knowledge is best realized through reflection, which assists in pattern appraisal. The nurse realizes that manifestations are not static but are partial perceptions of the synthesis of the past, present, and future. These perceptions provide the basis for reflection and intuitive knowing, which then further expands the appraisal. The manifestations, patterns, and rhythms are an indication of evolutionary emergence of the human field. Pattern appraisal, rhythm identification, and reflection provide the content for appraisal validation with the client.

Mutual Patterning

Once the client and nurse have consensus with respect to the appraisal, nursing action is centered around mutual patterning of the client human/environmental field. The goal of the nursing is promoting symphonic rhythms of the human/environmental field. This is done to "strengthen the coherence and integrity of the human field and to direct and redirect patterning of the human and environmental fields" (Rogers, 1970, p. 122). Patterning activities can be devised to address areas that are identified as dissonant and described as pain, discomfort, or anxiety. Through mutual patterning, manifestations of peace and enjoyment emerge as evidence of Barrett's knowing participation in change theory (Lutjens, 1991).

Mutual patterning emerges from the pattern appraisal and relates to areas of dissonance. Barrett (1990a) has outlined the components of the change process that are fundamental to formulating patterning processes. These components include awareness, choice, freedom, and involvement. Knowledge of the disease and various options for patterning are shared with the client. The knowledge shared is guided by the appraisal. Specific information relating to the illness and its treatments are included. The nurse must ensure that the client has adequate knowledge of the appraisal and implications of various options. The sharing of the appraisal empowers the client to participate in and direct the patterning process. Various therapeutic patterning activities are offered. Patterning activities instill hope and can be individualized. Modifications are made to allow the patterning activities to meet the limitations of the individual. The client must have the capacity to participate in the patterning.

The client is empowered by the process of patterning. Power is characterized by a continuously changing pattern. Power can be conceptualized as harmonious rhythmicity and as a consistent integration of the human and environmental field pattern. The "goal of patterning is substantive change in health dynamic and change in the direction of health as defined by the client" (Cowling, 1990, p. 51). The nurse's goal is to assist the client in reaching the maximum health potential and in fostering harmonious patterns, thereby reducing the perception of dissonance.

Barrett (1986) defines patterning as the continuous process whereby the nurse, with the client, patterns the environmental field to promote harmony related to the health event. Rogers (1970) contends that "[c]hange proceeds by the continuous patterning of both man and environment by resonating waves" (p. 102). Change is specific to an energy field and is perceived through manifestations. Increasing diversity of field patterning characterizes the process of change (Rogers, 1970). Each human possesses changing rhythmicities that have individual uniqueness. The goal is harmonious rhythmicities and pattern manifestations.

Human field patterning. Patterning activities revolve primarily around noninvasive modalities. However, all treatments and interactions are patterning activities because they are integral to the human/environmental field process. Practice modalities concern human life patterning and reflect the wholeness of the unitary human being in "continuous innovative change with the universe" (Barrett, 1990b, p. 35). The health-related change modalities allow for change; they do not require it. Nurses currently assist clients in the use of meditation, imagery, visualization, and therapeutic touch when there is a primary focus of the patterning of the human field. Additional practice modalities based on motion, sound, light and color, humor, relaxation, nutrition, affirmation, art and nature, bibliotherapy, and journal keeping are patterning modalities. The nurse is aware that the human/environmental field is one without boundaries. Awareness may center on the perception of the human field, but it too is a manifestation of the human/environmental field process. Centering is central to many of the modalities. With centering, the client focuses on his or her core or energy field. This centering is perceivable as a harmonious field manifestation. The purpose of patterning is to heal the physical body or to modify the perception of dissonance. All manifestations, including those called *illness*, emerge from the mutual human field and environmental field process. The patterning activities help the client move beyond the physical body to emergent patterns.

Environmental field patterning. Manifestations emerge from the human/environmental field process. The physical body is one manifestation of the human energy field. The environment, with its healing quality, or lack of dissonance, is a vital component of patterning. Wholeness implies concern with the totality of the human/environmental field manifestation. The key is interrelationship—energy patterns flowing through energy patterns. The nurse works with the client in the context of family, community, and cultural group. The nurse's concern for unitary human beings incorporates other nurses and healthcare providers as well as the family in the patterning. The nurse must recognize that the attitudes, intentions, and feelings of those with whom the client works are an integral part of the environmental field manifestation. A supportive environment is needed for harmonious patterning. Color, light, sound, and smell are manifestations of the environmental field. These manifestations can be perceived as dissonant or harmonious.

The nurse, in consensus with the client, introduces a combination of modalities based on the pattern appraisal. The proposed patterning activities allow the client's health patterns to manifest as harmonious rhythms or as a decrease in the perception of dissonance.

Evaluation

Evaluation is ongoing and encompasses a repetition of the appraisal process. Emphasis is placed on identifying perceptions of dissonance with respect to the initial pattern appraisal. The evaluation process is ongoing and fluid as the nurse reflects on his or her intuitive knowing. During the evaluation phase, the nurse repeats the pattern appraisal process to determine the level of perceived dissonance. The perceptions are then shared with the client and family/friends. Further mutual patterning is guided by the perceptions found during the evaluation process. This process continues as long as the nurse/client relationship continues.

Analysis and Synthesis

The Rogerian model provides a challenging and innovative means of planning and implementing client care. The abstract ideas presented in the Rogerian model are fertile for fostering theoretical application in the conceptualization of patient care. The concept of the unitary human being and the wholistic approach needed to provide care offer opportunities for nurses to design and implement healing environments that aid in the patterning of the unitary field during times of perceived dissonance or illness.

Care for the unitary human being must begin with a thorough pattern appraisal that leads to a comprehensive analysis. The validation of this analysis by the client is imperative before nursing strategies can be formulated. Appraisal is ongoing and active. The client directs and assists in pattern appraisal. The nurse provides the synthesis and the conceptual understanding of the unitary human being process.

Patterning activities that the nurse introduces are instrumental in field pattern evolution. The client experiences power as knowing participation in change. The nurse provides much of the knowledge that is necessary for this knowing participation, which becomes the springboard for innovative, noninvasive care of the unitary human being.

CASE HISTORY OF DEBBIE

Debbie is a 29-year-old woman who was recently admitted to the oncology nursing unit for evaluation after sensing pelvic "fullness" and noticing a watery, foul-smelling vaginal discharge. A Papanicolaou smear revealed class V cervical cancer. She was found to have a stage II squamous cell carcinoma of the cervix and underwent a radical hysterectomy with bilateral salpingoooophorectomy.

Her past health history revealed that physical examinations had been infrequent. She also reported that she had not performed breast self-examination. She is 5 feet, 4 inches tall and weights 89 pounds. Her usual weight is about 110 pounds. She has smoked approximately two packs of cigarettes a day for the past 16 years. She is gravida 2, para 2. Her first pregnancy was at age 16, and her second was at age 18. Since that time, she has taken oral contraceptives on a regular basis.

Debbie completed the eighth grade. She is married and lives with her husband and her two children in her mother's home, which she describes as less than sanitary. Her husband is unemployed. She describes him as emotionally distant and abusive at times.

She has done well following surgery except for being unable to completely empty her urinary bladder. She is having continued postoperative pain and nausea. It will be necessary for her to perform intermittent self-catheterization at home. Her medications are (1) an antibiotic, (2) an analgesic as needed for pain, and (3) an antiemetic as needed for nausea. In addition, she will be receiving radiation therapy on an outpatient basis.

Debbie is extremely tearful. She expresses great concern over her future and the future of her two children. She believes that this illness is a punishment for her past life.

NURSING CARE OF DEBBIE WITH ROGERS' MODEL

Within the Rogerian model, the process of caring for Debbie begins with pattern appraisal. Pattern appraisal is the most important component of the nursing process. Nursing care will involve pattern appraisal, mutual patterning, and evaluation.

Pattern Appraisal

The history is integral to the pattern appraisal. Debbie has a pattern of smoking, which has been associated with less than optimal health potential. This visible rhythmical pattern is a manifestation of evolution toward dissonance. In addition, Debbie has a pattern manifestation that has been labeled cervical cancer. This emergent pattern manifests as dissonant. Debbie has a low educational level, which is relevant as patterning activities are introduced. A pattern manifestation of healing is noted through reports of a positive-operative course.

Sensory data add to the pattern appraisal. Through language, Debbie identifies a perception of dissonance with her husband and with her environment, which she describes as "unsanitary." The nurse will explore with Debbie what perceptions and feelings she has with respect to her home environment. Can patterning be directed toward a reduction in perceived dissonance with her environmental field? Pain is a manifestation that needs to be further evaluated to determine the pattern of pain perception. Appraisal of pain as it relates to circadian rhythms and environmental field changes assist in this appraisal. Debbie is asked to reflect on characteristics of the pain, and together with the nurse, a pattern may emerge. Pain is a manifestation of dissonance.

The nurse has reported that Debbie has a manifestation of fear. Debbie reports the fear of inability to manage her life since this illness, and the nurse senses this manifestation of fear. Debbie's self-knowledge links the illness to her personal belief of being punished for past mistakes. History and focusing on the relative present to explore the pattern of punishment is imperative. It is important that the nurse appraise the environment of the hospital and of the others who share her existence. Debbie reports fear, a manifestation of dissonance. The pain and fear are dissonant manifestations. Appraisal of human/environmental factors as these perceptions emerge is needed.

Language provides a valuable addition to the pattern appraisal of Debbie. Appraisal concerning Debbie's sleep patterns, her nutritional status, and her perceptions of self and of what is a healthful or harmonious existence for her is needed. This appraisal can be grouped into exchanging patterns, communication patterns, and relating patterns, as discussed previously. Time with the nurse is needed to foster this comprehensive appraisal of Debbie. During this entire process, the nurse must rely heavily on personal intuition and insight regarding the pattern that is emergent with Debbie. All of the knowledge gained forms the unitary pattern of Debbie.

Dissonance can be perceived in many aspects of Debbie's appraisal. There is a lack of environmental harmony, as is noted in Debbie's perception of it as unsanitary. In addition, dissonance is perceived with respect to her relationship with her husband. Personal dissonance is noted in the manifestations of cancer, weight loss, pain, nausea, and tobacco use. This dissonance is also conceptualized as fear in Debbie's words and in the emotional distance that she feels.

On completion of the pattern appraisal, the analysis is presented to the client. Emphasis can be placed on areas in which dissonance and harmony are noted in the personal and environmental field manifestations. Consensus needs to be reached with Debbie before patterning activities can be suggested and implemented.

Mutual Patterning

Many patterning modalities can be introduced. The process is mutual between the nurse and the client. Surgery is a patterning activity. Manifestations will evolve from the surgical intervention and will require reconceptualization and validation with the patient. Medications are patterning modalities. Debbie is receiving medications. Decisions are made in conjunction with Debbie regarding the use of the medications and the patterning that emerges with the introduction of these modalities. Personal knowledge regarding the surgery and the medications empower Debbie to be integral in the selection of modalities. Debbie possesses freedom and involvement in the selection of modalities. Possible options include therapeutic touch, humor, meditation, visualization, and imagery. Debbie needs to be assessed fully regarding her ability to understand and select different patterning modalities.

Therapeutic touch can be introduced to Debbie. The touch is introduced and incorporated into the management of pain manifestations. Touch, in combination with medications, provides patterning that Debbie can direct. The nurse can introduce the process of touch to Debbie's husband and teach him how to incorporate touch into her care. This option would be acceptable only if Debbie felt safe being touched by her spouse. Another option would be to teach Debbie how to center her energy and channel her energy to the area in pain.

Patterning directed at the manifestation of fear is needed. Options that include imagery, music, light, and meditation can be discussed. Fear manifests as apprehension of self-catheterization. Emphasis needs to be placed on having Debbie direct how, where, when, and by whom the self-catheterization will be taught. Establishing a rhythm to the catheterization schedule that is harmonious with Debbie's life would reduce dissonance. Patterning of nutrition and catheterization based on the pattern appraisal can assist in empowering Debbie to learn self-catheterization. A rhythm that is harmonious with Debbie and her energy field rhythm will evolve. Specific actions of the nurse with respect to language and knowledge about the catheterization process empower Debbie to direct this phase of her treatment.

Human/environmental patterning needs to involve the other individuals who share Debbie's environment, including her husband, children, and mother. Options relating to increased communication and sanitation patterns are introduced. The entire family is involved in power as knowing participation in change. Language and the use of language is explored to determine what Debbie would prefer to change in her environment and sanitation. Options that allow pattern evolution that is not perceived as dissonant and is integral with her environment are introduced.

Evaluation

The evaluation process centers on the perceptions of dissonance and/or harmony that exist after the mutual patterning activities. The appraisal process is repeated. Specific emphasis is placed on emergent patterns of dissonance or harmony that are evident. Manifestations of pain, fear, and tension with family members are appraised. The nurse intuitively evaluates the amount of dissonance that is manifesting with respect to Debbie during care. A summary of the dissonance and/or harmony that is perceived is then shared with Debbie, and mutual patterning is modified or instituted as indicated based on the evaluation.

CASE HISTORY OF MARY

Mary is a 42-year-old woman who has been admitted to the oncology unit for pain management and testing. She becomes teary during the history taking and reports that she has had a recent recurrence of metastatic breast cancer and is here to determine future options for her care.

Mary is accompanied by her husband and two children, ages 15 and 10. Her husband and children appear anxious but supportive and attentive. She states she is employed as an interior decorator and is well respected in the community.

Mary reports that breast cancer was first diagnosed 5 years earlier. Initial therapy included 6 months of chemotherapy, followed by a mastectomy and radiation therapy. At the time of her mastectomy, she was found to have axillary lymph node involvement of the carcinoma. Four years ago, she underwent reconstructive surgery of the breast. At a routine follow-up examination 6 months ago, she was found to have two metastatic lesions of the spine and one of the hip, and fluid was noted around the liver. Chemotherapy was reinstituted. At the follow-up examination for the chemotherapy last week, she was informed that four new metastatic lesions had developed while she was on the chemotherapy and that her options are limited to palliative.

Mary reports that she has always remained hopeful during her journey with the cancer. She feels that she has learned a great deal about herself during her illness and has grown closer to her family and friends. After her initial treatment, Mary was instrumental in the formation of a local breast cancer support group and is currently the chairperson. She reports sadly that she has not been back to the group since the recurrence of the cancer because she does not want to discourage other group members.

Mary has read extensively on self-healing. She practices yoga and does weaving as a hobby. Her response after the mastectomy was to invite five close friends to share a ritual that involved burying a plaster replica of her diseased breast. She viewed this ceremony as a new beginning for her life as she prepared for reconstructive surgery. She denies any organized spiritual orientation.

Mary has a trusting, comfortable relationship with her oncologist and sadly reports that recently she has entertained the notion of consulting someone new since the disease has progressed. She says that for the first time, she is really frightened and is willing to do almost anything that might give her more time with her family.

Mary's weight is 140 pounds, and her height is 5 feet, 6 inches. She takes medications for pain and depression. Her general appearance is that of a teary-eyed woman in no acute distress. She sits quietly on the bed holding her husband's hand during the interview. She is articulate.

NURSING CARE OF MARY WITH ROGERS' MODEL

Nursing care for Mary offers the opportunity to incorporate many variations in patterning activities. Patterning activities will be directed by the knowledge gained during the appraisal phase. As Mary nears and prepares for the end of her life, many patterning concerns must be addressed for peaceful closure to her life and the change to another energy form. The steps involve pattern appraisal, mutual patterning modalities, and evaluation of the dissonance perceived before, during, and after patterning activities.

Pattern Appraisal

The pattern appraisal is ongoing. Mary is verbal and intuitive. She readily shares with others the story of her journey with cancer. A sense of sadness and communion with others is perceived. Dissonance is noted in the progression of the disease, in her pain, and in her confusion regarding how to proceed and whether to remain with her oncologist. Harmony is noted in her relationship with her husband and family and with her sense of how she has progressed through this disease process.

Mary has a great deal of knowledge about herself and about the disease. Mary, her family, and the nurse are aware that the pattern of breast cancer with multiple metastases is one of eventual death. The dissonance of the cancer is a rhythmical emergence that is pervasive to her wholeness.

Sensory data are gained through language, feelings, and perceptions. The nurse perceives that much attention to sensory information is needed because Mary has a great deal to share about her feelings regarding the disease and her thoughts and fears. Dissonance is perceived through her acknowledgment of fear and apprehension regarding her future.

Intuition is a major source of self-knowledge for Mary. She relates that it is hard for her to accept that she is terminal because she looks good and feels well. She states that intuitively her body tells her that she will be okay. However, all healthcare providers give her an entirely different perception of her health status. The intuitive knowing of the nurse is crucial in completing the pattern appraisal. Cognitive knowing tells the nurse that Mary's condition is grave; however, the addition of intuitive knowledge on the nurse's part may change the unitary perspective.

Knowledge gained through language is integral to the assessment. Mary and her family have a great deal of self-knowledge to share. Perceptions and beliefs regarding health and illness are important to the appraisal. Conversation with Mary flows easily and reveals a great deal. Mary is articulate and shares freely her perceptions about what is occurring to her and her family.

Valuable information regarding areas of dissonance can be gained through a field evaluation using therapeutic touch. During the initial examination, the nurse uses therapeutic touch to identify any irregularities of the energy field and also to channel energy for pain control. Energy field appraisal with the assessment of areas of pattern distortion adds critical information.

The unitary image that emerges is one of dissonance that manifests as metastatic breast cancer. The Rogerian model guides us to a field evaluation and analysis. Mary, her husband, and children are an emergent field pattern. The objective signs and symptoms are perceivable field pattern manifestations. The diagnosis of metastatic breast cancer is the label applied to the pattern manifestation.

Mutual Patterning

A sharing of the unitary pattern appraisal with Mary is imperative. Mary will confirm or reject the appraisal, and it will become the basis for the patterning recommendations. The nurse helps create an environment in which healing conditions are optimal and invites Mary to heal herself as she participates in various modalities used in deliberative mutual patterning.

Change is continuous and in the direction of increasing diversity of patterning. The varying forms of manifestation that are associated with change become somewhat predictable. In clinical practice, this means a consideration of the manifestations relative to the individual in developing therapeutic aims. As Mary deals with her emergent pattern, pain is a frequent perceivable manifestation. Assistance in options for the management of pain is needed.

The use of different-color light waves can be proposed to Mary. McDonald (1986) examined the relationship between visible light waves and the experience of pain. She reported that blue light waves decrease pain in individuals with rheumatoid arthritis. Trials of various colors and their patterning ability on the manifestation of pain could be offered. Mary, who is an interior decorator, has strong preferences and dislikes for various colors. Since the hospital walls are white, color can be introduced through blankets and/or sheets brought by the family. Mary can be asked whether she wishes to have certain art objects or flowers brought to her room. Every effort should be made to make the room environment consistent with Mary's preferences. Attention should also be given to the amount and type of light in Mary's room. Does she prefer natural, incandescent, or fluorescent light? The family can be encouraged to bring a bedside incandescent light if she prefers. The use of sound in the environment is also helpful for patterning. Mary is encouraged to have her family bring a tape player or CD player and music that she enjoys.

Therapeutic touch is introduced for assistance in the dissonant emergence of pain. Options relating to intermittent therapeutic touch are proposed. Modalities are taught to family members so they can continue the patterning in the absence of the nurse or after hospitalization. The family's comfort level with respect to administering therapeutic touch needs to be assessed. Families can be easily taught how to smooth the energy field and how to direct energy to areas of concern/pain. Therapeutic touch can be helpful to Mary and to her family as it allows closeness and the ability to nurture Mary through her pain.

Living/dying is a rhythmic manifestation of the life process. Unitary human and environmental rhythms find expression in the rhythmicities of the living/dying process. Death is a very real possibility for Mary. The nurses caring for Mary are concerned with dying as well as with living. Dying is a developmental process, during which there is continued actualization of potentials (Phillips, 1990). According to Rogers (1992), dying is moving beyond the pattern visible to human perception. Death is a transformation of energy (Rogers, 1970). At death, the human field ceases to exist, and identity as a living human being is gone. The process of dying is a period of transition in which the integrity of the human field as such diminishes and dies (Rogers, 1970). A transformation of energy occurs. As the pattern of cancer evolves for Mary, manifestations of pain will increase, and the reality of impending death will emerge. Nursing care will revolve around the introduction of several modalities that may assist Mary and her family as the human/environmental field evolves.

Uninterrupted time for Mary and her family to be together is imperative. Attention to visitation based on Mary's rhythm is implemented. Children, friends, and family can visit without restriction and are encouraged to bring items that help them feel harmonious in the hospital environment.

The power of humor in the patterning of chronic illness manifestation is proposed. Options include movies, books, or recordings. Sources for materials are shared with Mary and her family. Hospital volunteers are asked to search for and bring materials to Mary. She and her family are offered the option of bringing their VCR so that they may view humorous films if they so desire. The hospital medical library is consulted to see whether they have materials that Mary and her family could use. Nursing staff are encouraged to maintain their humor in their care for Mary. Often nursing staff members avoid terminally ill patients, and care should be taken to assign to Mary staff who are comfortable with terminally ill patients. Mary is offered some input into who is her nurse.

Meditation is introduced as a form of centering for Mary. She is asked to focus on a memory or a part of her body and slow down her breathing. She may choose to have her eyes open or closed. She may elect to center on an object in her room. Meditative music is introduced into the environment. Care is taken to place a sign that indicates "do not disturb" on Mary's door during meditation time.

Medication is also incorporated into the care of Mary's pain. Mary has identified that she is much more comfortable if she takes her pain medication every 4 hours and does not wait for it to "get bad." A routine is developed to allow Mary to receive her medication every 4 hours, and the family is involved in the administration of the dosage.

Mary and her family are close. The suggestion of journaling as a means of patterning her evolution into death is introduced. This journaling is used by Mary and by her family to record the relative present. This journal provides a forum for discussion of many issues regarding Mary's illness and her sadness regarding not seeing her children grow up. Nurses freely discuss their perceptions and share the joy they have in caring for Mary.

Because Mary is a professional interior decorator, the importance of color, light, and pattern are integral to her care. Options regarding how her physical space is oriented, decorated, and located are explored in the patterning of Mary. She and her family are given latitude in bringing personal effects, artwork, children's drawings, and photographs. The bed is turned to face the window at Mary's request. A favorite rocker and a bright rug for the floor are brought from home. Mary elects to place a beautiful cloth over her bedside table and has her small weaving loom placed in the room. The room radiates a sense of peace, and the feeling of the hospital is lost.

Evaluation

Frequent evaluation and pattern appraisal is needed as Mary approaches death. Intuition and family reflections assist the nurse in their knowing. A complete pattern appraisal is repeated with special attention to dissonance perceived in respect to pain. Therapeutic touch is administered to identify any field irregularities. A temporal recording of perceptions that surround the pain is reviewed. Perceptions of dissonance are identified and verified with Mary, and new patterning modalities are introduced. The care of Mary is most rewarding within a Rogerian model. She exemplifies a unitary human spirit that has been attuned to energy and intuition her entire life.

CRITICAL THINKING EXERCISES

1. Conduct a comprehensive pattern appraisal on yourself. Include cognitive, sensory, intuitive, and language as knowledge sources. Journal keeping and history provide additional sources of knowing. Keep the journal for 3 days. You may include photos as a source of pattern appraisal. Note harmonious and dissonant rhythms.
2. Conduct a comprehensive pattern appraisal of your environment. Focus on manifestations that are perceived as harmonious and those that seem dissonant. Record these observations in a journal. Note harmonious and dissonant rhythms.
3. Introduce one environmental patterning modality and record pattern appraisal evolution as the patterning activity is introduced. Follow the process of pattern appraisal, patterning, and evaluation. Center on rhythm evolution in the appraisal.
4. Select a friend or coworker and complete a comprehensive pattern appraisal, including a home visit and discussion with family members. Conceptualize a comprehensive appraisal, and review the appraisal with the person. Record the experience and the person's response to your appraisal.
5. Introduce a nursing plan for the above person following the steps outlined in knowing participation in change (awareness, choice, freedom, and involvement).

References

Alligood, M. (1991). Testing Rogers' Theory of Accelerating Change: The relationships among creativity, actualization, and empathy in persons 18-92 years of age. *Western Journal of Nursing Research, 13*(1), 84-96.

Alligood, M. (1994). Toward a unitary view of nursing practice. In M. Madrid and E. A. M. Barrett (Eds.), *Rogers' scientific art of nursing practice* (pp. 223-240). New York: National League for Nursing.

Barnum, B. (1994). *Nursing theory: Analysis, application, and evaluation* (4th ed.). Philadelphia: J. B. Lippincott.

Barrett, E. (1986). Investigation of the principle of helicy: The relationship of human field motion and power. In V. Malinski (Ed.), *Explorations on Martha Rogers' Science of Unitary Human Beings* (pp. 173-184). Norwalk, CT: Appleton-Century-Crofts.

Barrett, E. (1990a). Health patterning with clients in a private practice environment. In E. Barrett (Ed.), *Visions of Rogers' science-based nursing* (pp. 105-115). New York: National League for Nursing.

Barrett, E. (1990b). Rogers' science-based nursing practice. In E. Barrett (Ed.), *Visions of Rogers' science-based nursing* (pp. 31-44). New York: National League for Nursing.

Bultemeier, K. (1993). Photographic inquiry of the phenomenon premenstrual syndrome within the Rogerian-derived Theory of Perceived Dissonance. Unpublished doctoral dissertation, University of Tennessee—Knoxville; Knoxville, Tennessee.

Bultemeier, K. (1997). Photo-disclosure: A research methodology for investigating unitary human beings. In M. Madrid (Ed.), *Patterns of Rogerian knowing* (pp. 63-74). New York: National League for Nursing.

Butcher, H. (1998). Crystallizing the processes of the unitary field pattern portrait research method. *Visions, 6*(1), 13-26.

Cowling, W. (1990). A template for unitary pattern–based nursing practice. In E. Barrett (Ed.), *Visions of Rogers' science-based nursing* (pp. 45-65). New York: National League for Nursing.

Daily, J., Maupin, J., Satterly, M., Schnell, D., & Wallace, T. (1989). Unitary human beings. In A. Marriner-Tomey (Ed.), *Nursing theorists and their work* (2nd ed., pp. 402-419). St. Louis: Mosby.

Kim, M. J. & Moritz, D. A. (1982). *Classification of nursing diagnosis: Proceedings of the third and fourth national conferences.* New York: McGraw-Hill.

Lutjens, L. R. J. (1991). *Martha Rogers: The Science of Unitary Human Beings.* Thousand Oaks, CA: Sage.

Malinski, V. M. (1986a). Contemporary science and nursing: Parallels with Rogers. In V. Malinski (Ed.), *Explorations on Martha Rogers' Science of Unitary Human Beings* (pp. 15-23). Norwalk, CT: Appleton-Century-Crofts.

Malinski, V. M. (1986b). Further ideas from Martha Rogers. In V. Malinski (Ed.), *Explorations on Martha Rogers' Science of Unitary Human Beings* (pp. 9-14). Norwalk, CT: Appleton-Century-Crofts.

Malinski, V. M. (1986c). Nursing practice within the science of unitary human beings. In V. Malinski (Ed.), *Explorations on Martha Rogers' Science of Unitary Human Beings* (pp. 25-32). Norwalk, CT: Appleton-Century-Crofts.

McDonald, S. F. (1986). The relationship between visible lightwaves and the experience of pain. In V. Malinski (Ed.), *Explorations on Martha Rogers' Science of Unitary Human Beings* (pp. 119-130). Norwalk, CT: Appleton-Century-Crofts.

Parker, M. (1989). The theory of sentient evolution: A practice-level theory of sleeping, waking, and beyond-waking patterns based on the science of unitary human beings. *Rogerian Nursing Science News, 2*(1), 4-6.

Phillips, J. R. (1990). Changing human potentials and future visions of nursing: A human field image perspective. In E. A. Barrett (Ed.), *Visions of Rogers' science-based nursing* (pp. 13-25). New York: National League for Nursing.

Rogers, M. E. (1970). *An introduction to the theoretical basis of nursing.* Philadelphia: F. A. Davis.

Rogers, M. E. (1986). Science of unitary human beings. In V. Malinski (Ed.), *Explorations on Martha Rogers' Science of Unitary Human Beings* (pp. 3-8). Norwalk, CT: Appleton-Century-Crofts.

Rogers, M. E. (1990). Nursing: Science of unitary, irreducible, human beings: Update 1990. In E. Barrett (Ed.), *Visions of Rogers' science-based nursing* (pp. 5-11). New York: National League for Nursing.

Rogers, M. E. (1992). Nursing science and the space age. *Nursing Science Quarterly, 5*, 27-34. Quoted material copyright © 1992 by Sage Publications, Inc. Reprinted by permission of Sage Publications, Inc.

Roy's Adaptation Model in Nursing Practice

Kenneth D. Phillips

"The changing environment stimulates the person to make adaptive responses. For human beings, life is never the same. It is constantly changing and presenting new challenges. The person has the ability to make new responses to these changing conditions. As the environment changes, the person has the opportunity to continue to grow, to develop, and to enhance the meaning of life for everyone." (From Andrews, H. A. & Roy, Sr. C. [1991a]. Essentials of the Roy Adaptation Model. In Sr. C. Roy & H. A. Andrews [Eds.], The Roy Adaptation Model: The definitive statement [pp. 2-25]. Norwalk, CT: Appleton & Lange. Reprinted by permission of Pearson Education, Inc. Upper Saddle River, NJ 07458.)

Human beings are incessantly besieged by a host of internal and external environmental stimuli. A stimulus is any entity that provokes a response (Andrews & Roy, 1991a) and that serves as the point of interaction between the person and the environment (Roy & Andrews, 1999). Environmental stimuli either threaten or enhance the individual's ability to adapt. As an example, loving, supportive behaviors from a parent enhance a child's ability to successfully adapt, whereas a hostile, abusive parent poses a threat to a child's adaptation.

Nursing plays a vital role in assisting individuals who are sick or well to respond to a variety of new stressors, move toward optimal well-being, and improve the quality of their lives through adaptation. The Roy Adaptation Model (Roy & Andrews, 1991) provides an effective framework for addressing the adaptive needs of individuals, families, and groups.

As noted in Chapter 1, nursing's most pressing question is "What is the nature of the knowledge that is needed for the practice of nursing?" Nurses practicing within the Roy Adaptation Model seek the following: (1) greater knowledge of factors that either promote or hinder adaptation, (2) better methods and tools for assessing adaptation level, (3) specific nursing interventions that either promote or hinder adaptation, and (4) effective methods for evaluating adaptation as an outcome of nursing care.

HISTORY AND BACKGROUND

Sister Callista Roy, a Sister of Saint Joseph of Carondelet, developed the Roy Adaptation Model (RAM) in 1964 in response to a challenge by her professor, Dorothy E. Johnson. Since that time, the RAM has been reconceptualized for use in the twenty-first century. The development of the model has been a dynamic process. The preliminary ideas of this conceptual framework were first published in an article entitled "Adaptation: A Conceptual Framework for Nursing" (Roy, 1970). The RAM continues to be refined. The RAM is presented in its most complete and recent form in *The Roy Adaptation Model* (Roy & Andrews, 1999). Many nurses in the United States, Canada, and worldwide practice nursing from the perspective of the RAM. The RAM has stimulated other scholars to publish books of their own about adaptation nursing (Randell, Poush Tedrow, & Van Landingham, 1982; Rambo, 1984; Welsh & Clochesy, 1990). The RAM has been implemented in numerous hospitals and other healthcare settings. The RAM has been applied to diverse populations, adaptive needs, and developmental stages (Fawcett, 1995; Marriner-Tomey & Alligood, 1998).

OVERVIEW OF ROY'S ADAPTATION MODEL

The RAM provides a useful framework for providing nursing care for persons in health and in acute, chronic, and terminal illness. The RAM views the person as an adaptive system in constant interaction with an internal and external environment. The environment is the source of a variety of stimuli that either threaten or promote the person's unique wholeness. The person's major task is to maintain integrity in face of these environmental stimuli. Integrity is "the degree of wholeness achieved by adapting to changes in needs" (Roy & Andrews, 1999, p. 102). Roy, drawing on the work of Helson (1964), categorizes these stimuli as being either focal, contextual, or residual. The first type of stimulus—focal—is defined as the internal or external stimulus most immediately challenging the person's adaptation. The focal stimulus is the phenomenon that attracts the most of one's attention. Contextual stimuli are all other stimuli existing in a situation that strengthen the effect of the focal stimulus. Residual stimuli are any other phenomena arising from a person's internal or external environment that may affect the focal stimulus but whose effects are unclear (Roy & Andrews, 1999).

The three types of stimuli act together and influence the adaptation level, which is a person's "ability to respond positively in a situation" (Andrews & Roy, 1991a, p. 10). A person's adaptation level may be described as integrated, compensatory, or compromised (Roy & Andrews, 1999).

A person does not respond passively to environmental stimuli; the adaptation level is modulated by a person's coping mechanisms and control processes. Roy categorizes the coping mechanisms into either the regulator or the cognator subsystem. The coping mechanisms of the regulator subsystem occur through neural, chemical, and endocrine processes. The coping mechanisms of the cognator subsystem occur through cognitive-emotive processes. Roy has identified two control processes that coincide with the regulator and cognator subsystems when a person responds to a stimulus. The control processes identified by Roy are the stabilizer subsystem and the innovator subsystem. The stabilizer subsystem refers to "the established structures, values, and daily activities whereby participants accomplish the primary purpose of the group and contribute to common purposes of society" (Roy & Andrews, 1999, p. 47). The innovator subsystem refers to cognitive and emotional strategies that allow a person to change to higher levels of potential (Roy & Andrews, 1999).

Although direct observation of the processes of the regulator and cognator subsystems is not possible, Roy proposes that the behavioral responses of these two subsystems can be observed in any of the four adaptive modes: physiological, self-concept, role function, and interdependence adaptive modes. Roy and her associates describe the function of the adaptive modes in the Theory of the Person as an Adaptive System (Andrews & Roy, 1991a).

Roy's Theory of the Person as an Adaptive System postulates that the four adaptive modes are interrelated through perception. Either an adaptive response or an ineffective response in one mode influences adaptation in the other modes.

The physiological adaptive mode refers to the "way a person responds as a physical being to stimuli from the environment" (Andrews & Roy, 1991a, p. 15). The five physiological needs of this mode are oxygenation, nutrition, elimination, activity and rest, and protection. Four complex processes that mediate the regulatory activity of this mode are senses, fluids and electrolytes, neurological function, and endocrine function. Physiological integrity is the adaptive response of this adaptive mode (Andrews & Roy, 1991a, 1991c).

The self-concept adaptive mode refers to psychological and spiritual characteristics of the person (Andrews, 1991b; Andrews & Roy, 1991a; Roy & Andrews, 1999). A person's self-concept consists of all the beliefs and feelings that one has formed about oneself. The self-concept is formed both from internal perceptions and from the perceptions of others. The self-concept changes over time and guides one's actions. The self-concept incorporates two components: the physical self and the personal self. The physical self incorporates body sensation and body image (Buck, 1991b). The personal self incorporates self-consistency, self-ideal, and moral-ethical-spiritual self (Buck, 1991a). Psychic integrity is the goal of the self-concept mode (Andrews, 1991b; Andrews & Roy, 1991a).

The interdependence adaptive mode refers to coping mechanisms arising from close relationships that result in "the giving and receiving of love, respect, and value" (Andrews & Roy, 1991a, p. 17). In general, these contributive and receptive behaviors occur between the person and the most significant other or between the person and his or her support system. Affectional adequacy is the goal of the interdependence adaptive mode (Roy & Andrews, 1999; Tedrow, 1991).

The role function adaptive mode refers to the primary, secondary, or tertiary roles the person performs in society. According to Andrews and Roy (1991a), "A role, as the functioning unit of society, is defined as a set of expectations about how a person occupying one position behaves toward a person occupying another position" (p. 16). Social integrity is the goal of the role function mode (Andrews, 1991a; Nuwayhid, 1991; Roy & Andrews, 1999).

Adaptive or ineffective responses result from these coping mechanisms. Adaptive responses promote the integrity of the person and the goals of adaptation (Andrews & Roy, 1991a). The major task of a person is to adapt to environmental stimuli in order to achieve survival, growth, development, and mastery. Ineffective responses neither promote integrity nor contribute to the goals of adaptation (Andrews & Roy, 1991a).

As described earlier, adaptation is accomplished through two main coping subsystems: regulator and cognator. Roy has not explicated the mechanisms of regulator and cognator because the mechanisms of regulator and cognator cannot be directly observed and remain largely unknown. However, the behaviors of regulator and cognator are manifested in the four adaptive modes (Roy, 1981), and the behaviors of regulator and cognator can be observed and measured in the four adaptive modes.

Roy and Andrews (1999) define health as "a state and a process of being and becoming an integrated and whole person" (p. 31). Health is a reflection of how successfully an individual has adapted to environmental stimuli. The goal of nursing therefore is to help the person to achieve adaptation by helping the person to survive, grow, reproduce, and master. Adaptation leads to optimum health and well-being, to the highest quality of life possible, and to death with dignity (Andrews & Roy, 1991a). Adaptation enables the person to find meaning and purpose in life and to become an integrated whole.

CRITICAL THINKING IN NURSING PRACTICE WITH ROY'S MODEL

Nursing process is a goal-oriented, problem-solving approach to guide the provision of comprehensive, competent nursing care to a person or groups of persons. According to Andrews and Roy (1991b), nursing process "relates directly to the view of the person as an adaptive system" (p. 27). Roy has conceptualized the nursing process to comprise six simultaneous, ongoing, and dynamic steps. The steps of the nursing process are the following: (1) assessment of behavior, (2) assessment of stimuli, (3) nursing diagnosis, (4) goal setting, (5) intervention, and (6) evaluation (Roy & Andrews, 1999). Each of these phases of the nursing process is discussed within the RAM. The goal of nursing in the RAM is to promote adaptation in each of the four adaptive modes (Roy & Andrews, 1999).

The nursing process alone is limited in promoting critical thinking; however, nursing theory serves as a guide for nursing care. Nursing theory directs the practitioner toward important aspects of assessing, planning, goal setting, implementation, and evaluation. Furthermore, practice within a model allows the practitioner to ignore irrelevant considerations and to selectively choose among a variety of nursing strategies. Another way of saying this is that nursing theory promotes critical thinking. Table 14-1 illustrates how the RAM guides the nurse through the critical thinking process.

Assessment of Behavior

From Roy's perspective, behavior is an action or a reaction to a stimulus. A behavior may be observable or nonobservable. An example of an observable behavior is pulse rate; a nonobservable behavior is a feeling experienced by the person and reported to the nurse. Exploration of behaviors manifested in the four adaptive modes allows the nurse to achieve an understanding of the current adaptation level and to plan interventions that will promote adaptation. At the beginning of the nurse-client relationship, a thorough assessment of behavior must be performed (Roy & Andrews, 1999), and the assessment must be ongoing. Table 14-1 presents categories of behaviors that need to be assessed for each of the adaptive modes.

TABLE 14-1   Critical Thinking in the Roy Adaptation Model

Phases of Process	Physiological Adaptive Mode	Interdependence Adaptive Mode	Self-Concept Adaptive Mode	Role Function Adaptive Mode

Assessment of behavior	Oxygenation
	Nutrition
	Elimination
	Activity and rest
	Protection
	Senses
	Fluids and electrolytes
	Neurological function
	Endocrine function
		Significant other
		  Giving
		  Receiving
		Support system
		  Giving
		  Receiving
			Physical self
			  Body sensation
			  Body image
			Personal self
			  Self-consistency
			  Self-ideal
			  Moral-ethical-
			    spiritual self
				Instrumental
				  Primary role
				  Secondary roles
				  Tertiary roles
				Expressive
				  Primary role
				  Secondary roles
				  Tertiary roles

Assessment of stimuli	Focal stimulus Contextual stimuli Residual stimuli	Focal stimulus Contextual stimuli Residual stimuli	Focal stimulus Contextual stimuli Residual stimuli	Focal stimulus Contextual stimuli Residual stimuli
Nursing diagnosis	Statement of behaviors with most relevant stimuli	Statement of behaviors with most relevant stimuli	Statement of behaviors with most relevant stimuli	Statement of behaviors with most relevant stimuli
Goal setting	Behavior Change expected Time frame	Behavior Change expected Time frame	Behavior Change expected Time frame	Behavior Change expected Time frame

Intervention	Management of stimuli
	  Alter
	  Increase
	  Decrease
	  Remove
	  Maintain
		Management of stimuli
		  Alter
		  Increase
		  Decrease
		  Remove
		  Maintain
			Management of stimuli
			  Alter
			  Increase
			  Decrease
			  Remove
			  Maintain
				Management of stimuli
				  Alter
				  Increase
				  Decrease
				  Remove
				  Maintain

Evaluation	Observation of behaviors after interventions have been completed to see if goals have been obtained	Observation of behaviors after interventions have been completed to see if goals have been obtained	Observation of behaviors after interventions have been completed to see if goals have been obtained	Observation of behaviors after interventions have been completed to see if goals have been obtained

Assessment of Stimuli

A stimulus is any change in the internal or external environment that induces a response in the adaptive system. Stimuli that arise from the environment can be classified as focal, contextual, or residual. In this level of assessment, the nurse analyzes subjective and objective behaviors and looks more deeply for possible causes of a particular set of behaviors (Roy & Andrews, 1999).

Nursing Diagnosis

A nurse's education and experience enable him or her to make an expert judgment regarding healthcare and adaptive needs of the client. This judgment is expressed in a diagnostic statement that indicates an actual or a potential problem related to adaptation. The diagnostic statement specifies the behaviors that led to the diagnosis and a judgment regarding stimuli that threaten or promote adaptation (Roy & Andrews, 1999). The RAM defines nursing diagnosis "as a judgment process resulting in statements conveying the adaptation status of the human adaptive system" (Roy & Andrews, 1999, p. 77).

Goal Setting

Goal setting focuses on promoting adaptive behaviors. Together the nurse and the client agree on clear statements about desired behavioral outcomes of nursing care. The outcome statement should reflect a single adaptive behavior, be realistic, and be measurable. The goal statement should include the behavior to be changed, the change expected, and the timeframe in which the change in behavior should occur (Roy & Andrews, 1999).

Intervention

According to Andrews and Roy (1991b), "Intervention focuses on the manner in which goals are attained" (p. 44). A nursing intervention is any action taken by a professional nurse that he or she believes will promote adaptive behavior by a client. Nursing interventions arise from a solid knowledge base and are aimed at the focal stimulus whenever possible (Andrews & Roy, 1991b). Intervention is any nursing approach that is intended "to promote adaptation by changing stimuli or strengthening adaptive processes" (Roy & Andrews, 1999, p. 86).

Evaluation

In the RAM, evaluation consists of one question—"has the person moved toward adaptation?" Evaluation requires analysis and judgment to determine whether the behavioral changes desired in the goal statement have been achieved by the recipient of nursing care (Andrews & Roy, 1991b).

In the evaluation phase, the nurse judges the effectiveness of the nursing interventions that have been implemented and determines to what degree the mutually agreed upon goals have been achieved (Roy & Andrews, 1999).

CASE HISTORY OF DEBBIE

Debbie is a 29-year-old woman who was recently admitted to the oncology nursing unit for evaluation after sensing pelvic "fullness" and noticing a watery, foul-smelling vaginal discharge. A Papanicolaou smear revealed class V cervical cancer. She was found to have a stage II squamous cell carcinoma of the cervix and underwent a radical hysterectomy with bilateral salpingooophorectomy.

Her past health history revealed that physical examinations had been infrequent. She also reported that she had not performed breast self-examination. She is 5 feet, 4 inches tall and weights 89 pounds. Her usual weight is about 110 pounds. She has smoked approximately two packs of cigarettes a day for the past 16 years. She is gravida 2, para 2. Her first pregnancy was at age 16, and her second was at age 18. Since that time, she has taken oral contraceptives on a regular basis.

Debbie completed the eighth grade. She is married and lives with her husband and her two children in her mother's home, which she describes as less than sanitary. Her husband is unemployed. She describes him as emotionally distant and abusive at times.

She has done well following surgery except for being unable to completely empty her urinary bladder. She is having continued postoperative pain and nausea. It will be necessary for her to perform intermittent self-catheterization at home. Her medications are (1) an antibiotic, (2) an analgesic as needed for pain, and (3) an antiemetic as needed for nausea. In addition, she will be receiving radiation therapy on an outpatient basis.

Debbie is extremely tearful. She expresses great concern over her future and the future of her two children. She believes that this illness is a punishment for her past life.

NURSING CARE OF DEBBIE WITH ROY'S MODEL
Physiological Adaptive Mode

Debbie's health problems are complex. It is impossible to develop interventions for all of her health problems within this chapter. Therefore only representative examples are presented.

Assessment of behavior. Postoperatively, Debbie has been unable to completely empty her urinary bladder. She states that she is numb and unable to tell when she needs to void. Catheterization for residual urine revealed that she was retaining 300 ml of urine after voiding. It will be necessary for her to perform intermittent self-catheterization at home. Unsanitary conditions at Debbie's home place her at high risk for developing a urinary tract infection. She states that she is scared about performing self-catheterization.

Assessment of stimuli. In this phase of the nursing process, the nurse searches for stimuli responsible for the observed behavior. After stimuli have been identified, they are classified as focal, contextual, or residual.

The focal stimulus for Debbie's urinary retention is the disease process. Contextual stimuli include tissue trauma resulting from surgery and radiation therapy. Debbie verified anxiety as a residual stimulus.

Infection is a potential problem. The focal stimulus is the need for intermittent self-catheterization. Contextual stimuli include altered skin integrity related to surgical incision, poor understanding of aseptic principles, and unsanitary conditions at Debbie's home.

Nursing diagnosis. From the assessment of behaviors and the assessment of stimuli, the following nursing diagnoses were made:
1. Altered elimination: urinary retention related to surgical trauma, radiation therapy, and anxiety
2. Potential for infection related to intermittent self-catheterization, altered skin integrity related to surgical incision, poor under-standing of aseptic principles, and unsanitary conditions at Debbie's home

Goal setting. Goals were set mutually between the nurse and the client for each of the nursing diagnoses. The goals were the following:
1. Complete urinary elimination every 4 hours as evidenced by correct demonstration of the procedure for intermittent self-catheterization
2. Continued absence of signs of infection of the surgical incision and urinary tract

Intervention. To help Debbie attain these goals, the following nursing interventions were implemented:
1. *Altered elimination: urinary retention related to surgical trauma, radiation therapy, and anxiety*
Debbie was taught the importance of performing intermittent self-catheterization every 4 hours to prevent damage to the urinary bladder. She was taught to assess her abdomen for bladder distention and the proper procedure for intermittent self-catheterization. She was instructed to keep a record of the exact time and amount of voiding and catheteriza-

tions. In addition, Debbie was taught relaxation techniques to facilitate voiding so that it would not be necessary for her to catheterize herself as often.

    2. *Potential for infection related to intermittent self-catheterization, altered skin integrity related to surgical incision, poor understanding of aseptic principles, and unsanitary conditions at Debbie's home*

Debbie was taught the importance of washing hands before touching the surgical incision or doing incision care. The procedure for incision care was demonstrated by the nursing staff, and Debbie was asked to perform a return demonstration. After the intermittent self-catheterization procedure was explained and demonstrated, Debbie performed a return demonstration with good technique.

Evaluation. Evaluation of Debbie's adaptive level was performed each shift. Significant findings included the following:

    1. It will be necessary for her to perform intermittent self-catheterization at home. Debbie was able to state the importance of performing intermittent self-catheterization on a regular basis. She performed a return demonstration of intermittent self-catheterization before discharge, and she was able to adequately adhere to aseptic principles during the procedure. She accurately recorded the times and amount for each voiding and catheterization.

    2. Debbie was able to list the signs and symptoms of a wound and a urinary tract infection and to state appropriate steps to take if symptoms occur (i.e., notify physician or nurse practitioner). She was able to discuss the importance of maintaining adequate oral fluid intake. Debbie was given a thermometer and instructed in its use. She correctly demonstrated taking a temperature.

Interdependence Adaptive Mode

Assessment of behavior. *Significant other.* Debbie's most significant other is her husband. She describes her husband as emotionally distant and abusive at times. He has been at the bedside since Debbie was admitted to the hospital. He appears worried. In addition to these findings, it would be important to determine how Debbie and her husband give and receive love, value, and respect and how they express nurturing and caring behaviors to each other.

    Support system. Debbie's support system includes her mother and her two children. Debbie and her family live in her mother's home. It is important to know how Debbie and her support system give and receive love, value, and respect and how they express nurturing and caring behaviors to each other.

Assessment of stimuli. Assessment of stimuli within the interdependence adaptive mode reveals that Debbie's relationship needs with her husband are not being met. It is encouraging that her husband is displaying nurturing, caring behaviors while Debbie is in the hospital. Further evaluation of Debbie's self-esteem would be warranted. Debbie and her husband were married at an early age. Their knowledge regarding building friendships and relationships may be limited. It would be important to assess modes of communication as well. The developmental stage for Debbie and her husband is that of young adults. In this stage, the individual becomes independent and establishes his or her own family. Debbie and her family live with her mother. This may be creating a stress on interdependence. Debbie acknowledges that she and her husband have very little time alone.

The focal stimulus in the interdependence adaptive mode is an emotionally distant relationship with her husband. Contextual stimuli are the following: (1) Debbie and her husband were married at an early age following an unplanned pregnancy; (2) they exhibit ineffective communication skills; (3) they live with her mother; and (4) they have very little time alone.

Nursing diagnosis. The following nursing diagnoses of interdependence adaptive needs were made:

1. Affectional inadequacy related to emotionally distant relationship, marriage at an early age following an unplanned pregnancy, ineffective communication skills, living with a parent, and having very little time alone
2. Potential change in support system dynamics related to potential role changes and changes in health status

Goal setting. To help Debbie with these adaptive needs, she and the nurse agreed on the following goals:

1. Increased affectional adequacy between Debbie and her husband by discharge as manifested by verbalization of and a need for increased communication between Debbie and her husband
2. Support system dynamics to remain stable during Debbie's recovery period

Intervention. To help Debbie attain these goals, the following nursing interventions were implemented:

1. *Affectional inadequacy related to emotionally distant relationship, marriage at an early age following an unplanned pregnancy, ineffective communication skills, living with a parent, and having very little time alone*

Assessment of interdependence was begun while performing other routine care. Debbie was asked the following questions: (1) Can you tell me about your relationship? (2) Do you consider it a good relationship? (3) What do you think would make a good relationship? (4) How does your husband express to you that he loves you? (5) How do you express to your husband that you love him? (6) How do you and your husband talk about things important to you?

Debbie's husband has been with her much of the time she has been hospitalized, and he seemed worried. Her husband was encouraged to do back massage when Debbie was experiencing pain or to just hold her hand when she became tearful.

2. *Potential change in support system dynamics related to potential role changes and changes in health status*

With Debbie's permission, time was allocated to discuss important aspects of relationship building. Both Debbie and her husband were agreeable. Professional family counseling services were obtained through the parish nursing ministry of the hospital for Debbie's family.

Evaluation. Debbie was pleased that her husband was talking to her more and enjoyed the caring behaviors in which he was participating. They began their counseling sessions before Debbie's discharge. They both resolved to spend more time alone. They both felt the counseling was worthwhile and wanted to continue after discharge.

Self-Concept Adaptive Mode

Assessment of behavior. Debbie is extremely tearful. She expresses great concern over her future and the future of her children. Exploration of Debbie's tearfulness revealed that she was afraid of dying. She believes that this illness is a punishment for her past behavior. Debbie and her husband were married at a very young age after Debbie became pregnant with their first child.

Debbie has not asked the nurse any questions about sexuality. Her hesitancy to introduce the subject may be related to her cultural background. In this case, the nurse introduces the topic. Salient findings here are the following: (1) Debbie recently learned of a diagnosis of cervical cancer; (2) she has undergone a recent radical hysterectomy; (3) she is receiving radiation therapy in the hospital, and the need for this therapy will continue at home; (4) Debbie has a lack of information about the impact of cervical cancer, radical hysterectomy, and radiation therapy on sexuality; and (5) Debbie has unresolved guilt related to unplanned premarital pregnancy.

Assessment of stimuli. Debbie is a young adult, is married, and has two young children. Debbie has an eighth grade education. She is in an emotionally distant, sometimes abusive relationship. Being diagnosed with cervical cancer at an early age has resulted in a maturational crisis for Debbie. This is complicated by the fact that several of her relatives have died of cancer. It is important for the nurse to assess coping strategies. One coping strategy that is mentioned is that Debbie is frequently tearful; crying is therapeutic.

Nursing diagnosis. The following nursing diagnoses were made:
1. Fear and anxiety of dying related to medical diagnosis and witnessing other family members' deaths as a result of cancer
2. Spiritual distress related to severe life-threatening illness and unresolved guilt related to unplanned premarital pregnancy
3. Sexual dysfunction related to the disease process; recent radical hysterectomy; need for radiation therapy at home; loss of childbearing capacity; weakness; fatigue; pain; anxiety; hormonal changes; and a lack of information about the impact of cervical cancer, radical hysterectomy, and chemotherapy on sexuality
4. Grieving related to body image disturbance, loss of self-ideal, changes in roles, and potential for premature death

Goal setting. To help Debbie achieve adaptation in the self-concept adaptive mode, the following goals were mutually set:
1. Decreased fear and anxiety of dying as evidenced by less tearfulness, relaxed facial expression, relaxed body movements, verbalization of new coping strategies, and fewer verbalizations of fear and anxiety
2. Decreased spiritual distress, as evidenced by verbalization of positive feelings about self, verbalization about the value and meaning of her life, and less tearfulness
3. Resumed sexual relationship that is satisfying to both partners as evidenced by verbalization of self as sexually capable and acceptable, verbalization of alternative methods of sexual expression during the first 6 weeks following surgery, and verbalization of when to be able to resume vaginal intercourse
4. Progression through the grieving process as evidenced by verbalization of feelings regarding body image, self-ideal, changes in roles, and potential for premature death

Intervention. The following nursing interventions were implemented to help achieve these goals in the self-concept adaptive mode:
1. *Fear and anxiety of dying related to medical diagnosis and witnessing other family members' deaths as a result of cancer*
Although Debbie's prognosis appeared good, she remained fearful of

dying. Time was taken to sit with Debbie, to make eye contact, and to actively listen to her, especially when she began crying.

Debbie was asked to share an extremely difficult experience she had encountered in the past. She was asked how she coped with that experience. Once her present coping strategies were assessed, new coping strategies were suggested.

She was encouraged to express her feelings openly. After allowing Debbie adequate time to express her feelings, truthful and realistic hope based on Debbie's medical history was offered. A cancer support group met each Tuesday in the hospital where Debbie was a patient. Debbie was given a schedule of the meeting times and topics. She and her husband were encouraged to attend the cancer support group meetings.

2. *Spiritual distress related to severe life-threatening illness and unresolved guilt related to unplanned premarital pregnancy*

Debbie was encouraged to express her feelings openly about her illness. It was suggested that times of illness are good times to renew spiritual ties. Debbie was supported in positive aspects of her life (e.g., being a good mother). At Debbie's request, the parish nursing ministry was consulted, and a chaplain was asked to visit Debbie.

3. *Sexual dysfunction related to the disease process; recent radical hysterectomy; need for radiation therapy at home; loss of childbearing capacity; weakness; fatigue; pain; anxiety; hormonal changes; and a lack of information about the impact of cervical cancer, radical hysterectomy, and chemotherapy on sexuality*

A complete sexual assessment was conducted to evaluate the perceived adequacy of Debbie's sexual relationship and to elicit concerns or issues about sexuality before her diagnosis with cervical cancer. Private conversation with Debbie was initiated to gain an understanding of her sexual concerns resulting from her therapy and her beliefs about the effects of radical hysterectomy in regard to sexual functioning. Debbie was instructed regarding possible changes in sexual functioning, such as a temporary loss of vaginal sensation for up to several months, vaginal dryness, and dyspareunia resulting from vaginal dryness. Since vaginal intercourse would not be possible for up to 6 weeks, alternate forms of sexual expression were discussed. To facilitate communication and sexual expression between Debbie and her husband, long periods of uninterrupted privacy were provided.

4. *Grieving related to body image disturbance, loss of self-ideal, changes in roles, and potential for premature death*

Debbie's perceptions regarding the impact of the diagnosis of cervical cancer on her body image, self-ideal, roles, and her future were explored. Debbie was encouraged to verbally acknowledge the losses that she was experiencing. Debbie was observed to determine which stage of the grief process she was currently experiencing (denial, anger, bargaining, depression, or acceptance) (Kübler-Ross, 1969). The grieving process was explained to Debbie and to her family, and they were assured that grieving is a normal process. Family members were encouraged to allow Debbie to cry when she needed to cry and to talk about her fears and feelings of grief. The nursing staff offered realistic reassurance about Debbie's prognosis. Debbie was encouraged to attend the cancer support group so that she could talk to others who better understood her grief.

Evaluation. Debbie's behavior changed before discharge. At the cancer support group, Debbie met Marie, a survivor of cervical cancer. After meeting Marie, Debbie became more hopeful that she could conquer cancer. Less tearful, Debbie appeared more relaxed. Debbie verbalized a good understanding of sexual changes that would occur and ways to help her adapt to these changes.

Role Function Adaptive Mode

Assessment of behavior. Assessment in the role function adaptive mode requires the nurse to identify primary, secondary, and tertiary roles. When these roles have been identified, the nurse looks for instrumental and expressive behaviors related to each of these roles. An instrumental behavior is an actual physical act performed by the individual that helps achieve the goal of mastery of a primary, secondary, or tertiary role. An expressive behavior is the attitude or feeling a person holds about a primary, secondary, or tertiary role.

Assessment of behaviors in the role function adaptive mode revealed that Debbie loves her husband very much and want things to be better for them. She is a conscientious mother. She is a dutiful daughter who assists her mother as needed. She enjoys helping elders in her community because it makes her feel good to help others when they need it. She has been diagnosed with cervical cancer, undergone radical hysterectomy, and is being treated with radiation therapy.

Assessment of stimuli. The focal stimulus in the role function adaptive mode is the fear of not being able to care for herself or her children in the future. Contextual stimuli include severe illness, radiation therapy, weakness, fatigue, and increased dependency on others.

Nursing diagnosis. The following nursing diagnoses were made:
1. Ineffective primary role transition related to severe illness, radiation therapy, weakness, fatigue, and increased dependency on others
2. Ineffective secondary role transition related to fear of not being able to care for herself or her children in the future

Goal setting. To help Debbie achieve adaptation in the role function adaptive mode, the following goals were mutually set:

1. Effective primary role transition as manifested by less weakness, less fatigue, willingness to allow others to help her when she needs assistance, and desire to resume self-care activities as she becomes able
2. Effective secondary role transition as manifested by fewer verbalizations of anxiety over her ability to care for herself and her children in the future

Intervention. The following nursing interventions were implemented to help achieve these goals in the role function adaptive mode:

1. *Ineffective primary role transition related to severe illness, radiation therapy, weakness, fatigue, and increased dependency on others*

Debbie was monitored for factors that would hinder her from performing self-care activities. A daily routine was established that incorporates periods of activity and periods of rest. Measures were implemented to promote rest (e.g., activity restrictions, minimal noise, restricted visitation, a morning and afternoon nap time, assistance with personal care, needed items close to her bed, back massage, progressive relaxation, guided imagery, and soft music). However, maximum independence was encouraged. Family members were instructed regarding the importance of maintaining independence. She was given positive reinforcement for successful accomplishment of self-care behaviors.

Debbie was praised for her performance of her primary, secondary, and tertiary roles. Resumption of these roles was discussed with Debbie. Debbie was asked to identify her support system. She felt that she had adequate support at home with performing her roles. She was encouraged to rely on her support system for help when needed in maintaining these roles.

2. *Ineffective secondary role transition related to fear of not being able to care for herself or her children in the future*

A thorough assessment was performed to gain an understanding of Debbie's fears and misconceptions about the effects of cancer, radical hysterectomy, and radiation therapy on bodily functioning, her lifestyle, and her ability to perform roles. Debbie verbalized a fear of dying and leaving her children. Interventions to instill hope were implemented. For instance, Debbie was given realistic assurance about her expected prognosis.

Evaluation. Debbie's husband was exhibiting supportive behaviors in the hospital. Debbie's mother was at home to help Debbie when she arrived. As Debbie's energy level was increased, she became less anxious about her future. Before discharge, Debbie became increasingly anxious to return home to her children.

CASE HISTORY OF BOBBY

Bobby is a 27-year-old Caucasian, homosexual man. After experiencing severe diarrhea and pronounced weight loss, he scheduled an appointment with his family physician. Both enzyme-linked immunoassay (ELISA) and Western blot tests indicated that Bobby was infected with Human Immunodeficiency Virus (HIV).

Bobby has lost 31 pounds over the last 6 weeks. His weight loss has been rapid and unintentional. He complains of mouth soreness, dysphagia, and anorexia. Foods have less taste than usual. White patches are observed over the tongue, buccal mucosa, and palate. He reports poor nutritional habits.

Bobby began having infrequent episodes of diarrhea about 2 months ago. Both the frequency and amount of watery diarrhea have increased over time. This has led to a fluid volume deficit. A stool culture revealed the presence of Cryptosporidium muris.

Bobby's family consists of his partner of 5 years, his mother, his father, and his sister. By his acknowledgment, Bobby's most emotionally intimate relationship is with his sister. He states that he can share his deepest fears, thoughts, and wishes with her. Bobby relates well to his sister, her husband, and his two teenage nephews. She visits him daily and brings food and fresh flowers from the garden that they had planted together. She speaks gently to him and holds his hand when he is upset.

Bobby lives with his partner, Matt, in a small house on property owned by his sister and her husband. Matt has shown great concern about Bobby's health. Matt continues to work as a teacher and provides both emotional and financial support for Bobby. Matt is seronegative for HIV, and fear of contagion is a source of anxiety for both Bobby and Matt.

Bobby has a number of homosexual friends. None of them has visited. Bobby does not call his friends on the telephone because he does not "want to discuss AIDS with them." He communicates minimally with family and friends. Bobby states that he has had lots of friends in the past and that he has done many things for them. He asks, "Where are they when I need them?" He complains of being lonely much of the time.

Bobby's parents live in another city, and he has had a distant relationship with them for the past 10 years. His father is a minister in a fundamentalist, Protestant denomination. Bobby has been unable to discuss being homosexual with his parents because he knows they would disapprove. He fears being abandoned by his parents.

Bobby's primary role is that of a young adult. Bobby's secondary roles include partner, son, brother, brother-in-law, uncle, and friend. Bobby has always assumed the caretaker role where Matt is concerned. He is sad that Matt now has to do so many things for him. Bobby's sister has stated that she is not afraid, but she expresses some concern that her children might not be careful enough around Bobby to prevent becoming infected with HIV.

Bobby is a paramedic. He has enjoyed working as a paramedic for the past 8 years. He is questioning whether he will be able to work in this occupation in the future. Bobby's physician recommended that he resign his job. He talks about "all the adjustments" that he will have to make in his life. Bobby expresses guilt about all the responsibility that his illness has placed on Matt and other members of his family.

Bobby has always been concerned with his appearance. He has remained physically fit. He dresses neatly, but now his clothing is fitting more loosely. Bobby expresses concern about his deteriorating physical appearance and his lack of energy. Matt reports that he lies in bed most of the time, sighs often, and begins crying frequently. He asks, "Why is this happening to me? I don't deserve this. I am a good person." Things that he indicates make him feel better about himself are his job, regular physical workouts, and his friends.

NURSING CARE OF BOBBY WITH ROY'S MODEL
Physiological Adaptive Mode

Assessment of behavior. Bobby is a cachectic 27-year-old man. He has lost 31 pounds over the last 6 weeks. His weight loss has been rapid and unintentional. He complains of mouth soreness, dysphagia, and anorexia. Foods have less taste than usual. White patches are observed over the tongue, buccal mucosa, and palate. He reports poor nutritional habits.

Assessment of stimuli. It was determined by assessment of stimuli that the focal stimulus for Bobby's weight loss was increased metabolic demands as a result of HIV infection. Contextual stimuli contributing to the weight loss were mouth soreness, difficulty chewing and swallowing, decreased taste of foods, and poor dietary choices (Ungvarski & Flaskerud, 1999).

Nursing diagnosis. The following nursing diagnosis was made in the physiological adaptive mode:

1. Imbalanced nutrition: less than body requirements related to increased metabolic demands as the result of infection, mouth soreness, difficulty chewing and swallowing, and decreased taste of foods

Goal setting. The following goal was mutually established:

1. Improved nutritional status as evidenced by no further weight loss during the next week and improved appetite within 24 hours

Intervention. So that Bobby could achieve his goal for improved nutritional status, the following interventions were implemented:

1. *Imbalanced nutrition: less than body requirements related to increased metabolic demands as the result of infection, mouth soreness, difficulty chewing and swallowing, and decreased taste of foods*

Bobby was given verbal and written instructions on methods to increase his dietary intake of protein, carbohydrates, fats, and total calories. Bobby was advised to drink three cans of liquid nutritional supplements (e.g., Ensure, Advera) per day. A daily vitamin and a mineral supplement were recommended. Arrangements were made for a hot lunch to be delivered each day by the local AIDS support group. As suggested, Bobby began eating six small meals each day. Bobby's weight was measured each week (Ungvarski & Flaskerud, 1999).

Evaluation. Bobby's appetite was slowly improving. He gained one pound during the next week. Bobby reported less pain when chewing and swallowing. Bobby's intake and output averaged approximately 2400 ml per day during the next 3 days.

Interdependence Adaptive Mode

Assessment of behavior. Bobby's family consists of his partner, sister, brother-in-law, nephews, mother, and father. He has a good relationship with his partner, but his most emotionally intimate relationship is with his sister. He has a number of homosexual friends, but none of them has visited. He does not call his friends. Bobby has been unable to share with his parents that he is homosexual or that he has HIV infection.

Assessment of stimuli. Bobby is estranged from his parents and his homosexual friends. The focal stimulus for this estrangement is HIV infection. The contextual stimuli are related to his self-concept. These contextual stimuli are internalized stigma of AIDS (Phillips, 1994) (which prevents Bobby from contacting his homosexual friends) and internalized homophobia (Nungesser, 1978, 1979, 1983) (which prevents communication between Bobby and his parents).

Nursing diagnosis. The following nursing diagnosis of the interdependence adaptive needs was made:
1. Alienation or social isolation related to HIV infection, internalized stigma of AIDS, and internalized homophobia

Goal setting. To help Bobby experience a decreased sense of alienation or social isolation, the following goals were mutually set:
1. Maintenance of relationships with his family and friends
2. Talking to friends on the telephone by the end of the week
3. Verbalization of decreased feeling of loneliness
4. Participation in a diversional activity of his choice
5. Exploration of the possibility of attending the local AIDS support group next week

Intervention. To help Bobby attain these goals, the following nursing interventions were implemented:

1. *Alienation or social isolation related to HIV infection, internalized stigma of AIDS, internalized homophobia*

Bobby was assessed regularly for signs of increasing social isolation, such as decreased communication with family and friends. Bobby was encouraged to express his feelings of loneliness freely and openly. Because Bobby had a fear of contracting an infection from others, it was explained that contact with healthy adults was not a source of infection for him. Knowing Bobby's relationship with Matt, the nurse included Matt in discussions regarding Bobby's care. Bobby was urged to contact his friends by telephone. Bobby's gift at watercolor painting was obvious from his artwork displayed in his home, and he was encouraged to continue this hobby. Because Bobby was constantly concerned about telling his parents about his illness, role-playing was suggested. The nurse played the role of Bobby's father and asked him to tell her whatever he would like his father to know. Bobby was asked to think about where he would like to be when he tells his parents about his HIV infection and whom he would like to be with him for support when he tells his parents. He was encouraged to ask others in the AIDS support group how they handled this situation.

Evaluation. Bobby continued to be receptive to giving and receiving love and support from his sister and Matt. He remained hesitant to talk to his friends on the telephone. He spent a great deal of time watching the television. He felt that his energy level was too low for painting. At Bobby's request, a visitor from the local AIDS support group came to visit Bobby. Bobby stated later that he really enjoyed that visit. He indicated to the visitor that he would like to attend the support group sessions when he is discharged from the hospital. Bobby's parents came to visit him as soon as they heard that he was in the hospital. In the next few hours, they learned both that Bobby had HIV and that he was homosexual. They had suspected for many years that Bobby was homosexual. Bobby's father assured him that God loves him, that God would forgive him, and that God would change him.

Self-Concept Adaptive Mode

Assessment of behavior. Bobby has not shared with his parents that he is homosexual nor that he has HIV infection. He is concerned about his deteriorating physical appearance and his lack of energy. He lies in bed most of the time, sighs often, and begins crying frequently. He asks, "Why is this happening to me? I don't deserve this. I am a good person."

Assessment of stimuli. Bobby comes from a devoutly religious family and a religion that teaches that homosexuality is morally wrong. Bobby has found it difficult to tell his family that he is homosexual and has postponed telling them that he has HIV infection. The focal stimulus is HIV infection. Contextual stimuli are internalized stigma of AIDS (Phillips, 1994) and internalized homophobia (Nungesser, 1978, 1979, 1983). A residual stimulus was fear of losing his parents' support.

Nursing diagnosis. The following nursing diagnoses of self-concept adaptive needs were made:
1. Grief related to changes in current and anticipated physical appearance, lifestyle, sexual dysfunction, anticipated loss of health status, and probable impending death
2. Spiritual distress related to severe life-threatening illness and alternative lifestyle
3. Sexual dysfunction related to fear of transmitting HIV infection

Goal setting. To help Bobby meet self-concept adaptive needs, the following goals were mutually set:
1. A resolution of grief as manifested by verbalization of moving through the grief process
2. Increased experience of spirituality as manifested by verbalization of meaning and purpose of life and verbalization of connectedness with self, others, and God
3. Continuation of a mutually satisfying sexual relationship between Bobby and Matt and identification of methods to prevent the transmission of HIV

Intervention. To help Bobby achieve these goals, the following interventions were employed:
1. *Grief related to changes in current and anticipated physical appearance, lifestyle, sexual dysfunction, anticipated loss of health status, and probable impending death*

An assessment of Bobby's perception of the impact of AIDS on his physical appearance, sexual functioning, health status, and future was performed. Active listening skills and therapeutic communication techniques were used to assist Bobby in verbalizing his feelings and acknowledging losses he was experiencing. Bobby was asked to express a stressful event in the past and to discuss coping mechanisms that helped him get through that stressful event. Bobby and his partner had a good understanding of the stages of the normal grieving process. His behavior was observed to determine his current stage of the grieving process. Family members were encouraged to allow him to express his feelings freely.

2. *Spiritual distress related to severe life-threatening illness and alternative lifestyle*

Fear is a significant component of spiritual distress. Fear may be related to rejection and separation from others related to the diagnosis of HIV or a feeling of separation from God (Coward & Lewis, 1993). Bobby was encouraged to strengthen connections with old friends and to develop connections with new friends. Bobby was encouraged to experience connectedness with the universe through field trips, meditation, and guided imagery. Bobby's beliefs about a higher power (god-figure) were assessed. Bobby was encouraged to continue his belief in a loving god. Bobby was encouraged to spend time in meditation and prayer to discover more of this love.

Fear of the dying process may contribute to spiritual distress (Coward & Lewis, 1993). Bobby was encouraged to express his fears related to the dying process. Participation in the AIDS support group was recommended.

The fear of dying without making a lasting contribution to society is another element of spiritual distress (Coward & Lewis, 1993). When Bobby verbalized this fear, he was encouraged to look for ways to leave a lasting legacy. Bobby was encouraged to talk about his past events, interests, hobbies, occupation, and feelings. Bobby was prompted to focus on positive aspects of his life rather than on negative ones.

Bobby was encouraged to seek out new challenges and to do some of the things that he had always wanted to do (Coward & Lewis, 1993). Bobby's watercolor painting became an outlet for his feelings. As Bobby's health improved, he began a small gardening business. During the Christmas shopping season, he opened a shop in the shopping mall, where he sold his bonsai creations.

Hope and spirituality are intertwined. Bobby's sense of hope was assessed. He continued to be hopeful that a cure would be found. That hope was supported. However, his hope was tied to the present rather than to the future. He was encouraged to engage in self-care behaviors that would help him remain healthy. As the disease progressed, he was supported in his acceptance of his prognosis.

3. *Sexual dysfunction related to fear of transmitting HIV infection*

Active listening and therapeutic communication techniques were employed to facilitate expression of fears. Communication between Bobby and Matt was encouraged. Bobby and Matt were given factual information regarding HIV transmission. Instructions for the proper use of a latex condom during insertive sexual techniques were given. Bobby was instructed to wash his hands after toileting and after contact with body fluids such as semen, mucus, or blood. Matt was instructed to avoid contact with body fluids such as semen, mucus, or blood. Bobby and Matt were instructed to avoid sharing eating utensils, towels, washcloths, toothbrushes, razors, nail clippers, and sexual devices. Various forms of noninsertive sexual practices were discussed. Bobby and Matt were encouraged to attend the AIDS support group meetings to learn more about prevention.

Evaluation. Bobby moved appropriately through the stages of grief (Kübler-Ross, 1969). Although he has accepted the fact that his death is probably imminent, he continues to experience the fullness of life.

Bobby demonstrated increased spirituality. He has become very active and serves as a deacon in a church where he is readily accepted. He derives pleasure from helping others who have HIV infection. He has started two small businesses since he became ill.

Bobby and Matt are able to verbalize understanding of principles to prevent HIV transmission. Bobby and Matt report a mutually satisfying sexual relationship.

Role Function Adaptive Mode

Assessment of behavior. Bobby's primary role is that of a young adult. His secondary roles include partner, son, brother, brother-in-law, uncle, and friend. He is a paramedic. His physician has recommended that he resign from his job. Bobby talks about "all the adjustments" he will have to make in his life.

Assessment of stimuli. The focal stimulus in this adaptive mode is HIV infection. Contextual stimuli include the potential loss of employment and income and feeling guilty about the hardship his illness is causing others.

Nursing diagnosis. In nursing, the family is viewed as the client. HIV infection will greatly impact the lives of all those in Bobby's family. The following nursing diagnosis was made:
1. Ineffective role transition related to loss of employment, guilt about the responsibility his illness has placed on his family members, and the fear that he is not going to be able to "make it" financially

Goal setting. The following goals were mutually set:
1. Bobby: Effective primary role transition as evidenced by increased verbalization of his feelings about HIV infection and impending loss of independence
2. Bobby: Effective secondary role transition as evidenced by increased verbalization of his feelings regarding resignation from his job, increased verbalization of his feelings about the many changes in secondary roles that he is encountering, and by assumption of responsibility for applying for benefits to which he is entitled

3. Bobby's sister: Effective secondary role transition as evidenced by verbalization of less anxiety and fear about her children becoming infected with HIV

4. Bobby's family members: Effective secondary role transition as evidenced by participating in support group meetings, increased verbalization of their feelings regarding Bobby's illness, and taking time for personal and family needs

Intervention. Bobby was encouraged to freely express his feelings regarding the many changes in his life. Bobby was encouraged to attend the AIDS support group meetings. Time was allocated to just sit and talk with Bobby. Therapeutic communication techniques were used to facilitate Bobby's expression of his feelings.

His change in employment status was a major concern for Bobby. Bobby was encouraged to explore his feelings about resigning from his job. Work was begun to help Bobby find alternative sources of income. Supplemental Security Income (SSI) forms were obtained. Bobby and Matt were encouraged to complete the forms together.

By revealing that she was concerned that her children might become infected with HIV, Bobby's sister was sharing her fear of infection as well. Time was set aside for discussing these fears. Role-modeling by the nurse was an important intervention that was used. At Bobby's request, a session was arranged with his sister's family to discuss infection control principles. Age-appropriate written information about infection control principles was given to each of the family members. Bobby's sister, her husband, and Matt were encouraged to attend AIDS caregivers support group meetings.

HIV infection places enormous responsibilities on families. Family members were encouraged to maintain open communication and to share feelings with each other. Family members were encouraged to take time for themselves and for family activities.

Evaluation. Bobby increasingly verbalized his feelings and his fears. By attending support groups meetings, Bobby became aware of many services that were available to him in the community. He and Matt took an active role in "learning the system" for procuring resources from government agencies that Bobby needed. After Bobby resigned his job, he became a volunteer for the AIDS support group. After receiving information about how HIV is transmitted, Bobby's sister became less fearful. Bobby was able to maintain close relationships with his nephews. Many extra responsibilities were imposed on the family by Bobby's illness. Bobby's sister rearranged her busy schedule so that she could continue to help him and still spend time with her family.

CRITICAL THINKING EXERCISES

Critical thinking using Roy's model moves the nurse beyond the assessment phase of the nursing process to the following: (1) identifying stimuli that cause problems in adaptation, (2) making appropriate nursing diagnoses, (3) establishing meaningful goals, (4) applying innovative nursing interventions, and (5) evaluating the effectiveness of nursing care in moving the client toward adaptation. The following exercises demonstrate critical thinking from the perspective of the RAM.

1. In the case of Bobby under the role function adaptive mode, identify which goal is being met in the discussion of the intervention on page 304.
2. You have just been notified that you have won $30,000,000 in the Virginia State Lottery. Undoubtedly, this would lead to a significant change in your adaptive level. Using Roy's principles of a two-level assessment (assessment of behaviors and assessment of stimuli):
   a. List possible behaviors for each of the four adaptive modes.
   b. Identify focal, contextual, and residual stimuli for each of the four adaptive modes.
3. Your closest friend has just been diagnosed with breast cancer. She has undergone a radical mastectomy. She is receiving chemotherapy. She has just learned that the condition is terminal. She is single, and she has a daughter who is 6 years old.
   a. What would be her adaptive needs in the physiological adaptive mode? What interventions would you provide?
   b. What would be her adaptive needs in the self-concept mode? What interventions would you provide?
   c. What would be her adaptive needs in the interdependence adaptive mode? What interventions would you provide?
   d. What would be her adaptive needs in the role function adaptive mode? What interventions would you provide?
4. Your brother has just discovered that he is HIV positive. He was tested for HIV after his girlfriend told him that she was seropositive. Because you are a nurse, you are the first member of his family whom he has told.
   a. What would be his adaptive needs in the physiological adaptive mode? What interventions would you provide?
   b. What would be his adaptive needs in the self-concept adaptive mode? What interventions would you provide?
   c. What would be his adaptive needs in the interdependence adaptive mode? What interventions would you provide?
   d. What would be his adaptive needs in the role function adaptive mode? What interventions would you provide?

References

Andrews, H. A. (1991a). Overview of the role function mode. In Sr. C. Roy & H. A. Andrews (Eds.), *The Roy Adaptation Model: The definitive statement* (pp. 347-361). Norwalk, CT: Appleton & Lange.

Andrews, H. A. (1991b). Overview of the self-concept mode. In Sr. C. Roy & H. A. Andrews (Eds.), *The Roy Adaptation Model: The definitive statement* (pp. 269-279). Norwalk, CT: Appleton & Lange.

Andrews, H. A. & Roy, Sr. C. (1991a). Essentials of the Roy Adaptation Model. In Sr. C. Roy & H. A. Andrews (Eds.), *The Roy Adaptation Model: The definitive statement* (pp. 2-25). Norwalk, CT: Appleton & Lange.

Andrews, H. A. & Roy, Sr. C. (1991b). The nursing process according to the Roy Adaptation Model. In Sr. C. Roy & H. A. Andrews (Eds.), *The Roy Adaptation Model: The definitive statement* (pp. 27-54). Norwalk, CT: Appleton & Lange.

Andrews, H. A. & Roy, Sr. C. (1991c). Overview of the physiological adaptive mode. In Sr. C. Roy & H. A. Andrews (Eds.), *The Roy Adaptation Model: The definitive statement* (pp. 57-66). Norwalk, CT: Appleton & Lange.

Buck, M. H. (1991a). The personal self. In Sr. C. Roy & H. A. Andrews (Eds.), *The Roy Adaptation Model: The definitive statement* (pp. 311-335). Norwalk, CT: Appleton & Lange.

Buck, M. H. (1991b). The physical self. In Sr. C. Roy & H. A. Andrews (Eds.), *The Roy Adaptation Model: The definitive statement* (pp. 281-310). Norwalk, CT: Appleton & Lange.

Coward, D. D. & Lewis, F. M. (1993). The lived experience of self-transcendence in homosexual men with AIDS. *Oncology Nursing Forum, 9*(20), 1363-1368.

Fawcett, J. (1995). *Analysis and evaluation of conceptual models of nursing* (3rd ed.). Philadelphia: F. A. Davis.

Helson, H. (1964). *Adaptation-level theory.* New York: Harper & Row.

Kübler-Ross, E. (1969). *On death and dying.* New York: Macmillan.

Marriner-Tomey, A. & Alligood, M. R. (1998). *Nursing theorists and their work* (4th ed.). St. Louis: Mosby.

Nungesser, L. G. (1978). *Homophobia and speech disruptions.* Unpublished manuscript, Stanford University; Palo Alto, California.

Nungesser, L. G. (1979). *Homophobia prejudice in homosexual males.* Unpublished honors thesis, Stanford University; Palo Alto, California.

Nungesser, L. G. (1983). *Homosexual acts, actors, and identities.* New York: Praeger.

Nuwayhid, K. A. (1991). Role transition, distance and conflict. In Sr. C. Roy & H. A. Andrews (Eds.), *The Roy Adaptation Model: The definitive statement* (pp. 363-376). Norwalk, CT: Appleton & Lange.

Phillips, K. D. (1994). Testing biobehavioral adaptation in persons living with AIDS using Roy's Theory of the Person as an Adaptive System. Unpublished doctoral dissertation, University of Tennessee—Knoxville; Knoxville, Tennessee.

Rambo, B. (1984). *Adaptation nursing: Assessment and intervention.* Philadelphia: W. B. Saunders.

Randell, B., Poush Tedrow, M., & Van Landingham, J. (1982). *Adaptation nursing: The Roy conceptual model applied.* St. Louis: Mosby.

Roy, Sr. C. (1970). Adaptation: A conceptual framework for nursing. *Nursing Outlook, 18,* 43-45.

Roy, Sr. C. (1981). *Introduction to nursing: An adaptation model.* Englewood Cliffs, NJ: Prentice-Hall.

Roy, Sr. C. & Andrews, H. A. (1991). *The Roy Adaptation Model: The definitive statement.* Norwalk, CT: Appleton & Lange.

Roy, Sr. C. & Andrews, H. A. (1999). *The Roy Adaptation Model* (2nd ed.). Stamford, CT: Appleton & Lange.

Tedrow, M. P. (1991). Overview of the independence mode. In Sr. C. Roy & H. A. Andrews (Eds.), *The Roy Adaptation Model: The definitive statement* (pp. 385-403). Norwalk, CT: Appleton & Lange.

Ungvarski, P. J. & Flaskerud, J. H. (1999). *HIV/AIDS: A guide to primary HIV care* (4th ed.). Philadelphia: W. B. Saunders.

Welsh, M. D. & Clochesy, J. M. (Eds.). (1990). *Case studies in cardiovascular care nursing.* Rockville, MD: Aspen.

Orlando's Nursing Process Theory in Nursing Practice

Norma Jean Schmieding

"A deliberative nursing process has elements of continuous reflection as the nurse tries to understand the meaning to the patient of the behavior she observes and what he needs from her in order to be helped. Responses comprising this process are stimulated by the nurse's unfolding awareness of the particulars of the individual situation."(Orlando, 1961)

HISTORY AND BACKGROUND

For years, nursing education based its teaching on a medical model. In the 1950s, nursing leaders focused their attention toward defining its work and moving nursing education away from an apprentice model into higher education. At this same time, governmental grants were available to study nursing, including the integration of mental health concepts into the nursing curriculum. Yale University received a National Institute of Mental Health grant and hired Ida Orlando as project investigator. Whereas many nursing theories are developed deductively from other theories and adapted to nursing, Orlando was the first to develop a theory inductively through an empirical study of nursing practice. For 3 years, she observed and recorded what she heard and saw in contacts between patients and nurses (Pelletier, 1976).

When examining 2,000 records, Orlando was able to categorize them only as "good" and "bad" nursing. Recommendations by non-nurse researchers failed to establish mutually exclusive categories for these data. Finally, Orlando randomly selected records and asked nurses with dissimilar views, experience, and education to place each record into one of the categories she had initially identified. Remarkably, all the nurses agreed with Orlando's categorization. Then the light dawned! If they all agreed, then the record's anecdotal content contained "what made good and bad nursing happen" (Pelletier, 1976, p. 22).

According to Orlando, "In the records judged as good the nurse's focus was on the patient's immediate verbal and nonverbal behavior from the beginning through the end of the contact; whereas in those judged bad, the nurse's focus was on a prescribed activity or something that had nothing to do with the patient's behavior" (Pelletier, 1976, p. 23). When good nursing occurred, the nurse found out what was happening and identified the patient's distress. The nurse found out why the patient was distressed and recognized that without the nurse's help, the patient could not relieve the distress. Orlando concluded "that the function of professional nursing is to find out and meet the patient's immediate needs for HELP" (Pelletier, 1976, p. 24). Orlando's deliberative nursing theory was published in 1961.

Following this initial work, Orlando conducted research at McLean Hospital in Belmont, Massachusetts and was funded by a Mental Health Public Service grant. In this study, Orlando assessed the relevance of her earlier formulations, educated and evaluated nurses in the use of her formulations, and tested the validity of the theory formulations. Data were obtained through tape-recording verbalizations of nurses with patients and other healthcare members. Based on this research, her original formulations were validated and showed significant research results. She also extended her theory to include the entire nursing practice system (Orlando, 1972).

Orlando's theory remains one of the most effective practice theories. It is appealing because it clearly describes what nurses think is good nursing. Descriptions and analyses of the theory have been published by theory scholars, including Fawcett (1993), Meleis (1997), and Marriner-Tomey and Alligood (1998), as well as in articles related to its use in research (Olson & Hanchett, 1997; Reid-Ponte, 1992). It has been used for and by both clinical and administrative practice in two acute-care hospitals (Schmieding, 1984), in operating rooms (Rosenthal, 1996), and recently in a psychiatric hospital (Potter & Bockenhauer, 2000). Orlando's work has been translated into six languages. A web page on Orlando's theory by Schmieding (1999) contains extensive references (http://www.uri.edu/nursing/schmieding/orlando/).

OVERVIEW OF ORLANDO'S NURSING PROCESS THEORY

A theory organizes a phenomenon and identifies the salient features, separating the critical elements from the nonessential. It is like a road map that highlights important parts to guide the user (Barnum, 1994).

Each theory uses a different map. Different theories use alternate ways to categorize and make sense of the phenomenon. However, each nursing theory influences the nurse's thoughts and actions in his or her approach to nursing. Theory use changes the way one perceives and processes observations (Chinn & Jacobs, 1983).

Orlando's theory has been labeled differently by various theorists. Woolridge, Skipper, and Leonard (1968) classify it as a prescriptive theory. In using theory, few, if any, theories stand alone. Although nurses use one nursing theory as their organizing principle, nurses incorporate into their thoughts and actions dimensions of other theories to use in their nursing practice. Similarly, when using Orlando's theory, nurses draw on other knowledge and theory in their process of helping patients (Orlando, 1961). Orlando's theory is a reflective practice theory that is based on discovering and resolving problematic situations. If the problem is not discovered it cannot be solved. The centrality of the patient is ever-present in the use of Orlando's theory.

Framework of the Theory

As a reflective practice theory, Orlando's theory contains concepts that are interrelated but are described separately. These five interrelated concepts are addressed within the problematic framework derived from Schmieding's analysis (1983, 1987) of Orlando's theory using the works of John Dewey (1933, 1938) and Thomas Kuhn (1970). These include: (1) professional nursing function–organizing principle; (2) the patient's presenting behavior–problematic situation; (3) immediate reaction–internal response; (4) deliberative nursing process–reflective inquiry; and (5) improvement-resolution.

Professional nursing function–organizing principle. Orlando believed that without the authority derived from a distinct nursing function, nurses' practice could not be autonomous. From her research, she conceptualized the unique function as "finding out and meeting the patient's immediate needs for help" (Orlando, 1972, p. 20), which constitutes the theory's organizing principle. Thus the patient is the focal point of the nurse's investigation. Orlando states, "Nursing . . . is responsive to individuals who suffer or anticipate a sense of helplessness; it is focused on the process of care in an immediate experience; it is concerned with providing direct assistance to individuals in whatever setting they are found, for the purpose of avoiding, relieving, diminishing, or curing the individual's sense of helplessness" (Orlando, 1972, p. 12).

The patient's sense of helplessness, stress, or need originates from physical limitations, adverse reactions to the setting, and experiences that prevent a patient from communicating his or her needs. According to Orlando (1961), "Need is situationally defined as a requirement of the patient which, if supplied, relieves or diminishes his immediate distress or improves his immediate sense of adequacy or well-being" (p. 5). It is the nurse's responsibility to meet the patient's immediate needs for help either by supplying it directly or by calling in the services of others. The central core of the nurse's practice is to understand what is happening between the patient and the nurse, which provides the framework for the help the nurse gives the patient (Orlando, 1961).

At the first nurse-patient contact, the nurse does not know whether the patient is in need of help. However, information is available though exploration to achieve a correct understanding of the patient's presenting behavior and finding out if the patient is in need of help. This is not as easy as it appears. Orlando (1961) asserts, "First, the nurse must take the initiative in helping the patient express the specific meaning of his behavior in order to ascertain his distress. Second, she must help the patient explore the distress in order to ascertain the help he requires for his [immediate] need [for help] to be met"(p. 26). The nurse's focus of inquiry is always on the patient's immediate experience.

If the patient is in need and the need is fulfilled, the nursing function has been fulfilled. Orlando (1972) states, "The product of meeting the patient's immediate need for help is . . . 'improvement' in the immediate verbal and nonverbal behavior of the patient. This observable change allows the nurse to believe or disbelieve that her activity relieved, prevented, or diminished the patient's sense of helplessness" (p. 21).

The distinct function clarifies the nurse's role and guides the inquiry by directing it to the patient's immediate needs for help in the immediate situation. The function remains the same regardless of the patient's diagnosis, treatment, age, or whether the patient is hospitalized or at home (Orlando, 1972).

Repetitious use of this concept—to find out and meet the patient's immediate needs for help—becomes an acquired way of thinking. The nurse's subliminal thought in each patient contact is "Does the patient have an immediate need for help or not?" (Schmieding, 1987, p. 432). Thus this concept establishes the nurse's accountability to the patient and provides an evaluative framework for the nurse's action. Orlando's emphasis on the importance of the patient's immediate experience requires understanding the patient's behavior.

The patient's presenting behavior–problematic situation. Orlando focuses almost exclusively on understanding the complexities of problematic situations. Nursing practice is comprised of frequent patient-nurse contacts in which the patient manifests verbal and/or nonverbal behavior. These come in verbal forms (e.g., requests, comments, complaints, questions, moaning, crying, and wheezing), in nonverbal forms (e.g., skin color, silence, clinching fist, reddened face), or in physical forms (e.g., respirations or blood pressure). These situations disrupt the equilibrium and make the nurse take notice; they are cues to the nurse. It is unclear, however, whether the patient is experiencing a need for help. From her research, Orlando formulated the following statement to guide the nurse's observation: *"The presenting behavior of the patient, regardless of the form in which it appears, may be a plea for help"* (Orlando, 1961, p. 40). However, the need for help may not be what it appears to be. Therefore the initial behavior is not reliable for determining the meaning of the behavior or the help the patient requires, if any. Nonetheless, a nurse often makes assumptions about what help the patient needs and acts on the basis that his or her assumption is correct without first exploring the observation with the patient. This is a haphazard approach to nursing.

Orlando specifies that both the patient and the nurse participate in the exploratory process to identify the problem as well as the solution. Therefore the nurse-patient situation is a dynamic whole; each is affected by the behavior of the other. The interaction is unique for each situation. The patient's behavior stimulates the nurse's immediate reaction and becomes the starting point of the investigation.

Immediate reaction–internal response. The problematic situation, in the form of the patient's presenting behavior, triggers an automatic immediate reaction in the nurse that is both cognitive and affective. The reaction comprises the nurse's perceptions, thoughts about the perceptions, and the feelings evoked from the thoughts; they cannot be controlled. These items occur in an automatic, almost instantaneous sequence (Orlando, 1972). These data represent the only resource for understanding the meaning of the patient's behavior. The nurse's past experiences and knowledge combine with the nurse's understanding of the immediate situation to produce the nurse's unique reaction.

In any person's process of action, four distinct items occur sequentially. Orlando (1972) notes:

> These separate items reside within an individual and at any given moment occur in the following automatic, sometimes instantaneous, sequence: (1) The person perceives with any one of his five sense organs an object or objects; (2) The perceptions stimulate automatic thought; (3) Each thought stimulates an automatic feeling; and (4) Then the person acts (p. 25).

The interaction of these items is called the nursing process. The first three items cannot be observed; only the action can. The action is what the person says verbally or conveys nonverbally.

The nurse's immediate reaction is unique for each situation. What the nurse perceives, thinks, or feels reflects his or her individuality. The automatic thoughts come from the nurse's interpretation or meaning attached to the perception. It may or may not be correct from the patient's point of view (Orlando, 1961). Regardless of the extent of the nurse's accuracy, the perceptions that evoked the thoughts are communications from the patient and represent the raw data for the nurse to use in investigating or exploring the patient's behavior (Orlando, 1961). Orlando's deliberative nursing process guides nurses' use of their immediate reactions to understand the meaning of patients' behavior. In 1972, Orlando renamed the deliberative nursing process the *disciplined nursing process;* however, for consistency, the *deliberative nursing process* term will continue to be used throughout this chapter.

Deliberative nursing process–reflective inquiry. Orlando's deliberative nursing process (1961) views the nurse-patient situation as a dynamic whole. The nurse's behavior affects the patient, and the nurse is affected by the patient's behavior. Understanding the patient's behavior is a complex process in which observations and thoughts are used in a serial responsive way to get the "facts of the case." To be successful, the nurse's focus must be on the patient rather than on an assumption that he or she knows what the patient's problem is and on arbitrary decisions about what action to take.

The use of Orlando's deliberative process (1961) requires that there is a shared communication process between the nurse and patient to determine the following: (1) the meaning of the patient's behavior, (2) the help required by the patient, and (3) whether the patient was helped by the nurse's action. To understand this process, Orlando (1972) describes the components of a person's action process. In a person-to-person encounter, each experiences an immediate reaction. This contains the following: (1) the person's perception of the other person's behavior, (2) the thought about this perception, and (3) the feelings associated with the thought. Unless the content of a person's reaction is openly disclosed, it remains a secret from the other person. For example, if a nurse makes a statement to the patient and does not disclose what perceptions, thoughts, or feelings led to his or her action, the patient remains unaware of it because it was not expressed (Figure 15-1). Orlando (1972) notes this action process often functions in secret.

Although it is at first difficult to separate perceptions, thoughts, and feelings from one another, this activity will help a nurse visualize how one aspect of the reaction affects other aspects (Orlando, 1961). In 1972, Orlando developed specific guidelines that specify a person's use of the content or his or her reaction in a deliberative way. They include the following: "(a) in a situation a person verbally states to the other person any or all of the items of his or her immediate reaction; (b) the stated item must be expressed as self-designated; and (c) the person asks the other person to verify or correct the item verbally expressed"

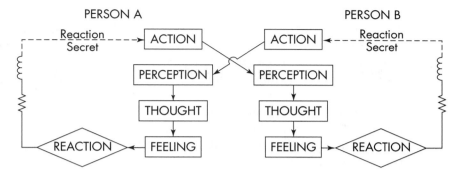

FIGURE 15-1

The action process in a person-to-person contact functioning in secret. The perceptions, thoughts, and feelings of each individual are not directly available to the perception of the other individual through the observable action. (From Orlando, I. J. [1972]. *The discipline and teaching of the nursing process: An evaluative study.* New York: G. P. Putnam. Reprinted with permission of Ida Orlando Pelletier; Belmont, MA.)

(Schmieding, 1993, p. 24). The deliberative nursing process is described as follows: "Whatever the nurse perceives about the patient with any one of the five sense organs and thinks and feels about the perception must, at least in part, be verbally expressed as self-designated to the patient and then asked about" (Schmieding, 1993, p. 25). This makes the origin of the remark explicit to the patient. Figure 15-2 provides its visual description of a communication process that operates by open disclosure (Orlando, 1972).

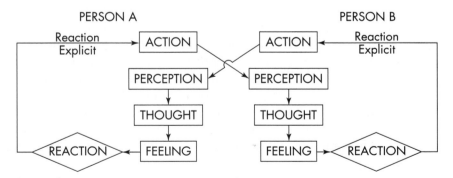

FIGURE 15-2

The action process in a person-to-person contact functioning by open disclosure. The perceptions, thoughts, and feelings of each individual are directly available to the perception of the other individual through the observable action. (From Orlando, I. J. [1972]. *The discipline and teaching of the nursing process: An evaluative study.* New York: G. P. Putnam. Reprinted with permission of Ida Orlando Pelletier; Belmont, MA.)

According to Orlando (1961), "The nurse does not assume that any aspect of her reaction to the patient is correct, helpful or appropriate until she *checks the validity of it* in exploration with the patient" (p. 56). The nurse will find it more efficient to find out what the patient's immediate need for help is by first exploring and understanding the meaning of his or her perception. The patient is more likely to agree with the correctness of the perception and often explains its meaning to the nurse. Efficiency is important because the longer it takes to find out the patient's immediate need for help, the more distressed the patient becomes (Orlando, 1961).

The nurse's automatic thought can also be used, but this approach is less efficient. However, if exploring perceptions is not successful, the nurse uses his or her thoughts to try to understand the nature of the patient's distress. Orlando (1961) cautions that the nurse's thoughts may not be valid. When using thoughts, the nurse must give the perception from which the thought was derived and ask the patient whether it is valid. Orlando (1961) cautions, however, that nurses are likely to assume that their thoughts are correct, unless they tentatively formulate them as a question or wondering. When the nurse states his or her thoughts as a tentative possibility, the patient is more likely to respond with his or her own negative reaction—for example: "I saw you close your eyes when I started to change your colostomy bag. I thought you might be frightened about having to learn how to do this yourself. Could that be so or not?" (Schmieding, 1993, p. 26). When nurses express their reactions, it minimizes the opportunity for nurses to make private interpretations about patients.

Feelings, either positive or negative, come from the thought about the perception. Feelings can also be used, but the nurse must state the perception that evoked the thought from which the feeling was derived. An example of this approach is the question "I get annoyed when you keep asking for the urinal because I don't think you really need it. Am I right or not?" The patient might respond, "Yes, but I'm afraid I might get short of breath and then I wouldn't be able to call for the nurse." If nurses do not resolve their feelings with patients, these same feelings occur each time they are in contact with the patients. Additionally, these unexpressed feelings may show in the nurse's verbal or nonverbal behavior.

Regardless of what aspect of his or her reaction the nurse uses, the patient is affected by the action; therefore "the nurse initiates a process of exploration to ascertain how the patient is affected by what she says or does. Only in this way can she be clearly aware of how and whether her actions are helping the patient" (Orlando, 1961, p. 67).

When nurses express their immediate actions to patients in a deliberative way, they are more likely to meet the patient's immediate needs for help because when they use it, patients are more likely to use it also. This approach minimizes the nurse's opportunity to make private interpretations about patients and maximizes the chance to correct or verify his or her private interpretation of the patient's action. Therefore both nurses and patients have a better understanding of how each experiences the immediate situation (Orlando, 1972). If this is not done, patients remain distressed because the communication between them is unclear since the nurse stated an automatic response to the patient (Orlando, 1961).

Orlando (1961) noted that automatic personal responses contribute to situational conflicts. Thus it is important to understand them so that problems associated with their use can be avoided. Basing her ideas on Orlando (1972), Schmieding (1993, p. 28) specifies the following reasons these responses are not helpful:

1. When a nurse withholds his or her immediate reaction, the patient cannot verify or correct it. The withholding of the nurse's perceptions, thoughts, or feelings allows the patient to make assumptions about the nurse's verbal and nonverbal behavior.
2. If the nurse's response is not stated as self-designated, the patient is allowed to make assumptions about the origin of what is heard (the use of "we" does not clearly provide the origin).
3. If the nurse's response is not in the form of a question, the other person may not feel free to correct or verify what she or he heard. As a result, neither person in the contact knows the immediate reaction of the other; therefore each is left with an unverified understanding of the other's action.

Actions based on the nurse's conclusion without the patient's participation are often not helpful. They are decided for reasons other than the meaning of the patient's behavior. Thus if actions are carried out automatically, even though they could be correct, they are ineffective in helping the patient because the patient was not involved (Orlando, 1961). A nurse's past experiences are not sufficient as the basis for understanding the patient's immediate behavior. Therefore in each nurse-patient experience a deliberative process of inquiry is required to prevent the use of automatic responses and arbitrary actions. When this occurs, the patient's immediate behavior improves.

Improvement-resolution. When a situation becomes clear, it loses its problematic character, and a new equilibrium is established. When the patient's immediate needs for help have been determined and met, there is improvement (Orlando, 1961). This change is observable in both the patient's verbal and nonverbal behavior. This allows the nurse to conclude that the patient's sense of helplessness has been relieved, prevented, or diminished (Orlando, 1972). If the patient's behavior has not changed, then the function of nursing has not been met, and the nurse continues with the inquiry process until there is improvement.

According to Orlando (1961), it is not the nurse's activity that is evaluated. Rather, it is the results—namely, whether the nurse's action helped the patient communicate his or her need for help and whether that need was met. Schmieding (1993) explains:

> Orlando's deliberative nursing process is *not* a linear process. . . . Rather the deliberative process is a 'muddy,' serial, back-and-forth process because it has elements of continuous reflection as the nurse attempts to understand the patient's meaning of the behavior and what help the patient needs from the nurse in order to be helped (p. 27).

Orlando's deliberative nursing process is an integral part of her theory, thus making it a practical theory to use. However, the theory's simplicity disguises the complexity of its use. Learning to use it requires its deliberate use, followed by a self-reflective analysis of one's action process. Practicing to separate one's perceptions, thoughts, and feelings will allow nurses to analyze their practice to see whether they have incorporated all or part of the immediate reaction into the action taken with the patient. If this is done, the nurse will include the patient as a reciprocal partner in both determining the immediate need for help and what will best meet the patient's need, thus relieving the patient's distress.

Schmieding (1993) explains:

> The nurse's *mind* is the major tool for helping patients. . . . Orlando regards the nurse's mind as the chief vehicle for converting mental processes, perceived from the immediate situation, into action. . . . The nurse's mind, therefore, is the intervening variable between the nurse's unique perception and its conversion into action (p. 14).

CRITICAL THINKING IN NURSING PRACTICE WITH ORLANDO'S THEORY

For more than a generation, the nursing process, based on the scientific method, has been the espoused method for nursing practice. Each component of the nursing process depends on the previous component before the next step is taken (Barnum, 1994). Although it systematizes and standardizes an approach to nursing practice, it is linear in design and, with few exceptions, patients have minimal involvement in any elements of the process. Nurses assess, determine a nursing diagnosis for each problem, establish goals and interventions, implement them, and evaluate the results. With the exception of assessment and implementation, other aspects of the nursing process are formulated out of the patient's sight. Because patients have minimal involvement in the process, there is little opportunity for patients to agree or disagree with any aspect of the nursing process. This is in contrast with medical practice, in which physicians generally share immediately their assessments, diagnoses, and plans with patients.

From an Orlando perspective, the espoused linear nursing process is fertile ground for operating on assumptions. The diagnostic classifications attached to patients generally lack patient participation and can readily lead to patient labeling and stereotyping. The nursing process offers little, if any, encouragement for nurses to use in their actions their thoughts about the situation. Rather, they tend to withhold their thoughts without verifying or correcting them, thus operating as if the thoughts, assumptions, and inferences, conceived in their minds, are factual and justifiable as the basis for nursing action. Consequently, patients cannot confirm or refute these assumptions. However, these thoughts, if stated, might be useful—even critical—in patient assessment, plans, goals, and interventions. Subsequently, many nurses have not fully developed the thinking processes that would enhance their effectiveness.

Leaders in nursing recognized the need to incorporate a nonlinear process—critical thinking—into the nurse's practice. There are numerous critical thinking definitions. As with theories, nurses select the description of critical thinking that best matches their conception of what will help them most in using a nonlinear thinking approach in all aspects of their patient care.

How to think is more important than what to think, as there is no one right answer (Jones & Brown, 1993). Regardless of the thoughts, they can be used in understanding any aspect of the patient's behavior (Orlando, 1961). Consequently, critical thinking requires a reflective process that is patient-centered (Daly, 1998) and also enhances nurses' functioning in the complex health environment. In contrast to the nursing process, critical thinking is characterized as a "unique, cognitive thought process that is grounded in reflection" (Jones & Brown, 1993, p. 73). Kataoka-Yahiro and Saylor (1994) stress attitudes toward critical thinking, knowledge fundamental to nursing practice, experience that leads to understanding complex situations, and cognitive competencies are needed for nursing judgment. Miller and Malcolm (1990) include similar criteria.

According to Dewey (1933), reflective thinking "involves (1) a state of doubt, hesitation, perplexity, mental difficulty, in which thinking originates; and (2) an act of searching, hunting, inquiring to find material that will resolve the doubt, settle and dispose of the perplexity" (p. 12). Dewey (1933) continues, "Any attempt to decide the matter by thinking will involve inquiring into other facts, whether brought to mind by memory, or by further observation, or by both" (pp. 13-14). The facts to which Dewey refers are not in one's mind but are only available in observable data. Thus Dewey (1933) emphasizes that conclusions must be based on existing evidence. In other words, both the problem and its solution require observable evidence. Thus critical thinking counteracts the tendency to base conclusions on assumptions.

In the Orlando theory, finding out the patient's immediate need for help underscores the importance Orlando gives to the first step of the critical thinking process. If the problem is inaccurately identified, the development of goals, strategies, and other components of the nursing process will not be effective, because they are based on a faulty foundation. In all aspects of the nursing process, Orlando's theory places high priority on patient involvement. Essentially, the nurse and patient are partners in the process. The Orlando theory also emphasizes that patient improvement, the evaluation component, is determined by positive changes in both the verbal and nonverbal behavior of the patient, which from Dewey's perspective, is the basis of evidence (Dewey, 1938).

Thus critical thinking is an integral part of Orlando's theory. Her work, a derivative of Dewey's theory of inquiry (1938), contains the basis elements of reflective inquiry (Schmieding, 1986). Orlando's work reflects her assumption that the nurse's mind is the most important tool in his or her armament and that the reflective process is recognized as critical in all phases of the deliberative nursing process used with patients. Our thoughts propel our actions, and therefore understanding the process by which we think is critical in any nursing situation. Patient situations are seldom as clear as they might appear. Each situation evokes in the nurse an immediate reaction in the nurse that is comprised of the present situation, previous knowledge and theories, and past nursing and other experiences. These elements combine to make the nurse's reaction unique for each situation. Within the nurse's reactions are tentative assumptions and inferences that the nurse will use to seek further evidence to refute or confirm them. This can be determined only by returning to the original source, namely the patient.

Assumptions are open to question; they are unvalidated conclusions about the nurse's perceptions. It is critical that the nurse recognize them as unverified thoughts.

In understanding and using the elements of the nurse's immediate reaction in a deliberative exploratory process, the nurse discovers, from the patient, information about the present situation. The nurse involves the patient in exploring alternative possibilities about the help the patient needs and exercises judgment in exploring with the patient to determine if the patient is capable of doing each intervention alone. If not, the nurse helps the patient as needed or does it on the patient's behalf. Nurses using Orlando's deliberative nursing process incorporate reflective elements of critical thinking into all phases of their practice. Patient involvement is a constant in the nurse's subliminal thinking and is manifested by nurses' focused actions with patients.

Nurses using Orlando's theory recognize the need to acquire new knowledge in multiple areas—such as physiological, psychosocial, political, and current research—in their specialty areas. By having more knowledge, nurses automatically retrieve it from their minds when it is relevant to the immediate patient situation. Additionally, they will question standardized practices for their relevance to current professional standards and knowledge and will seek out alternative approaches based on research and theory. The Orlando theory helps nurses see *that the patient is the source of the nurse's power* and, as such, it gives them the authority to use Orlando's guiding principle—the function of professional nursing—to negotiate on behalf of patients. Thus they engage in risk taking to benefit patients because they recognize their professional obligation to be accountable for their individual acts and also to work toward increasing collective professional accountability.

Because nurses using Orlando's theory have gained experience in articulating the thought processes that lead to their actions, they have a critical thinking frame of reference from which to propose and help make system changes. Consequently, they will question repetitive practices and rituals that consume their time and keep them from focusing on the real process of nursing—observing and making judgments about patients for whom they are both responsible and to whom they are professionally accountable, based on the authority of their position. Orlando nurses also know that they can use the content of their immediate reactions to help resolve interdisciplinary problematic situations. Using the content of their reactions in a disciplined way, they engage other professionals in dialogues to deal with practice issues that are of concern to each profession and are of critical importance to comprehensive integrated patient care. Changes in organizational practices and interdisciplinary collaboration enhances patient care and demonstrates the autonomy of the nurse's role. Using the Orlando Deliberative Nursing Process Theory is versatile, efficient, and effective. Most importantly, the patient is an active partner in the process. (Table 15-1.)

TABLE 15-1 Critical Thinking in Orlando's Theory

ASSESSING A PATIENT BY USING ORLANDO'S THEORY TO GUIDE THE NURSE'S PROCESS

Note: The nurse introduces himself or herself with full name and position, addresses the patient by title and last name (unless the patient prefers otherwise), and explains the nurse's role.

1. Guiding principle Finding out and meeting the patient's immediate need for help	The nurse's focus is on the patient. The nurse's mind is free of distracting thoughts.
2. Problematic situation and immediate reaction(s)	The nurse recognizes cues that a patient problem may exist before the next step in the process. The nurse identifies his or her immediate perception, thoughts, and feelings (immediate reaction).
3. Inquiry–problem determination	The nurse uses terms the patient can understand and explores immediate reactions with the patient to discover physical/nonphysical problems. As the problem is identified, the nurse asks the patient to confirm or refute its accuracy. The nurse explores the disagreement to determine its basis.
4. Identifying specific plans for each problem	With the patient, the nurse determines action(s) needed and develops plans for each problem. The nurse explores whether the patient agrees with or refutes the plan. The nurse explores and resolves the basis of disagreement. The patient verbally and/or nonverbally agrees. If not, the nurse continues the inquiry for the basis.
5. Implement	If the patient is unable, the nurse implements the plan and asks the patient whether the action is helpful. If it is not, the nurse explores the basis. The nurse helps the patient if he or she is unable to do it alone and explores whether the patient was helped. The nurse inquires about his or her results.
6. Improvement	The nurse asks the patient whether the action helped and observes the patient's verbal and nonverbal behavior. If he or she has improved, the need for help was met. If not, the nurse continues to use the content of immediate reaction to explore with the patient until a positive change is evident.

CASE HISTORY OF DEBBIE

Debbie is a 29-year-old woman who was recently admitted to the oncology nursing unit for evaluation after sensing pelvic "fullness" and noticing a watery, foul-smelling vaginal discharge. A Papanicolaou smear revealed class V cervical cancer. She was found to have a stage II squamous cell carcinoma of the cervix and underwent a radical hysterectomy with bilateral salpingooophorectomy.

Her past health history revealed that physical examinations had been infrequent. She also reported that she had not performed breast self-examination. She is 5 feet, 4 inches tall and weights 89 pounds. Her usual weight is about 110 pounds. She has smoked approximately two packs of cigarettes a day for the past 16 years. She is gravida 2, para 2. Her first pregnancy was at age 16, and her second was at age 18. Since that time, she has taken oral contraceptives on a regular basis.

Debbie completed the eighth grade. She is married and lives with her husband and her two children in her mother's home, which she describes as less than sanitary. Her husband is unemployed. She describes him as emotionally distant and abusive at times.

She has done well following surgery except for being unable to completely empty her urinary bladder. She is having continued postoperative pain and nausea. It will be necessary for her to perform intermittent self-catheterization at home. Her medications are (1) an antibiotic, (2) an analgesic as needed for pain, and (3) an antiemetic as needed for nausea. In addition, she will be receiving radiation therapy on an outpatient basis.

Debbie is extremely tearful. She expresses great concern over her future and the future of her two children. She believes that this illness is a punishment for her past life.

NURSING CARE OF DEBBIE WITH ORLANDO'S THEORY

The information presented about Debbie constitutes indirect information. Therefore the nursing care of Debbie with Orlando's theory is guided by Orlando's description of this type of information. Before discussing the nursing care of Debbie, this chapter offers some general remarks about Orlando's description of the use of various types of knowledge and information used in planning nursing care and provides the reader with additional information about how to use these sources.

Although general principles explain human behavior or foster health in general, it is within specific nursing situations that nurses must apply or use these principles. Therefore it is "exceedingly important for the nurse to distinguish between her understanding of general principles and the meanings which she must discover in the immediate nursing situation in order to help the patient" (Orlando, 1961, p. 1). If the nurse is preoccupied with application of principles, he or she will fail to find out what is happening to the patient (Orlando, 1961).

However, the greater the nurses' knowledge, the greater the resources upon which they can draw when necessary to help patients (Orlando, 1961). In any of these situations, determining the patient's need for help is the basis for applying principles rather than applying them automatically without patient involvement. Regardless of the types of data used, "the ultimate aim is to bring about improvement in the care of patients" (Orlando, 1961, p. 6).

Nurses often find that the only source of information available about a patient is indirect. Indirect observations come from comments made about a patient by colleagues—nurses, physicians, and other healthcare workers—and from such documents as progress reports, records, and nurses' notes (Orlando, 1961). Both comments and written material about the patient are second-hand information because they are not obtained in the nurse's presence of the patient. Direct information comes from nurses' observations of patients through direct contact with them.

The following description will not cover the routine activities done with and for the patient nor constitute a complete assessment. Rather, it will provide some examples of how Orlando's theory is used in practice.

Debbie's nurse is Bill, who graduated with a baccalaureate nursing degree 2 years ago. Bill will use words that are easy for Debbie to understand. Determining what indirect information Bill would use first in "real life" would depend on Bill's observing whether Debbie had either verbal or physical presenting behaviors that indicated a need for immediate exploration. For example, is Debbie crying, avoiding looking at Bill, or demonstrating evidence of physical trauma? When meeting Debbie, Bill introduces himself by his full name and tells her his type of position. He asks Debbie what she prefers to be called. Before Bill communicates anything else, he asks Debbie if she has any questions, concerns, or things she would like to ask or tell him. If Debbie does not raise any, Bill tells Debbie how long he will be her nurse. He explains that a staff nurse's responsibilities are to provide physical care as needed, explain anything that is new to her, and talk with her about any of her questions or concerns. He emphasizes that any question or concern is not too small or unusual to discuss with the nurse. By explicitly explaining what nurses provide, Debbie has a more comprehensive idea of how she can be a more sophisticated user of the nurse's service.

Bill informs Debbie that he will ask her some questions about her record to understand her needs better and to help her with anything that she thinks is important to her or her family. If Debbie does not raise any issues, Bill might say, "I read in your chart that you had major surgery.

Is there anything you think I should know about this so I can be more helpful to you?" Debbie's verbal or nonverbal behavior would help Bill determine whether he needs to explore Debbie's presenting behavior or to continue asking about information in the record.

The note on the chart about Debbie having pain and nausea is the next indirect data Bill explores. Bill informs Debbie, "In your record, I saw that you continue to have pain and nausea. I wonder—do you still have the same pain, or has it changed?" Bill would respond to Debbie based on his immediate reactions. Bill would also check to see if Debbie continued to have nausea or whether that had changed. His verbal question would be similar to the one about pain. It is critical that Bill explore both Debbie's verbal and nonverbal behavior to determine her need for help as well as whether she was helped by their verbal exchange.

Bill states he saw in the chart that she had gone from 110 pounds to 89 pounds. He tells her that, if she is able, she should eat foods that would help her gain strength as well as help the body heal. Bill asks Debbie what type of food she likes and tells her he can ask the dietitian to talk with her. He would say, "Debbie, would it be okay with you if I ask the dietitian to see you, or would you prefer not to?" If Debbie replied negatively, Bill would explore contents of his immediate reaction to understand her negative reply. This would help Bill find out that her basis was erroneous and end with her agreeing to see the dietitian. Orlando (1961) notes that by also stating a negative when asking a question, the patient is more likely to respond negatively.

After completing this area of investigation, Bill proceeds with additional data in the chart. He says, "It was noted in your chart that you were concerned about your children. It didn't state what your concerns were. Do you still have concerns?" If Debbie says she does, Bill would ask, "What type of concerns do you have?" If Debbie stated some, Bill would explore further to have a clearer understanding of what type of help Debbie might need. This would help Bill determine whether Debbie's concerns were related to areas with which nurses could help her; if not, as with the dietitian, Bill would say, "From what you say, I think it would be helpful for you to talk with the social worker. Would you like me to have one see you or not?" Depending on Debbie's reply, Bill would explore Debbie's presenting behavior to determine whether Debbie was no longer in need of immediate help with this by asking, "I think you are satisfied with these plans. Am I right or not?"

Another area Bill would explore pertains to Debbie's self-catheterization. He might say, "Debbie, I saw in your chart that you will be putting a tube into your bladder to drain your urine. I'd like to know if you have started to do this." If Debbie states that she has, Bill would ask, "Do you think you are learning how to do this more easily or not?"

Depending on Debbie's response, Bill would proceed with the next indirect information in the chart.

Although there is other information in the chart, the last area Bill explores in this contact with Debbie is about the statement in the chart that notes Debbie thinks her illness is a punishment for her past life. Bill brings this up by saying, "Another item in your record said you thought your illness was a punishment. Is that what you think now or not?" Bill responds according to Debbie's response. If it remains a source of distress to Debbie, Bill would use the content of his immediate reaction, such as "Debbie, I know there are various people, such as ministers, priests, and rabbis, from different religions that come to the hospital to see patients. Would you would like to talk about this with anyone, or not?" It may take more than one exploration with Debbie to determine whether this was a need for help. According to Orlando (1961), it is the nurse's responsibility to provide what help the patient needs for his or her need to be met, either by the nurse or by the services of others.

These are examples of how a nurse using Orlando's nursing process theory would approach the initial care of Debbie. Her theory emphasizes that nurses use whatever sources of patient information that are available to them in trying to find out whether the patient has an immediate need of help. These examples indicate how Bill states the information in a form that makes it easier for Debbie to respond, both positively or negatively. Certainly there are more areas that would need to be addressed. However, the ones addressed were clearly relevant to Debbie's immediate concerns and her state of health. Those that require additional exploration would, if necessary, draw on the theories and knowledge that are available to the nurse in the process of caring for Debbie.

CASE HISTORY OF VUALL*

Vuall, a 57-year-old Vietnamese immigrant, has been in the United States for 5 years and lives with his family, which is comprised of his wife, three daughters ranging in age from 16 to 23, and a son, age 25. Also living within the household are three members who are considered an extended family. Except for Vuall (who prefers to be called Vu), all members of the family speak English. Vu works part-time as a laborer. Recently, Vu tested positive on the Mantoux skin test and was diagnosed as having noninfectious tuberculosis (TB). He either has an active, noninfectious case or has been exposed to TB. Vu does not have pulmonary symptoms; however, his lymph nodes are enlarged. He is

*The author acknowledges the help of Martha Brown in the development of this section.

being treated at an occupational health clinic with the basic four frontline drugs. In addition to receiving care at the clinic for his TB, he also has had medical appointments for other health issues. These visits with physicians have not been very satisfying to Vu and his family. Vu has been treated for 4 months for TB and for 2 years for diabetes. Several nurses at the clinic say he is angry and that they find it difficult to care for him. When Vu sees his doctor, some of the staff are reluctant to be with him because he does not speak English.

Direct observation therapy for patients with TB is commonly used to assure that patients adhere to their treatment regimen. Therefore an agreed-upon place is arranged by the patient and healthcare worker to observe the taking of the prescribed medications and to assess for possible side-effects. Mary has been involved in the care of Vu since his first visit to the clinic.

NURSING CARE OF VUALL WITH ORLANDO'S THEORY

Several examples of situations with Vu illustrate how a nurse using Orlando's theory would provide deliberative nursing care. The nurse's name is Mary. She took a course in using Orlando's nursing process theory.

Many of the clients who come to this clinic do not speak English. Therefore observing such nonverbal behaviors as facial expression, eye contact, and types of body posture are of great importance with these patients. Orlando (1961) emphasizes the need to use the data in the immediate experience to explore its meaning. The physical behaviors are data that can be used to understand the patient's immediate needs for help.

Situation 1

Mary was told by a staff member that Vu was really "mad," but no one knew why. Mary thought to herself, "I'll listen to what the staff says, but I'll find out for myself what's going on rather than accepting the staff's conclusion about Vu."

Mary described that when she went to see Vu, his daughter Holly was there. When the doctor's examination was finished, Mary told Holly that Vu had to return for an appointment to have his eyes checked. She talked with Holly about the best time for an appointment. Instead of giving the appointment card to Holly, Mary handed it to Vu. He took the card and got a scowl and frown on his face, and Mary thought, "This is where the mad part that the staff had previously talked about comes from." However, Mary explored the meaning of his facial expression by asking "Holly, your father is really frowning. Is he upset about something?" Holly replied, "Oh, no. He's just trying to read what you wrote. He doesn't want people to think he can't read." Mary laughed and thought, "Mad, huh! Pretty simple to check out what you observe, but so many times nurses don't do it." Vu left the clinic with a smile on his face.

Analysis. Mary listens to the indirect data from the staff that includes an assumption about Vu. However, Mary does not base her actions with Vu on the staff's interpretation of his behavior. Rather, Mary relies on her own ability to discover whether Vu has unmet needs for help. She does this by exploring her perceptions with the patient through his daughter, the interpreter. Mary has developed a laser-sharp ability to use both obvious and subtle changes in the patient's behavior as cues that Vu might have an immediate need for help. Mary's exploring her perception first, from Orlando's perspective (1961), is the most efficient. She also used both her perception and her thoughts about it to explore Vu's behavior. Mary states the perception that gave rise to her thought, again an important part of Orlando's theory. Although this may appear to be a small problem, it is the type of problem that can lead to nonadherence to the treatment regimen. Without Mary's exploration of this situation, she would not have uncovered what the scowl and frown meant. Because Mary has known Vu and his family for some time, she does not always preface her statements as self-designated. As nurse and patient work together longer, using process elements becomes less critical. Orlando (1972) notes that although nurses may not use a self-designation in their actions, it is implied.

Situation 2

This problematic situation involves Vu and his son, Do. Mary was informed by the staff that his past appointments had ended with the doctor being frustrated. Mary was not present at this particular appointment, but she saw him after it was over.

Mary approached Vu to tell him that the doctor wanted to see him again in several weeks. Mary knew from previous experience that Vu needs to have the appointment when someone from his family can accompany him. This is very important because both Vu and his family need to know what treatment or recommendations the doctor makes to ensure that Vu can adhere to the plan.

Accompanying him on this visit was his son, Do. Mary said to Do, "Because your father isn't able to understand English, would it be possible for you to go with him to the doctor's office?" Do replied that he couldn't go. Mary explored her perception as well as some of her thoughts by asking, "Is there some reason you can't go, like the time of day or of the appointment?" Do repeated "no" and claimed that the doctor did not like him. When Mary asked, "What was that all about?", Do answered that the doctor had been concerned about Vu's "rung" and had shouted the word at him again and again. Do stated that he did not understand what the doctor meant. Recognizing that a person whose first language is not English might have difficulty understanding such words as *lung*, Mary explored her thought. Pointing to her lung area and breathing deeply, she said slowly, "Was it *lung*?" He confirmed that it was. Do then laughed and said that the doctor was speaking too quickly and that it sounded like "rung." He said, "If the doctor could slow down, I could understand better." Mary asked, "Do you think you could tell the doctor that?" Do agreed but asked the Mary also tell the doctor to slow down for him. Mary said, "I will tell the doctor's nurse about our conversation and will ask the nurse to tell the doctor that it would help you if the doctor would talk more slowly."

Analysis. On the surface, this appears to be a simple problem. However, because Mary explored her perceptions and thoughts with Do, he will be able to go to the appointment and participate in the process between his father and the doctor. In this situation both Vu and Do were helped. Do might be able to use the information Mary had discussed with him in other areas of his life.

Situation 3

Observation. Vu had his initial eye examination with the doctor, who wanted him to return in 1 year. When Mary asked, "Was another eye appointment scheduled for you?", Vu began to talk loudly in Vietnamese, but he had a smile on his face and a twinkle in his eyes. Mary asked his daughter Holly, "Your father is smiling but talking loudly. What is that all about?" Holly said, "He complains about the doctor's office because they say they will make an appointment, but they never do." Mary explored by saying, "Would it help you keep the appointment if I made the appointment for you?" Both Vu and Holly agreed and showed relief by expressing many thanks and smiling. Mary did not stop with this. She took the initiative to speak with the scheduler at the doctor's office and requested that Vu's next appointment be made at the time of his visit rather than having someone call for Vu.

Analysis. This is another case in which Mary, using a deliberative process, explores Vu's facial expression and his loud talking with Vu's daughter to find out what her father was saying. Because Vu has diabetes, it is critical that he has regular eye examinations. Not only will it benefit Vu but will also, by taking preventative actions, help avoid additional healthcare costs.

The nurse's use of Orlando's deliberative process is helpful to patients and rewarding to the nurse who uses it.

CRITICAL THINKING EXERCISES

1. Have you labeled some patients with such terms as *hostile, paranoid, depressed,* or *uncooperative*? Think about what you observed or heard that led you to these conclusions. Using a deliberative process approach, use some or all of the items in your reaction to explore the patient's behavior to find out the meaning of it, and explore what help the patient needs.
2. What assumptions (thoughts, not facts) have you had about a patient for whom you recently cared? What observable evidence from the patient do you need to support or refute your assumptions? How would you involve the patient in this exploratory process?
3. You recently heard a nurse use a stereotypical label of a person from a specific ethnic or racial group. What deliberative action would you take to investigate with the person the basis on which the person made the remark?
4. List some activities/procedures/practices that you routinely do for or with a patient. For each, what evidence do you need to continue or discontinue each? From where would you seek this evidence?
5. Think of examples when a colleague used a label (conclusion about someone) when discussing a patient or another staff member. What was your immediate reaction? With a deliberative exploratory process, use all or part of your reaction to understand your colleague's basis for the label.

References

Barnum, B. J. S. (1994). *Nursing theory: Analysis, application, evaluation* (4th ed.). Philadelphia: J. B. Lippincott.

Chinn, P. L. & Jacobs, M. K. (1983). *Theory and nursing: A systematic approach.* St. Louis: Mosby.

Daly, W. M. (1998). Critical thinking as an outcome of nursing education. What is it? Why is it important to nursing practice? *Journal of Advanced Nursing, 28*(2), 323-331.

Dewey, J. (1933). *How we think: A restatement of the relation of reflective thinking to the educative process.* Boston: D. C. Health.

Dewey, J. (1938). *Logic: The theory of inquiry.* New York: Holt, Rinehart, & Winston.

Fawcett, J. (1993). *Analysis and evaluation of nursing theories.* Philadelphia: F. A. Davis.

Jones, S. A. & Brown, L. N. (1993). Alternative views on defining critical thinking through the nursing process. *Holistic Nurse Practice, 7*(3), 71-76.

Kataoka-Yahiro, M. & Saylor, C. (1994). A critical thinking model from nursing judgment. *Journal of Nursing Education, 33*(8), 351-356.

Kuhn, T. S. (1970). *The structure of scientific revolutions* (2nd ed.). Chicago: University of Chicago.

Marriner-Tomey, A. & Alligood, M. R. (1998). *Nursing theorists and their work.* (4th ed.). St. Louis: Mosby.

Meleis, A. I. (1997). *Theoretical nursing: Development and progress* (3rd ed.). Philadelphia: J. B. Lippincott.

Miller, M. A. & Malcolm, N. S. (1990). Critical thinking in the nursing curriculum. *Nursing and Health Care, 11*(2), 67-73.

Olson, J. & Hanchett, E. (1997). Nurse-expressed empathy, patient outcomes, and development of a middle-range theory. *Image, 29*(1), 71-76.

Orlando, I. J. (1961). *The dynamic nurse-patient relationship, function, process, and principles.* New York: G. P. Putnam.

Orlando, I. J. (1972). *The discipline of teaching of nursing process: An evaluative study.* New York: G. P. Putnam.

Pelletier, I. O. (1976, August). Fundamental issues in professional nursing. Unpublished presentation, University of Tulsa College of Nursing; Tulsa, Oklahoma.

Potter, M. & Bockenhauer, B. (2000). Implementation of Orlando's nursing theory: A pilot study. *Journal of Psychosocial Nursing, 38*(3), 14-21.

Reid-Ponte, P. (1992). Distress in cancer patients and primary nurses' empathy skills. *Cancer Nursing, 15*(4), 283-292.

Rosenthal, B. C. (1996). An interactionist's approach to perioperative nursing. *Association of Operating Room Nurses Journal, 64*(2), 254-260.

Schmieding, N. J. (1983). The analysis of Orlando's nursing theory based on Kuhn's theory of science. In P. Chinn (Ed.), *Advances in nursing theory development* (pp. 63-87). Rockville, MD: Aspen Systems.

Schmieding, N. J. (1984). Putting Orlando's theory into practice. *American Journal Nursing, 84*(6), 759-761.

Schmieding, N. J. (1986). Orlando's theory. In P. Winstead-Fry (Ed.), *Case studies in nursing theory* (pp. 1-36). New York: National League for Nursing.

Schmieding, N. J. (1987). Problematic situations in nursing: Analysis of Orlando's theory based on Dewey's theory of inquiry. *Journal of Advanced Nursing, 12*(4), 431-440.

Schmieding, N. J. (1993). *Ida Jean Orlando: A nursing process theory.* Newbury Park, CA: Sage. Quoted material (from Schmieding pp. 14, 24-28) copyright © 1993 by Sage Publications, Inc. Reprinted by permission of Sage Publications, Inc.

Schmieding, N. J. (1999). URL www.uri.edu/nursing/schmieding/orlando/

Woolridge, P. J., Skipper, J. K., Jr., & Leonard, R. C. (1968). *Behavioral science, social practice, and the nursing profession.* Cleveland: Case Western Reserve University.

Additional Readings

Orlando, I. J. (1987, October). Nursing in the 21st century: Alternate paths. *Journal of Advanced Nursing, 12,* 405-412.

Orlando, I. J. & Dugan, A. B. (1989). Independent and dependent paths: The fundamental issue for the nursing profession. *Nursing and Health Care, 10*(2), 77-80.

Pelletier, I. O. (1967). The patient's predicament and nursing function. *Psychiatric Opinion, 4,* 25-29.

Schmieding, N. J. (1987). Face-to-face contacts: Exploring their meaning. *Nursing Management, 12*(11), 82-86.

Schmieding, N. J. (1992). Relationship between head nurse responses to staff nurses and staff nurse response to patients. *Western Journal of Nursing Research, 13*(6), 746-760.

Schmieding, N. J. (1993). Empowerment through context, structure, and process. *Journal of Professional Nursing, 9*(4), 239-245.

Modeling and Role-Modeling Theory in Nursing Practice

Margaret Erickson

"Modeling and Role-Modeling is based on the philosophy that all humans have the desire to live healthy, happy lives, to find meaning and purpose in their lives, and to become the most that they can be. This holds true across the lifespan. When we use strategies that focus on the strengths of our clients, help them become more fully alive (even as they approach physical death), and to live their lives to the fullest, then we are truly helping them grow, heal, and transcend. We help them discover the essence of their being, to find or reclaim their soul." (Erickson, 2000a)

HISTORY AND BACKGROUND

The Modeling and Role-Modeling (MRM) paradigm, conceived by Helen Erickson in the late 1950s, was an outcome of her exposure to the work of her father-in-law, Milton H. Erickson, coupled with her own experiences as a professional nurse. During the late 1940s and the 1950s, M. Erickson, M.D., developed an international reputation for his unorthodox methods, views on human nature, and clinical results (Rossi, O'Ryan, & Sharp, 1983; Rossi & O'Ryan, 1985, 1992). H. Erickson states she repeatedly asked him to tell her "what to do and how to do it" (Erickson, H. personal communication, February, 2000). She hoped for protocols, treatment recommendations, and quick fixes, but instead she was told that she must model the client's world and plan strategies within that context. He advised that each human has a unique view of the world and wishes to maintain roles in unique ways and that the practice of healthcare professionals was to help clients succeed in living quality lives and to grow to the maximum of their potential.

Over a period of approximately 16 years, H. Erickson came to understand the wisdom of her father-in-law's advice. As a result, by the mid-1970s, she had conceived and developed a practice framework that she called modeling and role-modeling. She began to label and articulate the theoretical components during her baccalaureate completion and master's study at the University of Michigan (1972-1976). Refinement of the concepts and their linkages continued as she worked with and was challenged by two colleagues, Mary Ann Swain and Evelyn Tomlin.

H. Erickson's first independent research attempt was during her master's study. This study, under the supervision of Swain, was designed to test the Adaptive Potential Assessment Model (APAM) (Erickson, 1976) which had been conceived, labeled, and articulated in the mid-1970s (Figure 16-1). About the same time, Swain and Erickson collaborated on another project designed to test the effects of MRM nursing interventions with persons who have hypertension (Erickson & Swain, 1982). This study led to a third, designed to explore the effects of using MRM with persons who have diabetes (Erickson & Swain, 1982). Tomlin joined the research team for this project.

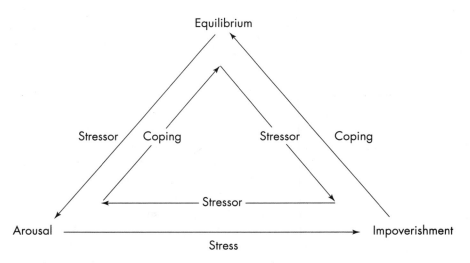

FIGURE 16-1

The dynamic relationship among the states of the APAM. (From Erickson, H., Tomlin, E., & Swain, M. (1983). *Modeling and role-modeling: A theory and paradigm for nursing.* Englewood Cliff, NJ: Appleton and Lange. Reprinted (1988, 1990, 1994, and 1999), Ann Arbor, MI: ETS. Reprinted with permission from Helen Erickson; Austin, TX.)

During these years, Erickson also expanded and tested the concept of self-care knowledge (Erickson, 1984, 1990) that had been conceived during the 1960s and early 1970s. She presented numerous papers, consulted in various agencies, taught at the University of Michigan, and continued her practice. Tomlin continued to explore ways to apply MRM in practice and to teach the theory and paradigm to undergraduate students while Swain supervised research, collaborated with Erickson on further elaboration of the theory, and launched the administrative phase of Erickson's career.

Finally, requests for written materials from practicing nurses, students, and faculty mandated that the book *Modeling and Role-Modeling: A Theory and Paradigm for Nursing* be produced. It was used as a text at the University of Michigan. Undergraduates were taught the basic premises; several university hospital units adopted it as a guide for practice (Walsh, Vandenbosch, & Boehm, 1989); a modified assessment form was developed at the University of Michigan Medical Center (Campbell, Finch, Allport, Erickson, & Swain, 1985); graduate students used it to guide their master's theses (Cain & Perzynski, 1986; Calvin, 1991; Clemintino & Lapinski, 1980; Doornbos, 1983; Finch, 1987; Hannon & McLaughlin, 1983; Kleinbeck, 1977; Smith, 1980; Walker, 1990); and doctoral students used it for their dissertations (Acton, 1993; Baas, 1992; Barnfather, 1987; Boodley, 1986; Bowman, 1998; Chen, 1996; Curl, 1992; Daniels, 1994; Darling-Fisher, 1987; M. E. Erickson, 1996; Hertz, 1991; Holl, 1992; Hopkins, 1994; Irvin, 1993; Jensen, 1995; Keck, 1989; Kennedy, 1991; Kline, 1988; Landis, 1991; MacLean, 1987; Miller, 1994; Miller, 1986; Raudonis, 1991; Robinson, 1992; Rosenow, 1991; Scheela, 1991; Sofhauser, 1996; Straub, 1993; Weber, 1995).

The Society for the Advancement of Modeling and Role-Modeling

In 1986, a website, www.mrm.globalmax.com (mrmlis@po.cwru.edu), was established by a cohort of students, faculty, and practitioners, and biennial conferences were initiated. The first conference was cosponsored by the University of Michigan in Ann Arbor in 1986, followed by the University of South Carolina at Hilton Head in 1988, the University of Texas at Austin in 1990, Brigham Women's Hospital in Boston in 1992, Humboldt State University in Eureka, California in 1994, Metro State University in Minneapolis in 1996, University of Cincinnati in Ohio in 1998, and again in Minnesota in 2000.

Schools including Humboldt State University in Eureka, California; Metro State University in St. Paul, Minnesota; St. Catherine's Hospital in Minneapolis, Minnesota; and the University of Texas at Austin have adopted MRM as the bases for either parts or all of their curricula, and various agencies have used it to guide nursing practice.

Continued research has provided support for several of the middle-range theories proposed in MRM. The three states of the APAM model have been tested and found to be independent of one another and predictors for stress (Barnfather, 1990; Barnfather, Swain, & Erickson, 1989a, 1989b; Erickson & Swain, 1982, 1990). Relations have been shown between the following: stress and needs status (Barnfather, 1990, 1993); need status and developmental residual and hope (as developmental residual) (Curl, 1992); burden and affiliated-individation in caretakers of persons with Alzheimer's disease (Acton, 1993); needs and affiliated-individuation (Acton & Miller, 1996); stress and affiliated-individuation (Irvin & Acton, 1996); stress, psychological resources, and physical well-being (Leidy, 1989, 1990); and needs satisfaction (Leidy, 1994).

Instruments have also been developed to enhance application of MRM in practice and research. Tools include those designed to measure the following: needs status (Leidy, 1994), developmental residual (Darling-Fisher & Leidy, 1988), the APAM stress states using content analysis (Hopkins, 1994), self-care resources of postcoronary patients (Baas, 1992), denial in postcoronary patients (Robinson, 1992), perceived enactment of autonomy in the elderly (Hertz, 1991), and the bonding-attachment process within the context of need satisfaction in teenage mothers (M.E. Erickson, 1996).

OVERVIEW OF MODELING AND ROLE-MODELING

Modeling and Role-Modeling (Erickson, Tomlin, & Swain, 1983), conceived within the context of numerous philosophical assumptions, was labeled and articulated by synthesizing several concepts from established theories. Concepts were drawn from the works of Maslow (1968, 1970), Bowlby (1969, 1973, 1980), Erikson (1963), Engel (1962, 1968), and Selye (1974) to create a new theory that described relations among needs, loss, grief, adaptation, developmental processes, growth and well-being of the holistic person (Figure 16-2). The practice paradigm was derived from integrating philosophical assumptions with theoretical underpinnings.

Philosophical Assumptions

Humans consist of cognitive, biophysical, social, and psychological subsystems permeated by genetic predispositions and a spiritual drive (Figure 16-3). The ongoing interaction of these multiple components creates a dynamic, holistic system that is greater than a sum of the parts (Erickson, Tomlin, & Swain, 1983). Health, which is affected by these dynamic interactions, is a perception of well-being. Although physical status influences perceptions of health, a person can perceive a high level

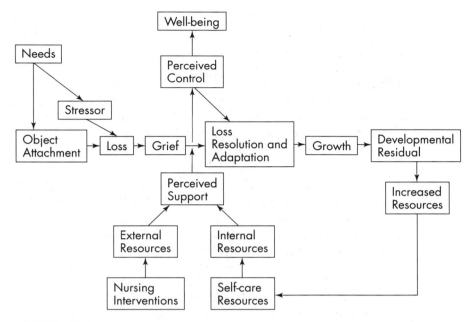

FIGURE 16-2

Relations among the constructs of the MRM theory. (From Erickson, M. E. [1996]. Relationships among support, needs satisfaction, and maternal attachment in adolescent mothers. Doctoral dissertation, University of Texas—Austin; Austin, Texas. Reprinted with permission of Margaret Erickson, Austin, TX.)

of well-being even as he or she takes his or her last breath. Therefore health can be defined as a dynamic, eudaemonistic sense of well-being (Erickson, Tomlin, & Swain, 1983) associated with self-fulfillment and transcendence beyond objective reality of the moment (Erickson, 2000a).

Humans are in a continual state of change and have inherent drives that motivate behavior. These include a drive for need satisfaction, adaptation, and growth sequential development. According to Erickson, Tomlin, and Swain (1983), "Growth is defined as the changes in body, mind, and spirit that occur over time" (p. 46) and facilitates an individual's development. Development is defined as "the holistic synthesis of the growth-produced . . . differentiations in a person's body, ideas, social relations, and so forth" (Erickson, Tomlin, & Swain, 1983, p. 47). When individuals are given necessary information and adequate emotional support and are empowered in making satisfactory decisions, growth and subsequent development occurs, and health is enhanced.

According to the MRM paradigm, the nurse facilitates an interactive, interpersonal relationship with the client. During this process, the nurse assists the client in identifying, developing, and mobilizing internal and

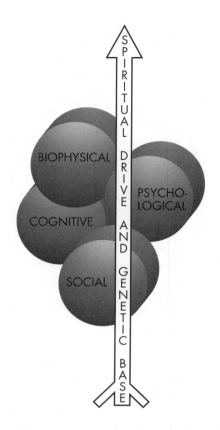

FIGURE 16-3

Relations among the human subsystems, genetic predispositions, and spiritual drive. (From Erickson, H., Tomlin, E., & Swain, M. (1983). *Modeling and role-modeling: A theory and paradigm for nursing.* Englewood Cliff, NJ: Appleton and Lange. Reprinted (1988, 1990, 1994, and 1999), Ann Arbor, MI: ETS. Reprinted with permission from Helen Erickson; Austin TX.)

external resources—resources needed to cope with life's stressors, to grow and heal. Essential to this process is the nurse's unconditional acceptance of the client. Erickson, Tomlin, and Swain (1983) argue that "[b]eing accepted as a unique, worthwhile, important individual—with no strings attached—is imperative if the individual is to be facilitated in developing his or her own potential" (p. 49).

In a supportive and caring environment, the nurse attempts to understand "the client's personal model of his or her world and to appreciate its value and significance for the client from the client's perspective" (Erickson, Tomlin, & Swain, 1983, p. 49). The act of developing an image and understanding of the clients' worldviews from within their perspectives and frameworks is called *modeling.* "The way an individual communicates, thinks, feels, acts, and reacts—all of these factors comprise the individual's *model of his or her world*" (Erickson, Tomlin, & Swain, 1983, p. 84). After the client's world has been modeled, the nurse facilitates and nurtures the individual "in attaining, maintaining, or promoting health through purposeful interventions" (Erickson, Tomlin, & Swain, 1983, p. 254). This is known as *role-modeling*. In role-modeling the client's world, the nurse plans interventions that do the following: (a) identify mutual nurse-client goals, (b) promote client strengths, control, and positive orientation, and (c) build trust. These interventions are aimed at helping the client "achieve an optimal state of perceived health and contentment " (Erickson, Tomlin, & Swain, 1983, p. 49).

Nursing interventions are designed based on the belief that all individuals at some level understand what has interfered with their growth and development and altered their health status. Accordingly, people also know what they need to improve and optimize their state of health, facilitate their growth and development, and maximize their quality of life. This inherent knowledge is called *self-care knowledge*. Individuals also have internal and external self-care resources. *Internal self-care resources* (or *self-strengths*) refer to all of the "internal resources that an individual can use to promote health and growth" (Erickson, Tomlin, & Swain, 1983, p. 128). These strengths are defined by the nurse and the client's perceptions and can include attitudes, endurance, patterns, or whatever else is perceived to be a personal strength and resource of that individual. *External self-care resources* include the client's social network and support systems. The social network is a set of individuals with whom the client is socially acquainted, and support systems are a set of individuals who are perceived to support, energize, and provide resources for the client.

Development and utilization of self-care knowledge and self-care resources is known as *self-care action*. "Through self-care action the individual mobilizes internal resources and acquires additional resources that will help the individual gain, maintain, and promote an optimal level of holistic health" (Erickson, Tomlin, & Swain, 1983, p. 49). Finally, an individual's potential for mobilizing resources and achieving a state of coping is directly related to his or her level of need satisfaction (Erickson, Tomlin, & Swain, 1983). Individuals who have a high level of need satisfaction have a greater ability to positively cope with life's stressors and to achieve a state of equilibrium. However, individuals who have a high level of unmet needs have less ability to mobilize resources and are at risk when confronted with stressors.

Nursing interventions are designed to facilitate the client in utilizing self-care actions that will help them meet their physiological, psychological, social, cognitive, and spiritual needs. Repeated need satisfaction results in growth; continued growth produces healthy developmental residual. Crucial to this theory is the understanding that an individual's needs are only met when the individual perceives that they are met.

Theoretical Underpinnings

Developmental processes are sequential tasks, strengths, and virtues that are associated with biological time (Figure 16-4). Each stage has a central focus and related life task to be accomplished. The manner in which this task is completed will determine what type of developmental residual results. Residual from stage one serves as a resource (or hindrance) for task resolution of the stage two, and so forth across the lifespan. Because of the epigenetic nature of the developmental processes, people are constantly reworking earlier residual. One's ability to resolve developmental tasks in a healthy manner (and to rework earlier residual) are dependent upon resources accrued from having one's needs met across the lifespan.

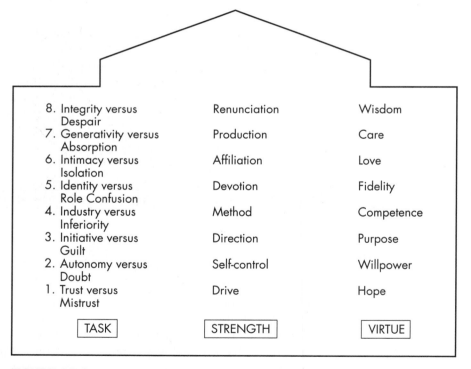

TASK	STRENGTH	VIRTUE
8. Integrity versus Despair	Renunciation	Wisdom
7. Generativity versus Absorption	Production	Care
6. Intimacy versus Isolation	Affiliation	Love
5. Identity versus Role Confusion	Devotion	Fidelity
4. Industry versus Inferiority	Method	Competence
3. Initiative versus Guilt	Direction	Purpose
2. Autonomy versus Doubt	Self-control	Willpower
1. Trust versus Mistrust	Drive	Hope

FIGURE 16-4

Erikson's developmental tasks, strengths, and virtues. (From Erickson, H., Tomlin, E., & Swain, M. (1983). *Modeling and role-modeling: A theory and paradigm for nursing.* Englewood Cliff, NJ: Appleton and Lange. Reprinted (1988, 1990, 1994, and 1999), Ann Arbor, MI: ETS. Reprinted with permission from Helen Erickson; Austin, TX.)

Inherent needs, classified as survival, affiliated-individuation (AI), or growth-related, emerge in a quasi-ordered manner. Lower-level needs must be satisfied to some degree before higher-level needs emerge (Figure 16-5). Minimal lower and mid-level need satisfaction is necessary for survival; repeated need satisfaction facilitates growth. Lower and mid-level need deficits create tension and drive behaviors aimed at meeting those unmet needs; satisfaction of these needs dissipate the tension. Higher-level need satisfaction creates tension and desire for additional growth experiences. People who repeatedly experience unmet needs during the early years of life develop a deficit motivation toward relationships. Those who repeatedly experience need satisfaction during early years of life develop a being motivation.

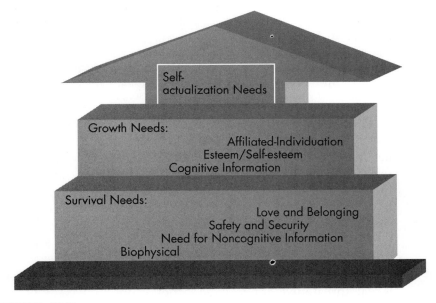

FIGURE 16-5

Needs across the lifespan. (Adapted from Erickson, H., Tomlin, E., & Swain, M. (1983). *Modeling and role-modeling: A theory and paradigm for nursing.* Englewood Cliff, NJ: Appleton and Lange. Reprinted (1988, 1990, 1994, and 1999), Ann Arbor, MI: ETS. Reprinted with permission from Helen Erickson; Austin, TX.)

Unmet needs are *stressors;* stressors produce *stress responses.* Resolution of stress requires adequate resources; one's ability to mobilize adequate resources determines the outcome of the stress response. Stressors, stress responses, and resources may be within the same subsystem; however, they are not limited to a single subsystem.

There are two types of stress-response states: *arousal* and *impoverishment.* When adequate resources are available and readily mobilized, arousal occurs (Figure 16-6). When inadequate (or diminished) resources are available, impoverishment occurs. Those in impoverishment are at greatest risk for continued stress, depletion of resources and resulting illness, disease, and/or physical death than those in arousal (see Figure 16-6).

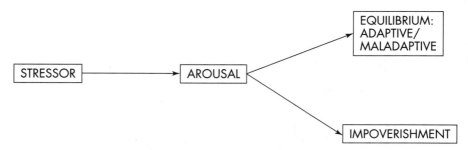

FIGURE 16-6

The Adaptive Potential Assessment Model. (From Erickson, H., Tomlin, E., & Swain, M. (1983). *Modeling and role-modeling: A theory and paradigm for nursing.* Englewood Cliff, NJ: Appleton and Lange. Reprinted (1988, 1990, 1994, and 1999), Ann Arbor, MI: ETS. Reprinted with permission from Helen Erickson; Austin, TX.)

Adaptation occurs as needs are met, stress responses are diminished, and new resources are built. Those objects that meet needs repeatedly become *attachment objects*. Such objects change as people move through various developmental stages. When attachment occurs, loss of attachment objects will result. Loss can be situational and/or developmental. Loss is real, threatened, or perceived. Examples of situational losses are the loss of a favored item, perceived rejection by a loved one, a major flooding of one's home, etc. Developmental losses are aspects of movement through the developmental sequence, such as weaning during infancy, going to school, leaving home, etc. When loss occurs—whether it is real, threatened, or perceived—grief results.

The grief process has sequential phases; movement through the grief process requires mobilization of resources. One's ability to mobilize adequate resources determines the outcome of the grief response. Inadequate resources results in morbid grief (Lindemann, 1942); morbid grief affects future developmental processes, as Figure 16-1 illustrates. A synthesis of these multiple theories provided the bases for the MRM theory. Major theoretical linkages are shown in Box 16-1.

CRITICAL THINKING IN NURSING PRACTICE WITH THE MODELING AND ROLE-MODELING THEORY

The MRM practice paradigm is guided by five related nursing principles, intervention aims, and outcome goals for the nursing process (Table 16-1). There are interview guidelines that influence the type of data

> **BOX 16-1   MAJOR THEORETICAL LINKAGES IN MODELING AND ROLE-MODELING**
>
> 1. There is a relationship between adaptive potential and need satisfaction.
> 2. There is a relationship between developmental task resolution and need satisfaction.
> 3. There is a relationship between developmental task resolution and developmental residual.
> 4. There is a relationship between developmental residual and self-care resources.
> 5. There is a relationship among basic need satisfaction, object attachment, loss, grief, growth, and development.
>
> From Erickson, H., Tomlin, E., & Swain, M. (1983). *Modeling and role-modeling: A theory and paradigm for nursing.* Englewood Cliff, NJ: Appleton and Lange. Reprinted (1988, 1990, 1994, and 1999), Ann Arbor, MI: ETS. Reprinted with permission from Helen Erickson; Austin, TX.

TABLE 16-1   Nursing Principals, Aims, and Goals

Intervention Goal	Principle	Aim
1. Develop a trusting and functional relationship between yourself and your client.	The nursing process requires that a trusting and functional relationship exist between the nurse and the client.	Build trust.
2. Facilitate a self-projection that is futuristic and positive.	Affiliated-individuation is contingent on the individual's perceiving that he or she has some control.	Promote client's positive orientation.
3. Promote affiliated-individuation with the minimum degree of ambivalence possible.	Human development is dependent on the individual's perceiving that he or she has some control over life while concurrently sensing a state of affiliation.	Promote client's control.
4. Promote a dynamic, adaptive, and holistic state of health.	There is an innate drive toward holistic health that is facilitated by consistent and systematic nurturance.	Affirm and promote client's strengths.
5. (a) Promote (and nurture) coping mechanisms that satisfy basic needs and permit growth-need satisfaction. (b) Facilitate congruent actual and chronological developmental stages.	Human growth is dependent on satisfaction of basic needs and is facilitated by growth-need satisfaction.	Set mutual goals that are health-directed.

From Erickson, H., Tomlin, E., & Swain, M. (1983). *Modeling and role-modeling: A theory and paradigm for nursing.* Englewood Cliff, NJ: Appleton and Lange. Reprinted (1988, 1990, 1994, and 1999), Ann Arbor, MI: ETS. Reprinted with permission from Helen Erickson; Austin, TX.

collected and specify the purpose of the data (Table 16-2). Table 16-3 illustrates the process for each phase of assessment. It discusses the data interpretation and analysis that lead to nursing impressions.

TABLE 16-2 Interview Guidelines and Purpose for Data Collection	
Category and Subcategories	**Purpose of Data Collection**
DESCRIPTION OF THE SITUATION	
1. Overview of the situation	1. To develop an overview of the client's situation from his or her perspective
2. Etiology Stressors and distressors	2. To identify the etiological factors involved
3. Therapeutic needs	3. To identify possible therapeutic interventions
EXPECTATIONS	
1. Immediate 2. Long-term	1. To understand the client's personal orientation in terms of the client's expectations for the present and the future
RESOURCE POTENTIAL	

1. External
     Social network
     support system
     Healthcare system
	1. To determine the nature of the external support system

2. Internal
     Strengths
     Adaptive potential
     Feeling states
     Physiological data
	2. (a) To determine the client's strengths and virtues
	    (b) To determine the client's current available internal resources

GOALS AND LIFE TASKS	
1. Current 2. Future	1. To determine the current developmental status in order to understand the client's personal model and to utilize maximum communication skills

Adapted by H. Erickson (2001), from Erickson, H., Tomlin, E., & Swain, M. (1983). *Modeling and role-modeling: A theory and paradigm for nursing.* Englewood Cliff, NJ: Appleton and Lange. Reprinted (1988, 1990, 1994, and 1999), Ann Arbor, MI: ETS. Reprinted with permission from Helen Erickson; Austin, TX.

Critical thinking occurs continuously in the process as the following steps occur: data are collected, interpreted, analyzed, and synthesized; strategies are planned and used to facilitate growth and healing; and the caring process is evaluated to determine whether a healing process has been initiated. The primary source of information is the client; secondary sources include the family's view and the nurse's observations. Tertiary sources are all others, including medical information. The client's self-care knowledge is considered primary information and is the initial focus of the nursing assessment. As the nurse uses an unstructured interview to collect self-care knowledge (primary data), both verbal and nonverbal

TABLE 16-3 Data Analysis Methods, Interpretation, and Nursing Impressions

Assessment Phase	Nursing Interventions	Nursing Impressions
DESCRIPTION	Write a paragraph on the relationship among the factors. Include comments that state client's perceptions, identified stressors, distressors, perceptions of loss, congruency of this perception with that of secondary and tertiary resources, mind-body relationships, and associated subsystems. Identify possible therapeutic interventions, desire for information; include congruency with family and healthcare providers.	Basic need assets/deficits Growth need assets/deficits Attachment/loss status Affiliation status
Expectations	Write a paragraph regarding client's positive orientation. Include expectations for immediate nurse-client relationship, projection of self into future, extent of projection and nature of projection, sense of self as worthwhile, valued person, role of self in future.	Self-futurity
Resource Potential External	Write a paragraph on client-family relationship in their social network. State whether the relationship is invigorating or draining; comment on the availability of a significant other and the mode of communication with other. Comment on perceived control in respect to others (i.e., ability to satisfy needs and resolve problems and dependency on others). Comment on past use of healthcare providers and perceptions of healthcare providers.	Affiliation Individuation Perceived control
Resource Potential Internal	Write a paragraph on the client's strengths and virtues, which includes both universal and unique individual strengths and virtues. Describe feelings and patterns, length of time of feeling pattern.	Assets, APAM, developmental status, psychological, cognitive
Goals	Write a paragraph on planned goals, factors that facilitate, and barriers that inhibit. State the chronological/current task. Note the type of cognitive processing used.	

Copyright Helen Erickson, 2001. Reprinted with permission from Helen Erickson; Austin, TX.

communications are noted. A continuous appraisal of the congruence between the two are determined when nonverbal messages indicate lack of congruence with verbal statements; the interviewer needs to store this information for further consideration (Erickson, 1990; Erickson, Tomlin, & Swain, 1983). Secondary data are collected from the family or significant others and, when needed, additional data are collected from other sources, such as the medical record, physicians, or other healthcare providers. These data are interpreted individually and then integrated to determine congruency among the sources, differing views, and other information. The primary source of data (self-care knowledge) always serves as the primary focus of nursing care. When there are differences in views, information, and orientation among the data sources, the nurse accepts the responsibility of working with the secondary client after first addressing the needs of the primary client. The MRM nurse also provides leadership for the interface between these three sources (primary, secondary, and tertiary) of information. That is, MRM nurses serve to facilitate better understanding of the client's self-care knowledge and vice versa among other members of the team.

Although critical thinking is usually considered a scientific process, MRM practitioners also use critical thinking during the artistic phase of the caring process. That is, practitioners use critical thinking during the strategy implementation phase as well as during the previous phases of the process. Although there are specific strategies that can be used to facilitate growth and healing, they are always applied within the context of the client's worldview (Erickson, 2000a, 2000b). That is the artistic aspect of MRM.

CASE HISTORY OF DEBBIE

Debbie is a 29-year-old woman who was recently admitted to the oncology nursing unit for evaluation after sensing pelvic "fullness" and noticing a watery, foul-smelling vaginal discharge. A Papanicolaou smear revealed class V cervical cancer. She was found to have a stage II squamous cell carcinoma of the cervix and underwent a radical hysterectomy with bilateral salpingooophorectomy.

Her past health history revealed that physical examinations had been infrequent. She also reported that she had not performed breast self-examination. She is 5 feet, 4 inches tall and weights 89 pounds. Her usual weight is about 110 pounds. She has smoked approximately two packs of cigarettes a day for the past 16 years. She is gravida 2, para 2. Her first pregnancy was at age 16, and her second was at age 18. Since that time, she has taken oral contraceptives on a regular basis.

Debbie completed the eighth grade. She is married and lives with her husband and her two children in her mother's home, which she describes as less than sanitary. Her husband is unemployed. She describes him as emotionally distant and abusive at times.

She has done well following surgery except for being unable to completely empty her urinary bladder. She is having continued postoperative pain and nausea. It will be necessary for her to perform intermittent self-catheterization at home. Her medications are (1) an antibiotic, (2) an analgesic as needed for pain, and (3) an antiemetic as needed for nausea. In addition, she will be receiving radiation therapy on an outpatient basis.

Debbie is extremely tearful. She expresses great concern over her future and the future of her two children. She believes that this illness is a punishment for her past life.

NURSING CARE OF DEBBIE WITH MODELING AND ROLE-MODELING

Data Aggregation and Interpretation

Primary data. Debbie's self-care knowledge is not discussed. Therefore the logical first step would be to return to Debbie and ask for her description of the situation, related factors, expectations, resources, and goals. These data would then be integrated with secondary and tertiary data to determine the appropriate course of action. However, since there are "reported" comments made by Debbie, these can be integrated with obvious secondary and tertiary data.

Secondary and tertiary data. Description of the situation. According to report, Debbie is distressed and depressed about her current life situation. Physically, she has just undergone major surgery, is experiencing postoperative pain, nausea, difficulty emptying her bladder, and a recent significant weight loss. No data are provided regarding Debbie's ability to complete self-catheterization or her feelings about the multiple losses associated with her altered body image, need for self-catheterization, inability to have children in the future, discomfort associated with postoperative pain and nausea, and fear of the future regarding her radiation treatment and the potential for reoccurrence of the cancer. Furthermore, no information is provided on personal or professional resources available to help her meet these needs.

Psychologically, Debbie is depressed and blames her current life situation on her past life transgressions. She believes that this illness is punishment for her past life. It is difficult to know if Debbie is referring to having been an adolescent mother, having smoked cigarettes since she was 16 years old, or other past perceived transgressions. It would be important to ask her if she could share more information regarding this statement so that relevant data could be collected.

Debbie has experienced multiple losses recently and over the last several years that have resulted in need deficits related to unmet love and belonging needs. As an adolescent mother, Debbie had little time to care for herself. At a time in her life when she needed to focus on who she was and on meeting her own needs, her resources were directed toward the care of two small children (M. Erickson, 1996). This conflict of interest might have resulted in feelings of loss and related unmet needs (M. Erickson, 1996). In addition, she describes her marital relationship as emotionally distant and at times abusive. Consequently, she has received little if any social support from her husband. No data concerning her relationship with her mother and children are available. Further information is needed before it can be determined whether these individuals are perceived as supportive and help meet her basic love and belonging needs.

Debbie has multiple stressors and distressors in her life. She is the mother of a preadolescent and an adolescent; her husband is unemployed; her housing accommodations are unsanitary and unacceptable. She has had surgery, is nauseated, is in pain, is unable to void normally, and must learn intermittent self-catheterization. Her husband's unemployment and her low educational level both affect their ability to achieve financial freedom and security. Subsequently, they are dependent on her mother for a place to live. Inability to provide a home for her children and one in which she feels safe to live are additional losses she faces. These losses indicate basic physiological, safety and security, and self-esteem need deficits. Furthermore, surgery and related costs will only exacerbate an already difficult financial situation. Under the circumstances, it is highly possible that Debbie does not have health insurance, which is an additional stressor. Major physical alterations in her body, weight loss, surgery, nausea, pain, and problems with voiding are all real losses.

Expectations. Debbie has not offered any immediate or long-term expectations. However, she has expressed great concern over her future and the future of her children. These findings suggest impoverishment, unresolved losses, and threatened future loss. Because we do not have primary data (self-care knowledge), we do not know whether these are related to basic physiological, safety and security, or love and belonging needs secondary to her current health status, living situation, or interpersonal relationships. No information from the other sources regarding her expectations is provided. The healthcare providers have identified their expectations for her as follows: (a) take her medications for pain and nausea, (b) perform self-catheterization as needed, and (c) undergo radiation therapy on an outpatient basis.

Resource potential. Debbie's social network includes her mother, husband, and two children, who are approximately 13 and 11 years old. No information regarding her support system is provided except that her husband is emotionally distant and abusive. Debbie currently is receiving postoperative care in an oncology unit. She has not provided any data on the care she has received during her hospitalization or on the nurse-client relationship, nor has data been provided regarding her interpersonal family dynamics and whether her family members are physically and emotionally accessible for her needs.

Debbie, who is extremely tearful, shares that she has not been performing breast self-examinations and has completed the eighth grade. She has not identified any personal strengths. Debbie has demonstrated some responsibility. She has cared for her children and practiced birth control for the last 11 years.

Goals and life tasks. Debbie has not identified any goals, although she has expressed concern about herself and the future of her children. Future goals will need to focus on helping Debbie get her basic needs met and helping her work on the developmental task of autonomy. The nurses' goals for Debbie include antibiotic therapy to prevent an infection, an antiemetic to help control nausea, and radiation therapy to destroy any remaining cancerous cells. No interventions to help her meet her basic or growth needs are identified.

Data Integration and Analysis

Debbie has recently experienced multiple losses that have affected her basic and growth needs satisfaction. Unfortunately, she has minimal resources, so her ability to adapt to her current circumstances and achieve health and well-being is unlikely; she is impoverished. She is at high risk for further decline in her health status because of her inability to mobilize resources. Nursing interventions need to focus on helping Debbie achieve affiliated-individuation and basic and growth need satisfaction.

Living at home, being married to a distant and abusive husband, having quit school after eighth grade, and lack of physical care of self all suggest that Debbie may be working on the developmental stage of autonomy versus doubt. Her life situation indicates that Debbie is having difficulty with affiliated-individuation. She has been unable to complete the education necessary to become financially independent. Her family is residing with her mother. She is married to a man who does not meet her financial or emotional needs. She was an adolescent mother. All of these factors indicate her difficulty in being autonomous and simultaneously having healthy connections (or feelings or affiliation) with her significant others.

Nursing impressions. Debbie has multiple survival, growth, and self-actualization need deficits. She is in morbid grief, probably secondary to early life experiences. These are compounded by her recent and current life situation. She lacks a secure attachment object and thus suffers from inadequate affiliated-individuation. She cannot positively project herself into the future and has diminished resources; therefore she is impoverished. Her aggregate situation suggests that she has minimal trust and (developmental) residual, unhealthy shame and doubt, guilt, and inferiority. She probably has difficulty with role confusion as well. She is currently confronted with the task of intimacy and appears to have more isolation (developmental) residual than intimacy.

Nursing interventions. The aim of MRM nursing interventions are to build trust, affirm and promote client strengths, promote positive orientation, facilitate perceived control, and set health-directed mutual goals. The first step in the process for this client is to collect self-care knowledge. This will help the nurse confirm, revise, and/or adapt nursing interpretations and impressions. Because the MRM nurse also approaches the interview process with unconditional acceptance and with a belief that all humans have the potential to grow, the nurse's attitude will promote a sense of positive orientation in the client. (Note that this approach is used to facilitate the developmental stage of trust.) As an MRM nurse, you will want to explore your client's perceived strengths and goals. It will also help you building a trusting, *functional* relationship with Debbie and help Debbie perceive a sense of control. (Note that this approach is used to facilitate the resolution of the developmental stage of autonomy.)

Remember that Debbie is impoverished. Thus she will not be able to project herself very far into the future. Perhaps the most that will be possible will be setting goals for increased physical comfort (basic physical needs) and sense of being connected to you (belonging needs). By reinforcing her perceived strengths and helping her identify additional internal resources, she will continue to rework the tasks of trust and autonomy. She will also develop a sense of affiliated-individuation.

You can inform Debbie that we sometimes have life experiences that interfere with our ability to grow, that the miracle in life is that we always have new opportunities, and that it is never too late. Although it may seem that life is nothing but a cloudy storm, there usually is a rainbow if we can just learn how to find it. It might also be important to tell her that sometimes we do things to meet our needs. These actions seem right at the time but later we realize that they did not work very well. These actions make us neither bad nor wrong; they just alter our lives. It is never too late to start anew.

You can also ask Debbie what kind of information she would like to have. Tell her what information you can offer. (Start with survival needs and move up the hierarchy.) Let her choose whether she wants information and, if so, what information she wants. In this discussion, you would probably offer to talk about how she could help herself be more comfortable or to quiet and calm her stomach when she is receiving chemotherapy or is feeling uncomfortable. It is important that we use language such as *comfort*—language that reflects health—rather than words that reflect illness, such as *pain*. You could also mention that when she is ready, you could teach her how to empty her bladder so she would be more comfortable.

To provide physical care, it is essential that the approach include unconditional acceptance of the person and her body. Through soft voice tones, gentle and soothing touch, and eye contact, the nurse projects unconditional acceptance, love, and respect for the holistic person. Comments that identify her physical strengths are also important. Debbie needs to be assisted to discover what is right with her; with such discoveries she will be better able to handle her limitations.

Debbie also needs help with external resources. She has a social network, but she may not see them as her support system. Although the nurse will want to keep this in mind, Debbie probably will not want to talk about her family until she has developed new internal resources. Impoverished people have difficulty viewing the world from another person's eyes. Instead they often see the other as a part of their problems. However, Debbie will need help in planning for her chemotherapy. Thus you might inform Debbie that you are there to talk and to help her problem solve and that Debbie should be encouraged to think about how she can meet her own needs when she is ready, but there is no rush. Right now, the focus is on helping her rest and find comfort.

When Debbie indicates she is ready, she may need time to simply tell her story. Although we can only imagine that she has had a difficult childhood and marriage, only Debbie can relate it in such a way as to express her real feelings. Informing her that all people deserve to be loved and respected but that it doesn't always happen is one way to initiate such a discussion.

Debbie will also want to discuss how she can care for her children and what will happen to them. To facilitate this discussion, you might comment about the children, their beauty, and how they are like their mother. When Debbie is ready and has built sufficient trust, she will raise the issue.

Remember that each of the above topics is related to unmet needs, loss, and grief. Therefore the nurse should expect to see behaviors that represent the grieving process, such as denial, shock, anger, bargaining, and sadness. Until Debbie has worked through the grieving process, you will not see acceptance with attachment to new objects or attachment to old objects in new ways. Do not be fooled by behaviors that suggest giving up; giving up is not the same as letting go. Giving up represents continued morbid grief (with unresolved losses); letting go represents moving on, attaching in new ways.

As Debbie continues to rework the tasks related to the first two stages of life, she will begin to work on initiative, followed by industry, identity, and intimacy. Throughout these processes, it is important to help her begin to think about her life, what it has meant, and what her purpose in life might be. These processes are especially important for Debbie because she may be facing physical death. If this is the case, it is essential that she have an opportunity to develop a sense of positive orientation, meaning in life, and be able to express her purpose for being. This will help her develop a sense of spiritual well-being.

CASE HISTORY OF JOHN

Background

John, a 70-year-old male, was admitted to the hospital for shortness of breath secondary to exacerbation of his emphysema. After a few days, he was ready for discharge. John's medical records indicate that he has been admitted 16 times in the last 18 months. John is referred to the community case manager to see "if something can be done about this." The following report was provided at that time.

Secondary and Tertiary Data

John is well known by the nurse, who states, "John's a regular here. It seems he is here all the time. That's fine. John really doesn't require much care once he is stabilized. It gives us a break. He often comes in drunk, but he isn't a mean drunk. Once his breathing gets better, he'll leave so he can smoke. He smokes like a chimney!"

John's past medical history indicates that he is 5 feet, 11 inches and weighs 160 pounds. He has cirrhosis of the liver, emphysema, mild anemia; has a history of chronic alcohol use; and smokes three packs of cigarettes a day. His doctor documented that he will not take care of himself and is noncompliant. Following his admission, John is started on oxygen therapy 2L per nasal cannula and is given respiratory treatments. The respiratory therapist greets John by his first name and asks how he is doing. After 3 days, John says he is "feeling better and ready to be discharged."

Primary Data
Description of the Situation

The nurse asked if she could speak with John before his discharge. He replied, "Sure. I'd be happy to help however I can." She asked him to tell her why he feels he has had so many admissions in the last 18 months. He replied, "I live alone in an apartment building for senior citizens. My daughter lives 400 miles away, and we don't see each other very often. I wish she was closer. I miss her. I don't have any other family. My wife divorced me years ago because of my drinking. It was my own fault. I wish there was somebody in my life that cared about me. I don't do much anymore, because my breathing won't let me. I don't get out and see people or go bowling like I used to. Too bad. I was pretty good. My only real enjoyment comes when I'm drinking or having a smoke. Sometimes, I have a smoke with some of the other guys who live in my building. It's good to get together and talk. I don't eat much anymore. It's too much work for just me. I know I should quit smoking and drinking, but why bother?"

John was asked what would help him feel better. He responded "I guess if I knew somebody cared and was there when I needed him or her, but that probably isn't going to happen. Everybody is pretty busy at the hospital. I expect that I will just continue to see them when I have problems breathing."

Expectations
When asked what he thought was going to happen, John stated that he expected that some day, he would come in with shortness of breath, be put on a ventilator, and never be able to get off.

Resource Potential
When John was asked about his ability to help himself, he said that he could be compliant but commented that he probably could not stop smoking and drinking even though that would make the doctors feel better. When asked what he thought about the care he had received while he was in the hospital, he said, "They do okay. Some of the nurses really care and take a few minutes to talk. I like that. It is always kind of nice to see people. My doctor doesn't want to be bothered. He is frustrated because he says I don't take care of myself and it's a waste of his time."

Goals and Life Tasks
He was then asked what he would like to see happen. He stated that he wanted to have fewer hospitalizations, be able to breathe more easily, and would like to quit smoking and drinking, but he didn't think these were very realistic.

NURSING CARE OF JOHN WITH MODELING AND ROLE-MODELING

Data Interpretation and Analysis

Description of situation. John is friendly and interested in sharing his story. He seeks affiliation and hopes to find someone that will care for him and take care of him. His coping mechanisms (smoking and drinking) reflect oral, stage one developmental processes with related unmet needs and developmental residual. His perception of his health status is congruent with that of his healthcare providers. He knows that he is physically compromised, that he drinks and smokes too much, that he has not followed his physician's advice, and that this makes the doctors unhappy. He also recognizes that it would help his physical health if he quit smoking and drinking, but he expresses inability to give up these coping strategies at this time. This is because he does not have adequate developmental residual from the first two stages of life; he lacks drive, self-control, and willpower.

His living conditions facilitate some sense of affiliated-individuation, but it is not growth-directed. Although he lives alone in an apartment in a senior housing unit, his shortness of breath limits his daily activities. He is no longer able to bowl or carry out a number of activities that he enjoyed in the past. His recreational activities include visiting with other residents, smoking, and drinking. He recognizes that he is not eating enough but states that he lacks the interest or energy to cook for himself.

John has experienced many losses in his life and probably has morbid grief with multiple related need deficits. The changes that he has had to make, the activities that he has had to give up, and his inability to breathe without assistance and to complete his activities of daily living are all regular occurrences in his life. These have created perceived and real loss. He is also divorced, lives alone and does not have children who visit regularly. Although his daughter lives 400 miles away, he commented that she probably would not come very often because of his drinking. He expressed feelings of sadness related to his divorce, that his daughter was distant, and that he could no longer get out and see people because of his breathing problems.

Expectations. John does not see his life situation changing much. He believes that if he had people who cared about him that were available for him when he needed them to be, his health situation would improve. He does not believe, however, that this is a realistic expectation. The nurse expected that caring for John would be easy while he was hospitalized and that he would leave as soon as he was stable. No other expectations for John were identified by the nurse or by the other healthcare providers. They had given up on his ability to stop smoking or quit drinking.

Resources. When he was asked why he thought he had so many frequent hospitalizations, John talked about the lack of a social network and support system. His statements that he has a daughter whom he rarely sees indicated his feelings of loneliness. He also stated, "I wish she was closer. I miss her. I don't have any other family. My wife divorced me years ago because of my drinking." In addition, he talked about visiting with the nurses who "cared" about him and took the time to visit with him and about his regrets that he no longer got out to see people. In regards to his relationship with his physician, he perceived that the doctor was frustrated with him and that he did not want to waste his time working with him. These feelings were corroborated by the physician.

John's limited social network includes his friends with whom he smokes and drinks, the hospital staff he sees when he is admitted for hospitalization, (the respiratory therapist greets him by his first name upon admission and asks how he is doing), and his daughter. He does not seem to have a support system, but he communicates easily and openly with the nurse.

Goals and life tasks. His current goals include continuing to live independently and to experience minimal episodes of respiratory distress. His desired future goal would be to have a caring relationship with someone. The nurse's goals for John include the following: (1) less frequent hospitalizations, (2) improved nutritional status, (3) cessation of smoking and drinking, and (4) decreased episodes of respiratory distress. The physician would like John to be "compliant" with the medical plan. These goals are not compatible because John cannot stop smoking and drinking and will not be motivated to eat better until he feels loved, cared for and about, and connected.

Nursing impressions. John has multiple survival, growth, and self-actualization need deficits. He probably has a deficit motivation for relationships. This means that he has probably developed relationships to meet his own needs without much consideration of the needs of the other member in the relationship, as is evidenced by the fact that he is divorced, his daughter is estranged, and his "friends" drink and smoke with him.

He lacks a sense of affiliated-individuation. Because of his strong need to be connected (affiliated) with someone who will care for him and because he has no such relationship, he has difficulty taking health-directed self-care actions. Instead, his actions are aimed at getting his basic, oral needs met. He cannot positively project himself into the future and has diminished internal and external resources; he is impoverished. John is at the age of generativity but is having trouble projecting into the future. He has trouble with the task of initiative, which is most likely secondary to issues that deal with the tasks of trust and autonomy.

Thus John's survival and growth need deficits are related to early life experiences. He has unmet physical, safety and security, love and belonging, and self-esteem needs as well as unresolved losses. His psychosocial and physical subsystems interface in a way that jeopardizes his physical health.

Nursing interventions. Because the aims of interventions are to build trust, promote positive orientation and a sense of control, affirm and build strengths, and set goals, initial interventions were designed to meet survival needs, facilitate secure attachment (related to developmental trust), and encourage autonomy following secure attachment. This would result in survival and growth need satisfaction and would facilitate growth and new trust and autonomy residual.

To accomplish these outcomes, weekly visits were made to his home for the first month. During these visits, John and the nurse identified his strengths, reaffirmed his worth, and talked about his concerns, how he was feeling, what would help him feel better. The nurse gave him a business card and told him that he could call whenever he wanted to talk with someone or needed help. She also called him about once a week to see how he was doing. During their phone calls and visits, John and the nurse also talked about generativity issues such as what his life had been about, what he had contributed, and what he could continue to contribute.

To help him continue work on meeting his survival and growth needs (related to trust, autonomy, etc.), John was invited to join a support group every other week. The focus of the group was to help him build a support system and to have people with whom to connect. Group members were encouraged to discuss their feelings first and then to talk objectively about possible solutions to their problems. Then they were encouraged to think about the differences between their feelings and their thinking.

Finally, the nurse served as an advocate for him with the rest of the healthcare team and other agencies. She discussed his need deficits, developmental processes, and relationships with the healthcare team. She also discussed the difference between compliance and adherence and the importance of facilitating adherence with clients like John. Adherence comes from goals set by the client, within the context of his or her world. Work with adherence rather than compliance is based on the assumption that all people want to grow, be the best they can be, and will grow when they have repeated *perceived* need satisfaction. Although this did not seem to change the team members' goals, it did help alter their attitudes. They seemed more interested in John's view of the world.

Summary

John was seen by the nurse for 2 and a half years. Shortly after she initiated the interventions, which were based on MRM, John quit smoking. He attended regular meetings and called the nurse regularly. He began to take his medication as prescribed and had no additional side-effects. His hospitalizations decreased to once a year. Later, he quit drinking as well.

After about 2 and a half years, the nurse left the hospital. Later, the nurse who had replaced her position decided that John was doing so well that he no longer needed to be called, attend the support group, or have special attention from the healthcare team. Within 6 months, John had an acute respiratory episode, was hospitalized, and died.

CRITICAL THINKING EXERCISES

1. Select a movie of your choice, view it, and then analyze it using the MRM theory.

2. Using the MRM guidelines, interview a client. Organize the data according to the four categories for data collection. Compare the data with the purpose for data collection. Is anything missing?
3. Based on the client interview, interpret the data and then review the records for data derived from secondary and tertiary sources. Compare the three sets of data for similarities and discrepancies. Note the influence of the discipline's philosophy on their interpretation of data and expectation for client outcome. Notice also how these affect approval or disapproval of the client's behaviors.
4. Review your client interview and sort out self-care actions and self-care resources. Note how self-care actions are sometimes directed toward meeting our dependent (or affiliation) needs. Notice also how most healthcare providers reinforce self-care actions that are directed toward independent (or individuation) needs. Consider the consequences of focusing on individuation needs without first considering affiliation needs.
5. List nursing impressions based on the interpreted data from your client interview.
6. Based on the data interpretations from your client interview, list the aims of your interventions, and link them to the nursing impressions and anticipated interventions. Specify outcome goals that can be used to evaluate the caring process.

References

Acton, G. (1993). Relationships among stressors, stress, affiliated-individuation, burden, and well-being in caregivers of adults with dementia: A test of the theory and paradigm for nursing, modeling, and role-modeling. Doctoral dissertation, University of Texas—Austin; Austin, Texas. *Dissertation Abstracts International, 54/05-B.*

Acton, G. & Miller, E. (1996). Affiliated-individuation in caregivers of adults with dementia. *Issues in Mental Health Nursing, 17,* 245-260.

Baas, L. (1992). The relationships among self-care knowledge, self-care resources, activity level and life satisfaction in persons 3 to 6 months after a myocardial infarction. Doctoral dissertation, University of Texas—Austin; Austin, Texas. *Dissertation Abstracts International,* 53, 1780B.

Barnfather, J. (1987). Mobilizing coping resources related to basic need status in healthy, young adults. Doctoral dissertation, University of Michigan—Ann Arbor; Ann Arbor, Michigan. *Dissertation Abstracts International,* 49, 0360B.

Barnfather, J. (1990). Mobilizing coping resources related to basic need status. In H. Erickson & C. Kinney (Eds.), *Modeling and role-modeling: Theory, practice and research,* 1(1), 156-169. Austin, TX: Society for Advancement of Modeling and Role-Modeling.

Barnfather, J. (1993). Testing a theoretical proposition for modeling and role-modeling: Basic needs and adaptive potential status. *Issues in Mental Health Nursing, 13,* 1-18.

Barnfather, J., Swain, M., & Erickson, H. (1989a). Construct validity of an aspect of the coping process: Potential adaptation to stress. *Issues in Mental Health Nursing, 10,* 23-40.

Barnfather, J., Swain, M., & Erickson, H. (1989b). Evaluation of two assessment techniques. *Nursing Science Quarterly, 4,* 172-182.

Boodley, C. (1986). A nursing study of the experience of having a health examination. Doctoral dissertation, University of Michigan—Ann Arbor; Ann Arbor, Michigan. *Dissertation Abstracts International, 47,* 992-B.

Bowlby, J. (1969). *Attachment.* New York: Basic Books.

Bowlby, J. (1973). *Separation.* New York: Basic Books.

Bowlby, J. (1980). *Loss.* New York: Basic Books.

Bowman, S. (1998). The human-environment relationship in self-care when healing from episodic illness. Doctoral dissertation, University of Texas—Austin; Austin, Texas. *Dissertation Abstracts International, 60/07-B.*

Cain, E. & Perzynski, K. (1986). Utilization of the self-care knowledge model with wife caregivers. Unpublished master's thesis, University of Michigan—Ann Arbor; Ann Arbor, Michigan.

Calvin, A. (1991). Personal control: Conceptual analysis and its role in the nursing theory of modeling and role-modeling. Unpublished master's thesis, University of Texas—Austin; Austin, Texas.

Campbell, J., Finch, D., Allport, C., Erickson, H., & Swain, M. (1985). A theoretical approach to nursing assessment. *Journal of Advanced Nursing, 14,* 111-115.

Chen, Y. (1996). Relationships among health control orientation, self efficacy, self-care, and subjective well-being in the elderly with hypertension. Doctoral dissertation, University of Texas—Austin; Austin, Texas. *Dissertation Abstracts International,* 5706-B.

Clemintino, D. & Lapinski, M. (1980). The effects of different preparatory messages on distress from a bronchoscopy. Unpublished master's thesis, University of Michigan—Ann Arbor; Ann Arbor, Michigan.

Curl, E. (1992). Hope in the elderly: Exploring the relationship between psychosocial developmental residual and hope. Doctoral dissertation, University of Texas—Austin; Austin, Texas. *Dissertation Abstracts International, 47,* 992B.

Daniels, R. (1994). Exploring the self-care variables that explains a wellness lifestyle in spinal cord–injured wheelchair basketball athletes. Doctoral dissertation, University of Texas—Austin; Austin, Texas. *Dissertation Abstracts International,* 55/07-B.

Darling-Fisher, C. (1987). The relationship between mothers' and fathers' Eriksonian psychosocial attributes, perceptions of family support, and adaptation to parenthood. Doctoral dissertation, University of Michigan—Ann Arbor; Ann Arbor, Michigan. *Dissertation Abstracts International, 48,* 1640B.

Darling-Fisher, C. & Leidy, N. (1988). Measuring Eriksonian development of the adult: The modified Erickson psychosocial stage inventory. *Psychological Reports, 62,* 747-754.

Doornbos, M. (1983). The relationship of the social network to emotional health in the aged. Unpublished master's thesis, University of Michigan—Ann Arbor; Ann Arbor, Michigan.

Engel, G. (1962). *Psychological development in health and disease.* Philadelphia: W. B. Saunders.

Engel, G. (1968). A life setting conducive to illness: The giving-up, given-up complex. *Annuals of Internal Medicine, 69*(2), 293-300.

Erikson, E. (1963). *Childhood and society.* New York: W. W. Norton.

Erickson, H. (1976). Identification of states of coping utilizing physiological and psychological data. Unpublished master's thesis, University of Michigan—Ann Arbor; Ann Arbor, Michigan.

Erickson, H. (1984). Self-care knowledge: Relations among the concepts support, hope, control, satisfaction with life, and physical health. Doctoral dissertation, University of Michigan—Ann Arbor; Ann Arbor, Michigan.

Erickson, H. (1990). Self-care knowledge: An exploratory study. In H. Erickson & C. Kinney, (Eds.). *Modeling and role-modeling: Theory, practice, and research, 1,* 178-202. Austin, TX: Society for Advancement of Modeling and Role-Modeling.

Erickson, H. Personal Communication. February, 2000.

Erickson, H. (2000a). Facilitating generativity and ego integrity: Applying Ericksonian methods to the aging population. In J. Zeig & B. Geary (Eds.), *The handbook of Ericksonian pychotherapy.* Phoenix: Zeig, Tucker, & Theisen, Incorporated.

Erickson, H. (2000b). Complementary health strategies and modalities. In C. Clark (Ed.), *Health and wellness promotion in nursing.* Philadelphia: Lippincott, Williams, & Wilkins.

Erickson, H. & Swain, M. (1982). A model for assessing potential adaptation to stress. *Research in Nursing and Health, 5,* 93-101.

Erickson, H. & Swain, M. (1990). Mobilizing self-care resources: A nursing intervention for hypertension. *Issues in Mental Health Nursing, 17,* 185-200.

Erickson, H., Tomlin, E., & Swain, M. (1983). *Modeling and role-modeling: A theory and paradigm for nursing.* Englewood Cliffs, NJ: Appleton & Lange. Reprinted (1988, 1990, 1994, and 1999), Ann Arbor, MI: ETS.

Erickson, M. E. (1996). Relationships among support, needs satisfaction, and maternal attachment in adolescent mothers. Doctoral dissertation, University of Texas—Austin; Austin, Texas. *Dissertation Abstracts International, 57/06-B.*

Finch, D. (1987). Testing a theoretically based nursing assessment. Unpublished master's thesis, University of Michigan—Ann Arbor; Ann Arbor, Michigan.

Hannon, J. & McLaughlin, K. (1983). Relationship between interpersonal trust and compliance in the adolescent with diabetes. Unpublished Master's thesis, University of Michigan—Ann Arbor; Ann Arbor, Michigan.

Hertz, J. (1991). The perceived enactment of autonomy scale: Measuring the potential for self-care action in the elderly. Doctoral dissertation, University of Texas—Austin; Austin, Texas. *Dissertation Abstracts International, 52,* 1953B.

Holl, R. (1992). The effect of role-modeled visiting in comparison to restricted visiting on the well-being of clients who had open heart surgery and their significant family members in the critical care unit. Doctoral dissertation, University of Texas—Austin; Austin, Texas. *Dissertation Abstracts International, 53,* 4030B.

Hopkins, B. (1994). Assessment of adaptive potential. Doctoral dissertation: University of Texas—Austin; Austin, Texas. *Dissertation Abstracts International, 55/06-B.*

Irvin, B. (1993). Social support, self-worth, and hope as self-care resources for coping with caregiver stress. Doctoral dissertation, University of Texas—Austin; Austin, Texas. *Dissertation Abstracts International, 54(06),* B2995.

Irvin, B. & Acton, G. (1996). Stress mediation in caregivers of cognitively impaired adults: Theoretical model testing. *Nursing Research, 45(3),* 160-166.

Jensen, B. (1995). Caregiver responses to a theoretically based intervention program: Case study analysis. Doctoral dissertation, University of Texas—Austin; Austin, Texas. *Dissertation Abstracts International, 56/06-B.*

Keck, V. (1989). Perceived social support, basic needs satisfaction, and coping strategies of the chronically ill. Doctoral dissertation, University of Michigan—Ann Arbor; Ann Arbor, Michigan. *Dissertation Abstracts International, 54,* 3921B.

Kennedy, G. (1991). A nursing investigation of comfort and comforting care of the acutely ill patient. Doctoral dissertation, University of Texas—Austin; Austin, Texas. *Dissertation Abstracts International, 52,* 6318B.

Kline, N. (1988). Psychophysiological processes of stress in people with a chronic physical illness. Doctoral dissertation, University of Michigan—Ann Arbor; Ann Arbor, Michigan. *Dissertation Abstracts International, 49,* 2129B.

Kleinbeck, S. (1977). *Coping states of stress.* Unpublished master's thesis, University of Michigan—Ann Arbor; Ann Arbor, Michigan.

Landis, B. (1991). Uncertainty, spiritual well-being, and psychosocial adjustment to chronic illness. Doctoral dissertation, University of Texas—Austin; Austin, Texas. *Dissertation Abstracts International, 52,* 4124B.

Leidy, N. (1989). A physiological analysis of stress and chronic illness. *Journal of Advanced Nursing, 14,* 868-876.

Leidy, N. (1990). A structural model of stress, psychological resources and symptomatic experience in chronic physical illness. *Nursing Research, 39,* 230-236.

Leidy, N. (1994). Operationalizing Maslow's theory: Development and testing of the basic needs satisfaction inventory. *Issues in Mental Health Nursing, 15,* 277-295.

Lindemann, E. (1942). Symptomatology and management of acute grief. *American Journal of Psychiatry, 101*(1944), 141-148.

MacLean, T. (1987). Eriksonian development and stressors as factors in healthy lifestyle. Doctoral dissertation, University of Michigan—Ann Arbor; Ann Arbor, Michigan. *Dissertation Abstracts International, 48,* 1710A.

Maslow, A. (1968). *Toward a psychology of being* (2nd ed.). New York: D. Von Nostrand.

Maslow, A. (1970). *Motivation and personality* (2nd ed.). New York: Harper & Row.

Miller, E. (1994). The meaning of encouragement and its connection to the inner-spirit as perceived by caregivers of the cognitively impaired. Doctoral dissertation, University of Texas—Austin; Austin, Texas. *Dissertation Abstracts International, 55/06-B.*

Miller, S. (1986). The relationship between psychosocial development and coping ability among disabled teenagers. Doctoral dissertation, University of Michigan—Ann Arbor; Ann Arbor, Michigan. *Dissertation Abstracts International, 47,* 4113B.

Raudonis, B. (1991). A nursing study of empathy from the hospice patient's perspective. Doctoral dissertation, University of Texas—Austin; Austin, Texas. *Dissertation Abstracts International, 52/07-B.*

Robinson, K. (1992). Developing a scale to measure responses of clients with actual or potential myocardial infarctions. Doctoral dissertation, University of Texas—Austin; Austin, Texas. *Dissertation Abstracts International, 53,* 6226B.

Rosenow, D. (1991). Multidimensional scaling analysis of self-care actions for reintegrating holistic health after a myocardial infarction: Implications for nursing. Doctoral dissertation, University of Texas—Austin; Austin, Texas. *Dissertation Abstracts International, 53,* 1789B.

Rossi, E. & O'Ryan, M. (1985). *Life reframing in hypnosis by Milton H. Erickson.* New York: Irvington Publishers, Inc.

Rossi, E. & O'Ryan, M. (1992). *Creative choice in hypnosis by Milton H. Erickson.* New York: Irvington Publishers, Inc.

Rossi, E., O'Ryan, M., & Sharp, F. (1983). *Healing in hypnosis by Milton H. Erickson.* New York: Irvington Publishers, Inc.

Scheela, R. (1991). The remodeling process: A grounded study of adult male incest offenders' perceptions of the treatment process. Doctoral dissertation, University of Texas—Austin; Austin, Texas. *Dissertation Abstracts International, 92,* 12628.

Selye, H. (1974). *Stress without distress.* Philadelphia: J. B. Lippincott.

Smith, K. (1980). Relationship between social support and goal attainment. Unpublished master's thesis: University of Michigan, Ann Arbor, Michigan.

Sofhauser, C. (1996). The relationships among self-esteem, psychosocial residual, self-concept, and hostility in persons with coronary heart disease. Doctoral dissertation, University of Texas—Austin; Austin, Texas. *Dissertation Abstracts International, 58/01-B.*

Straub, H. (1993). The relationship among intellectual, psychosocial, and ego development of nursing students in associate, baccalaureate, and baccalaureate-completion programs. Doctoral dissertation, University of Texas—Austin; Austin, Texas. *Dissertation Abstracts International, 55/02-B.*

Walker, M. (1990). Modeling and role-modeling and quantum physics. Unpublished master's thesis. University of Texas—Austin; Austin, Texas.

Walsh, K., Vandenbosch, T., & Boehm, S. (1989). Modeling and role-modeling: Integrating nursing theory into practice. *Journal of Advanced Nursing, 14,* 775-761.

Weber, G. (1995). Employed mothers with preschool aged children: An exploration of their lived experiences and the nature of their well-being. Doctoral dissertation, University of Texas—Austin; Austin, Texas. *Dissertation Abstracts International, 56/06-B.*

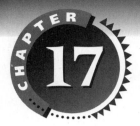

Mercer's Maternal Role Attainment Theory in Nursing Practice

Molly Meighan

"Women becoming mothers face increasingly complex situations with fewer role models. The period of transition into the new identity, from pregnancy and over the first year, is a time of much uncertainty that motivates the woman to seek out information and help. The kind of help or care she receives can have long-term effects for her and for her child. For that help or care to be relevant, the caregiver must understand the woman's experience in this process." (*From* Becoming a mother, *R. T. Mercer, copyright ©️ 1995, Springer Publishing Company, Inc. New York 10012. Used by permission.)*

"The need for a shift in society's priorities to place a greater value on mothers and their children by providing more extensive support and healthcare during childbearing and child rearing has never been more urgent." (*From* Becoming a mother, *R. T. Mercer, copyright ©️ 1995, Springer Publishing Company, Inc. New York 10012. Used by permission.)*

The study of parental role attainment is extremely complex because of the many variables influencing the process. Table 17-1 lists variables identified as having a direct impact on the maternal role. Despite the efforts of researchers to identify and study these and other variables, understanding the transition to the parental role remains elusive. However, research on this process has been beneficial in improving the nursing care of families in a wide variety of settings. Mercer is among the researchers contributing most greatly to understanding this process.

HISTORY AND BACKGROUND

Mercer's Theory of Maternal Role Attainment is based on her extensive research on the topic beginning in the late 1960s and early 1970s. The

TABLE 17-1   Factors Influencing Maternal Role Attainment

Variables	Impact on the Maternal Role
Maternal age	*Adolescent mothers* are at increased risk for preterm birth and low birth weight infants, as well as increased risk for long-range financial, educational, and family structural problems. *Older mothers* (>30 years) are at an increased risk of fetal/infant and maternal health problems, as well as increased risk of depression.
Birth experience	Birth is seen as a formal entry into motherhood. The mother's experience during birth is related to knowledge, her self-concept, and her perceived control over the process.
Early separation from infant	Early separation of mother and infant decreases opportunities for bonding or attachment to the child. Therefore it may delay the process of maternal role attainment.
Social stress/social support	Stress has been associated with increased illness, but the impact of stress can be mediated by effective social support. The emotional support from a mate appears to be the most helpful support in the transition to the maternal role.
Personality traits	Temperament and learned traits of flexibility and empathy influence maternal role-taking. Empathy is especially important to the maternal role.
Self-concept	A positive self-concept influences an individual's ability to relate to another, thus facilitating the process of maternal role attainment.
Child-rearing attitudes	Maternal attitudes about child-rearing have a direct effect on mothering behavior and are believed to have a direct effect on the child's socialization.
Health status	Maternal illness decreases self-esteem and produces fatigue, which interferes with mothering. Illness may delay the process of maternal role transition.
Infant temperament	An infant who is not easily consoled or comforted can make the transition to motherhood more difficult by decreasing the women's perception of competence and her confidence in being a mother.
Infant health status	Health status is directly related to the infant's ability to respond to the mother. The separation of mother and infant due to poor health delays the attachment process. The mother may be reluctant to begin transition to the maternal role for fear that the infant may die.

Reference: Mercer, R. T. (1986). *First-time motherhood: Experiences from teens to forties.* New York: Springer.

stimulus for both research and the development of theory came from her admiration of Reva Rubin, who was her professor and mentor at the University of Pittsburgh, where Mercer earned a Ph.D. (Bee, Legge, & Oetting, 1994). Rubin's work (1961, 1967a, 1967b) in defining and understanding maternal role attainment is well known by nurses who practice in obstetrical settings. Rubin (1977) described maternal role attainment as a process of "binding-in," (being attached to the child) and "maternal role identity" (seeing oneself in the role and having a sense of comfort about it) (p. 67). Rubin's concepts and assertions about the variables influencing maternal role attainment served as the basis of Mercer's research. Whereas Rubin focused on maternal role attainment during pregnancy and the first month after birth, Mercer expanded her concepts to include the first year following birth (Meighan, Bee, Legge, & Oetting, 1998; Mercer, 1995). In addition, she has considered the parents, the influence of high-risk pregnancy, and maternal illness in her Theory of Role Attainment.

The mother's ability to cope with having an infant with a congenital defect was among Mercer's earliest research interests. In addition, she has studied the needs and concerns of breastfeeding mothers, adolescent mothers, and mothers with postpartum illness as well as the response of fathers to stress and complications during the child-bearing process. In 1981, Mercer introduced a framework for studying factors that impact the maternal role. The framework was more clearly defined in her book *First-Time Motherhood: Experiences from Teens to Forties* (Mercer, 1986). Her Maternal Role Attainment theory and descriptive model were proposed in 1991 during a symposium at the International Research Conference, sponsored by the Council of Nurse Researchers and the American Nurses Association, Los Angeles, California (Bee, Legge, & Oetting, 1994; Mercer, Personal Communication, January 4, 2000). Her theory and the theoretical framework for research were presented in her latest book, *Becoming a Mother* (Mercer, 1995).

OVERVIEW OF MERCER'S THEORY

Mercer not only relied on the previous works of Rubin but also based her research on both role and developmental theories. In addition, she selected study variables from an extensive review of the literature, borrowed from several disciplines, and used a variety of research tools. Her studies served as the platform for the design and development of her Theory of Maternal Role Attainment. Many of the assumptions, definitions, and concepts are based on Reva Rubin's work, transition theories, and the role theories of Thorton and Nardi (1975).

Mercer's definition of maternal role attainment, which is based on the process described by Rubin is as follows (Mercer, 1979):

> The maternal role may be considered . . . attained when the mother feels internal harmony with the role and its expectations. Her behavioral responses to the role's expectations are reflexive and are seen in her concern for and competency in caring for her infant, in her love and affection for and pleasure in her infant, and [in] her acceptance of the responsibilities posed by the role. (p. 374)

According to Mercer (1986, 1995), "the major components of the mothering role are: (1) attachment to the infant, (2) gaining competence in mothering behaviors, and (3) expressing gratification in maternal-infant interactions" (1986, p. 6; 1995, p.13). Borrowing from transition theory, Mercer (1995) described the following concepts as having to do with maternal role attainment: "(1) pregnancy is a marker event upsetting the woman's status quo, (2) pregnancy requires the woman to move from one reality to another, and (3) pregnancy requires a new role identity" (pp. 13-14). Mercer (1986) stated that a woman who becomes a mother must do the following: "(1) recognize the permanency of the required change, (2) seek out information, (3) seek role models, and (4) test herself for competency" (p. 14).

Four stages of maternal role attainment adapted from Thorton and Nardi (1975)—anticipatory, formal (role-taking), informal (role-making), and personal (role identity)—are part of Mercer's theory (1979, 1981, 1985a, 1986, 1990). Table 17-2 lists and describes these stages. The anticipatory stage is closely related to Rubin's cognitive operations and fantasy stages (Rubin, 1967a, 1967b), which included the mother's acceptance of the fetus as a separate individual and fantasizing about the new baby. Mercer's definition of the anticipatory stage included the initial social and psychological adjustments to pregnancy. Expectations of the maternal role are learned during this stage by seeking information from others in the role and by visualizing oneself in the role of mother. The formal (role-taking) stage begins with the birth of the infant. Professionals and others in the woman's social environment often guide this stage. Maternal behavior is learned and replicated in this early stage. The informal (role-making) stage begins as the woman structures the maternal role to fit herself based on past experiences and future goals. In the informal stage, she learns infant cues and develops her own unique style of mothering. The final stage is the personal (role identity) stage. The woman integrates mothering into her self-system. The role is internalized, and she views herself as a competent mother (Mercer, 1981).

TABLE 17-2 Stages of Maternal Role Attainment	
Stage	**Description**
A. Anticipatory stage	Begins during pregnancy and includes the social and psychological adjustments to pregnancy. Expectations of the maternal role are explored. The woman seeks information from others in the role and visualizes herself as a mother.
B. Formal stage (Role-taking)	Begins with the birth of the infant. In this role-taking stage, the woman learns from others in the role or from professionals and replicates their behavior.
C. Informal stage (Role-making)	Begins as the woman structures the maternal role to fit herself based on past experiences and future goals. The woman learns infant cues and develops her own unique style of mothering.
D. Personal stage (Role identity)	Begins as the woman integrates mothering into her self-system. The role is internalized, and she views herself as a competent mother.

Modified from Mercer, R. T. (1981). A theoretical framework for studying factors that impact on the maternal role. *Nursing Research, 30*, 73-77.

Stages of maternal role attainment and corresponding behaviors overlap and are often readjusted as the infant grows and develops. Maternal role identity may be achieved in a month or may require several months (Mercer, 1995). Several factors, including stress, social support, family functioning, and the mother's relationship with the father may have indirect or direct effects on role identity. Table 17-1 lists some of the variables related to maternal role identity.

Mercer (1995) expanded her earlier concepts to emphasize the importance of the role of the father or significant other. According to Mercer (Personal Communication, January 4, 2000), the father (or the mother's intimate partner) contributes to the process of role attainment in a way that cannot be duplicated by any other supportive person. As described by Donley (1993), maternal attachment to the infant develops within the emotional field of the parents' relationship. Figure 17-1 depicts the interaction between father, mother, and infant. The previously described stages of maternal role attainment are represented in layers a through d. Infant developmental stages are displayed in a similar fashion.

The father's interactions help diffuse tension and facilitate maternal role identity (Donley, 1993; Mercer, 1995). Although it is not depicted by the model in Figure 17-1, the father's role identity also occurs and enlarges with infant development and maternal role identity (Mercer,

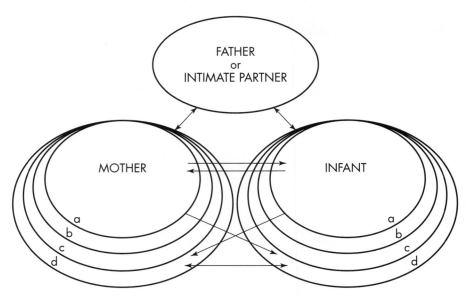

FIGURE 17-1

A microsystem within the evolving model of maternal role attainment. (From *Becoming a mother*, R. T. Mercer, copyright © 1995, Springer Publishing Company, Inc. New York 10012. Used by permission.)

1995). The interaction of mother, father (or significant other), and infant is an important concept and has been added to the larger model first presented by Mercer (1991) and described by Bee, Legge, and Oetting (1994) (Figure 17-2).

Mercer used a general systems approach in her model of maternal role attainment. The model is displayed in Figure 17-2. Bronfenbrenner's nested circles (1979) provide the overall framework. The original model proposed by Mercer in 1991 during the International Research Conference in Los Angeles, California was revised on the basis of her most recent writings in her fifth book, *Becoming a Mother* (Mercer, 1995). The term *exosystem* originally found in the second circle, was replaced with the term *mesosystem* in a personal communication (January 4, 2000). Mercer explained that this change makes the model more consistent with Bronfenbrenner's model, on which it is based.

The mother's microsystem, which is the most influential on her maternal role attainment includes the mother, her infant, her partner, and intimate relationships within her family (Mercer, personal communication, January 14, 2000). Maternal role attainment is achieved within this microsystem of father-mother-infant interaction (see Figure 17-1). The mesosystem includes extended family, school, work, church, and other systems within her more immediate community that directly influence the mother and her microsystem. The exosystem is an exten-

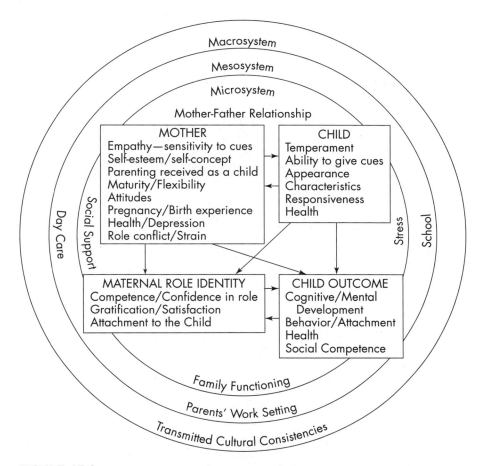

FIGURE 17-2

Model of maternal role attainment. (From Mercer, R. T. [1991]. Paper presented at the "Maternal Role: Models and Consequences" Symposium, International Research Conference, Council of Nurse Researchers and the American Nurses Association, Los Angeles. *Note:* The figure has been modified based on personal communication with Mercer [January 4, 2000]. The word *mesosystem* has replaced *exosystem*, consistent with Bronfenbrenner's model [1979].)

sion of the mesosystem and is described by Mercer (1995; Personal Communication, January 4, 2000) as interrelationships of two or more settings (subsystems) that influence the mother more indirectly. Examples of the mesosystem (formerly exosystem) are interactions between the woman's work setting, day care, local laws/rules, or church. The outer circle, or macrosystem, includes the social, political, and cultural influences on all of the systems.

Traits and behaviors influencing maternal role identity are included in the model. Maternal characteristics are empathy or sensitivity to infant cues, self-esteem or self-concept, parenting received as a child, maturity and flexibility, attitudes, pregnancy and birth experience, overall health, and role conflict or strain. Infant characteristics that influence maternal role attainment include temperament, ability to give cues, appearance, responsiveness, and health. The outcomes of maternal role identity include competence and confidence in the role, gratification in the role, and attachment to the child. Child outcomes are cognitive and mental development, behavior, attachment, health, and social competence.

CRITICAL THINKING IN NURSING PRACTICE WITH MERCER'S THEORY

The use of Mercer's theory and model for maternal role attainment directs you to consider many of the variables identified by Mercer that have an impact on maternal role identity. Table 17-3 illustrates how the theory and model guide your thinking in nursing practice. During your assessment of the microsystem, you should determine both the health and the responses of mother, infant, and father (or mother's intimate partner). The direct involvement of other immediate family members should also be considered so that you can include them in teaching infant care as needed.

According to Mercer (1995), the relationship between the mother and father (or her intimate partner) is of utmost importance. The initial interaction between mother, father, and infant and other immediate family members most often begins in the hospital and can be influenced by nurses. Helping the father or significant other to understand the importance of the role as a caregiver and as a support to the mother should begin immediately after delivery. An assessment of the availability of a support person for single mothers or for mothers separated from their mates for any reason is also an important consideration.

The stages of maternal role attainment—including the anticipatory, formal, informal, and personal stages—are also taken into account during the assessment of the microsystem. You should continue this assessment during subsequent visits or contacts with the mother. As her nurse, you can lead her through many of the steps associated with these stages. The infant's developmental stage and ability to send cues or elicit responses from the parents should also be considered. This is represented in Figure 17-1 as the infant's a through d levels. Many first-time parents are unaware of their infants' capabilities. You can assist them in learning to recognize infant cues soon after delivery. The parents also need to understand how infant behavior and cues change as the infant grows and develops.

Healthcare professionals—and in particular, nurses—play a role in all stages of maternal role attainment. Prenatal education, either formal

TABLE 17-3	Applying Mercer's Theory in Practice
Assessment	**Nursing Considerations**
Microsystem	
Mother	Has the mother recuperated from childbirth, and is she free from illness, discomfort, or extreme stress?
Infant	Is the infant free from illness and able to respond to the parents as expected?
Father or intimate partner	Is the father or significant other present, supportive, and actively involved with the mother and infant?
	Are other family members supportive? Do they live nearby?
Stages of Maternal Role Attainment	
Anticipatory	Did the couple attend prenatal classes or receive information about infant care before delivery?
Formal	Since childbirth, has the mother asked for information or assistance about providing care and nourishment for the infant?
	Does the mother perform infant care appropriately?
	Does the mother display empathy and attachment toward her infant?
Informal	Does the mother seek advice from others in the role?
	Does the mother have role models in the home environment to emulate?
	Has the woman adjusted her lifestyle and patterns for her infant?
Personal	Is there evidence that the woman is committed to and willing to make personal sacrifices for the well-being of her child?
	Does the woman see herself as a mother?
Mesosystem	
	Does the mother have close friends nearby on whom she can depend if needed?
	Does the mother plan to go back to work outside the home?
	Does the family need advice or assistance regarding childcare?
	What resources in the community, at work, in schools, or in the church are immediately available for the new family?
Macrosystem	
	Are there cultural influences on chilbirth or childcare that need to be addressed?
	Are there social or political issues that directly impact the new family?
	Will changes within the healthcare system, such as short hospital stays, access to nearby services, or limited services, impact the new family?

classes or informal teaching, assists the woman in the anticipatory stage of role attainment. Nurses in any childbirth setting are usually the teachers and role models during the formal stage. The mother relies heavily on the nurse to provide immediate postpartum care to begin her journey toward role identity. Both the informal stage (role-making) and the personal stage (role identity) are influenced by professional role models, such as home care nurses and nurses in clinics and in pediatric settings.

Your assessment of the mesosystem, including the mother's influence on the microsystem, is essential in preparing the new family for discharge from the hospital. Look at some of the nursing considerations listed in Table 17-3 during the assessment. After returning home, the new mother's need for experienced role models is fulfilled by extended family, neighbors, and friends. Many young couples relocate away from family and friends, have few resources, and need help in locating someone on whom they can rely. The new family may need your assistance in finding resources within the community. Some local agencies may be available to help with breastfeeding, housekeeping, childcare, and other concerns. Because reliance on two incomes has become the trend in American families, returning to work and day care arrangements have become major issues for new parents. Therefore they may seek your advice regarding childcare options.

Cultural and societal factors that may affect the new family include beliefs and traditions surrounding childbearing. Table 17-3 can guide you in assessing the macrosystem's impact on the new family. You should not only be aware of cultural differences and expectations of new families but also of the social status and even the larger healthcare system. A major influence has been the trend toward shorter hospital stays and, in some situations, limited access to healthcare services. You must assist the new mother and father to become acquainted with their newborn and to learn how to provide care before hospital discharge, which takes place in a shorter period of time. It is also important to consider and provide information to families about available healthcare resources within the larger macrosystem. Assistance in applying for state or federal financial assistance, supplemental food programs such as Women, Infants, and Children (WIC), or Department of Health and Human Services–sponsored follow-up programs are examples.

Nursing goals and patient care outcomes are included in Mercer's model (see Figure 17-2). Nursing care can be evaluated based on the woman's achievement of maternal role identity and on child outcomes. Maternal role identity is determined by the woman's feelings of confidence and competence in the role, her satisfaction in the role, and her attachment to her child. You can evaluate these goals based on the mother's statements about her role, her ability to provide infant care, and her behavior toward her child. Showing genuine concern for the child, responding to the child's needs, providing competent care, and demonstrating affection for the child are behaviors that you might observe as indications of maternal role identity. Outcomes for the child that indicate maternal role identity include continued cognitive or mental development, attachment behaviors, health state, and social competence. Although there may be some exceptions, even infants who are born small, sick, or premature continue to grow and develop physically and cognitively and eventually gain some social ability. Maternal role identity in these situations is determined by the response of the woman to the unique needs of her infant and by her infant's continued growth and development to his or her fullest capability.

Variables that influence both maternal and child outcomes are also included in Mercer's model (see Figure 17-2). The mother's empathy or sensitivity to infant cues; her self-esteem; the parenting she received as a child; her maturity and flexibility; her attitude; her experiences during pregnancy and birth; and the presence of health, depression; and role conflict affect maternal role identity and child outcome. In turn, the child's temperament, ability to give cues, appearance, characteristics, responsiveness, and health also impact maternal role attainment and child outcome. You can help the mother and child move toward more positive outcomes by considering these variables in your nursing care plan. An example of using this information is to increase the mother's empathy by helping her understand her infant's cues and needs and how to respond appropriately. You can provide support and give information to the mother to help her overcome problems associated with most of the variables listed. Although some of these factors cannot be changed, many of them can be influenced by your teaching, guidance, and role-modeling.

CASE HISTORY OF JANIE

Janie is a 20-year-old primipara who is 6 days postpartum. She and her husband live on a nearby military base. Her husband was present at the delivery but was required to leave for duty overseas before Janie's discharge from the hospital. He will be away for at least 6 months.

A friend who also lives on the base has brought Janie to the clinic this morning with her baby. Janie's temperature is 101.6° F, and she is complaining of a severe headache and pain on urination. During your assessment, you note that the baby is crying and irritable and is gnawing on her fist. However, she appears healthy, and you note a weight gain of six ounces over her birth weight. Janie appears tired, anxious, and depressed. She begins to cry and says, "I just can't seem to feed her enough. She cries all the time. I'm just not a very good mother. I wanted to breastfeed her, but my nipples are sore, and I don't think she is getting enough. I don't know what to do. I just can't do this."

Based on Janie's urinalysis, antibiotics and an analgesic are prescribed. Janie is told that she has a urinary tract infection (UTI) and is instructed to drink extra fluids. All other findings are within normal limits.

NURSING CARE OF JANIE WITH MERCER'S THEORY

Assessment

Using Mercer's Maternal Role Attainment Theory, both Janie and her baby are considered as separate entities within the microsystem. Therefore a complete assessment of both of them is in order. UTIs following childbirth are not uncommon and are usually treated successfully with antibiotics. You should provide information about the prescribed antibiotic and forcing fluids, and you should reinforce discharge instructions regarding perineal care and personal hygiene. There are several possible causes of nipple soreness. Improper grasping of the nipple by the infant is one common cause. The infant's weight gain suggests that she is getting nourishment. Because Janie's baby is breastfeeding, it is not uncommon for her to be hungry every 2 to 3 hours. Frequent crying can indicate hunger, but it can also indicate frustration or simply a desire to be held. You should perform a physical assessment on the infant including the frequency of voiding and the consistency and number of stools.

In addition to assessing both Janie and her infant individually, you should assess the microsystem and the interaction between them. The source of difficulty with breastfeeding is identified while observing the process. In addition, Janie's ability to read infant cues and the infant's reaction to her mothering attempts can be assessed. In assessing the microsystem, a major problem for Janie is revealed. She does not have the immediate emotional support and assistance from her husband, which makes her situation even more difficult.

According to Mercer's theory, Janie is in the formal stage of role attainment, but there is some informal stage activity (role-making). She is still seeking information and needs the support of role models while she attempts to take on the role she has learned thus far. Because they live several hundred miles away, there are no immediate role models available to Janie from her own family. You should consider Janie's mesosystem in search of someone to provide emotional support and serve as a role model. A close friend or neighbor could provide some support to Janie as she adapts to her new role. Janie needs enough help at home to rest and to recover from her present illness and general fatigue following the birth.

An assessment of the macrosystem will assist Janie in obtaining help with healthcare needs. Follow-up telephone calls and—if the service is available—a home visit would be beneficial. She needs more information to help her move from the formal stage to the informal stage. Ensuring that Janie knows whom to call and when to ask for help is essential. Therefore you need to help Janie determine what resources are available to her as she works toward maternal role identity.

Nursing Care Plan

The goals for nursing care of Janie are to recover from her present illness, regain confidence in her ability to be a mother, and reach the stage of maternal role identity. To help accomplish these goals, you should provide information about UTIs and about some of the difficulties that she is facing. By pointing out the weight gain and general health of her infant, you can assure Janie that she has been taking good care of her infant. It may be helpful to explain to Janie that she and her infant are responding in a normal fashion and that she has done very well in caring for her baby alone thus far. Making arrangements for a family member or friend to help Janie at home is needed, at least temporarily. Although more teaching and guidance regarding breastfeeding would be helpful, assistance from a breastfeeding support person, such as a lactational nursing consultant, is also needed over a longer period of time. La Leche League or a local childbirth educator may be available to help Janie.

Evaluation

Follow-up care should be arranged for both Janie and her infant to determine the effectiveness of her treatment for the UTI, her infant's growth and development, and her progress toward maternal role attainment. Therefore you should determine whether appointments have been made with the clinic or physician's office and when. You should give Janie a list of phone numbers and information about when and whom to call in an emergency.

CASE HISTORY OF LISA

Lisa is a 16-year-old single mother who has just delivered prematurely. Her infant is about 31 weeks' gestation. Lisa's mother was with her during the delivery and plans to provide a home for Lisa and her son after he is discharged from the Neonatal Intensive Care Unit (NICU). The infant's father has not participated in Lisa's care during pregnancy and did not come to the hospital when she was in labor.

Lisa and her mother were permitted to see and hold the baby immediately after delivery before he was taken to the NICU. Since his admission to the nursery, he has been intubated and is on a ventilator. The neonatologist has determined that the baby's condition is serious but stable. Lisa is able to visit the nursery for the first time since delivery to see her son, whom she has named Clarence after her maternal grandfather, and she has asked you to take her to the NICU to see him. Her mother is present and wants to accompany Lisa.

NURSING CARE OF LISA WITH MERCER'S THEORY
Assessment of the Microsystem

A physical assessment of Lisa will determine her immediate needs and potential problems before visiting the nursery. An assessment of her expectations of seeing her son on a ventilator and the general environment of the NICU is also needed. An assessment of the condition of and prognosis for the infant to realistically prepare Lisa and her mother before the visit is also warranted.

Lisa's mother has served as her significant other throughout the pregnancy and the delivery. Although the infant's father has not been present, an assessment of any of his future interactions with the infant should take place. You can ask Lisa whether the father knows about the birth and whether he knows that Clarence is in the NICU. If the father is planning on being involved with the infant, an assessment of his understanding about Clarence's birth and present condition would be beneficial. In the absence of the father, Lisa's mother is her primary support and should be included in Lisa's care.

According to Rubin (1984), a woman's mother is the strongest maternal role model. Having a good relationship with her mother is extremely important to Lisa. Thus including Lisa's mother in teaching and caring for Lisa and Clarence and in trips to the NICU is important. In studying the relationship between mother and daughter during pregnancy and childbirth, Mercer (1985b) noted that mother-daughter relationships appear most critical during the early transition to the maternal role and become less essential over time as the daughter gains confidence and competence in the role.

Assessment of the Mesosystem

An interview with Lisa and her mother may provide answers about school plans, work, friends, and other factors that may impact role identity for Lisa. Adolescents often have difficulty with maternal role identity because of their own developmental stage and basic needs. The presence of both supportive and/or nonsupportive situations may be identified within Lisa's mesosystem. Mercer (1986) noted that not all social support networks are helpful in the transition to the maternal role. Lisa's adolescent peers would not likely encourage the self-sacrifice necessary for taking on the maternal role. However, some schools have developed special programs to help adolescent mothers continue their education while they fill the role requirements of motherhood. Seeking this support for Lisa would be beneficial.

Assessment of the Macrosystem

You can help determine what additional resources are available for Lisa and Clarence. Financial resources may be available through federal and/or state-funded assistance. Food resources are available to many women through the WIC program and are based on income. Additional resources for Clarence that are based on special needs may also be available.

Nursing Care Plan

Lisa's situation is extremely complex because of the impact of the baby's preterm birth, her infant's condition, her age, and her lack of support from the infant's father. The nursing care goals for Lisa are to become well-acquainted with and attached to her son, demonstrate concern for his well-being, seek information about his care, and begin the stages of maternal role identity. Interventions for Lisa include preparing her and her mother for a visit to the NICU, providing opportunities for her to touch and hold Clarence, teaching her about his condition and care, and assisting in finding needed resources for Lisa and her family.

Evaluation of Nursing Care for Lisa

Preterm birth is especially troublesome for new mothers in adjusting to the maternal role. Feelings of anxiety, depression, guilt, and shame are not uncommon. There is an uncertainty about the infant's general health and survival. In addition, the infant's immature state prevents many of the normal responses that encourage parental attachment. According to Mercer (1990), the formal stage of maternal role attainment may be delayed beyond the expected 6 to 8 weeks prescribed by most experts. Discharge from the hospital without her infant, who must remain in the NICU, compounds the problem, delays role attainment, and increases the woman's feelings of sadness. All of these factors should be considered in evaluating Lisa's progress toward maternal role attainment.

Often, adolescents fail to recognize the permanency of becoming a mother and rely too heavily on their own mothers to fill the role requirements. Inconsistent responses are characteristic of teenage mothers and reflect their immaturity. Ambivalence is common and is present in many forms (Mercer, 1990). An adolescent mother may be happy about being a mother yet sorry that she often feels tied down with the responsibility of parenthood. Secondly, adolescents are often reluctant to ask questions or seek solutions to problems; they tend to wait for information to be provided. Finally, negative self-concept and decreased self-esteem are common problems for adolescents and prevent them from gaining confidence and competence in the maternal role (Mercer, 1986).

Keeping in mind the major components of the maternal role as stated by Mercer (1986), namely "(1) attachment to the infant, (2) gaining competence in mothering behaviors, and (3) expressing gratification in maternal-infant interactions" (p. 6), you should assess Lisa's response to Clarence on each visit to the nursery. Because teenagers tend to have poor self-concepts as persons, Lisa may benefit from being praised for her attempts at mothering Clarence. The complexity of Lisa's case requires continued support and follow-up within the healthcare system.

CONCLUSION

Mercer's theory and Model of Maternal Role Attainment is very useful in assessing, planning, implementing, and evaluating nursing care. The theory is applicable in a wide variety of settings and with diverse populations. Finally, Mercer's theory not only provides a framework for practice but also provides a frame of reference for nursing research. Because of the influence of numerous variables, the attainment of the maternal role is complex. Mercer has studied the impact of many of these variables and has laid the foundation for continued research in this area to improve nursing practice.

CRITICAL THINKING EXERCISES

1. In what situations is Mercer's Theory of Maternal Role Attainment most useful? Are there situations involving maternal role attainment in which Mercer's theory would not be helpful?
2. How does Mercer's model and Theory of Role Attainment apply to working with new fathers?
3. Discuss with your classmates how the Theory of Maternal Role Attainment might be applied to help families deal with cases of neglect and abuse.
4. You are responsible for setting up parenting classes for first-time parents beginning in the last trimester of pregnancy and meeting every other month for a year (six times). Using Mercer's theory as a guide, what topics would be most important and in what order?
5. You are working in a pediatric primary care clinic. In assessing a 9-month-old infant, you notice a severe diaper rash. The infant's clothes are soiled, and he does not appear to have been bathed recently. When asking the mother what she has been doing to clear up the rash, you find that she seems disinterested and is not very knowledgeable about diaper rash or general care of her infant. Further assessment reveals that her husband works many hours and is seldom at home to help. Her mother and an older sister live about 60 miles away. Would Mercer's theory be applicable in planning nursing care in this situation? What factors may be impeding the maternal role? What nursing interventions would be helpful?

References

Bee, A. M., Legge, D., & Oetting, S. (1994). Ramona T. Mercer: Maternal role attainment. In A. Marriner-Tomey (Ed.), *Nursing theorists and their work* (3rd ed., pp. 390-405). St. Louis: Mosby.

Bronfenbrenner, U. (1979). *The ecology of human development: Experiment by nature and design.* Cambridge, MA: Harvard University Press.

Donley, M. G. (1993). Attachment and the emotional unit. *Family Process, 32,* 3-20.

Meighan, M. M., Bee, A. M., Legge, D., & Oetting, S. (1998). Ramona T. Mercer: Maternal Role Attainment. In A. Marriner-Tomey & M. R. Alligood (Eds.), *Nursing theorists and their work* (4th ed., pp. 407-422). St. Louis: Mosby.

Mercer, R. T. (1979). *Perspectives on adolescent healthcare.* Philadelphia: J. B. Lippincott.

Mercer, R. T. (1981). A theoretical framework for studying factors that impact on the maternal role. *Nursing Research, 30,* 73-77.

Mercer, R. T. (1985a). The process of maternal role attainment over the first year. *Nursing Research, 34,* 198-204.

Mercer, R. T. (1985b). The relationship of age and other variables to gratification in mothering. *Healthcare for Women International, 6,* 295-308.

Mercer, R. T. (1986). *First-time motherhood: Experiences from teens to forties.* New York: Springer.

Mercer, R. T. (1990). *Parents at risk.* New York: Springer.

Mercer, R. T. (1991). Paper presented at the "Maternal Role: Models and Consequences" Symposium, International Research Conference, Council of Nurse Researchers and the American Nurses Association, Los Angeles.

Mercer, R. T. (1995). *Becoming a mother.* New York: Springer.

Mercer, R. T. Personal Communication. January 4, 2000.

Rubin, R. (1961). Basic maternal behavior. *Nursing Outlook, 9,* 683-686.

Rubin, R. (1967a). Attainment of the maternal role: Part I, processes. *Nursing Research, 16,* 237-245.

Rubin, R. (1967b). Attainment of the maternal role: Part II, models and referrants. *Nursing Research, 16,* 342-346.

Rubin, R. (1977). Binding-in in the postpartum period. *Maternal Child Nursing Journal, 6,* 67-75.

Rubin, R. (1984). *Maternal identity and the maternal experience.* New York: Springer.

Thorton, R. & Nardi, P. M. (1975). The dynamics of role acquisition. *American Journal of Sociology, 80,* 870-885.

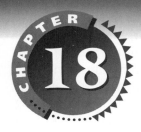

CHAPTER 18

Leininger's Theory of Culture Care Diversity and Universality in Nursing Practice

Marjorie G. Morgan

"The purpose of transcultural nursing [is] to discover and establish a body of knowledge and skills focused on transcultural care, health [or well-being] and illness in order to assist nurses giving culturally competent, safe, and congruent care to people of diverse cultures worldwide." (From Leininger, M. M. [Ed.]. [1995]. Transcultural nursing: Concepts, theories, research, and practices *[ed. 2, p. 11]. New York: McGraw-Hill. Used by permission of The McGraw-Hill Companies.)*

HISTORY AND BACKGROUND

Leininger began formulating her ideas related to nursing in light of her background in anthropology. In the late 1950s, she envisioned that the world was becoming one in which humans interact on a global level. She realized that she needed to go beyond anthropology, with its emphasis on groups of people in different parts of the world, to bring her thoughts into a nursing perspective. At that time, nursing was centered primarily on a medical model. Practice was usually in hospitals or in public health nursing. Leininger had a more holistic view of nursing that would incorporate some anthropological concepts but also a strong nursing component. This would be a new kind of nursing that would focus on human beings in a multicultural world. Leininger (1995a) stated, "I envisioned that transcultural nursing was different from anthropology in that the focus was on *comparative health care, health, and well-being in different environmental contexts and cultures"* (p. 26). Her vision met a deficiency in healthcare—the absence of cultural knowledge.

Even before Leininger formulated her theory of transcultural nursing, she had begun to believe that care was the most important component of nursing. She later stated, "Care is the essence and the central, unifying, and dominant domain to characterize nursing" (Leininger, 1984, p. 3). The theorist needed to meld culture and care together and did so, averring that "[h]uman caring is a universal phenomenon, but the expressions, processes, and patterns vary among cultures" (Leininger, 1984, p. 5). The combination of culture and care can also be seen in some of the language within transcultural nursing. For example, Leininger refers to culture-specific care and culturally congruent care as integral parts of the theory and of the model based on the theory. She further avers that her Theory of Culture Care Diversity and Universality provides the overriding framework for the study of transcultural nursing.

The first research study of transcultural nursing was Leininger's study of the Gadsup people in Papua New Guinea in the early 1960s. In 1965, the first formal courses in transcultural nursing were established at the University of Colorado School of Nursing, and the first doctoral graduate in the field came from the same school in 1974. Since then, approximately 70 nurses have completed doctorates in transcultural nursing under Leininger's tutelage and mentorship as she taught at the University of Colorado, University of Washington, and University of Utah and at Wayne State University in Detroit. The first book published on the theory was *Nursing and Anthropology: Two Worlds to Blend,* written by Leininger and published in 1970. Leininger's most recent theory-based book is the second edition of *Transcultural Nursing: Concepts, Theories, Research, and Practices* (1995b).

In 1974, the Transcultural Nursing Society was founded to serve nurses worldwide. An annual meeting in which research studies are presented is held by the society. Most of the research in transcultural work is done with qualitative research methods. These methods allow for more holistic study of cultural areas rather than reduction to parts as in quantitative research. The *Journal of Transcultural Nursing* began publication in 1989 as the official organ of the society. Since 1988, when a mechanism for certification of transcultural nurses (CTN) was developed, over 90 nurses have been designated as CTNs by passing the written and oral examinations to become certified as experts in the field (Leininger, 1995a).

OVERVIEW OF LEININGER'S TRANSCULTURAL NURSING THEORY

To enlarge on the brief quote that gave the purpose of transcultural nursing at the opening of this chapter, Leininger (1995c) identifies the essential features of the Theory of Cultural Diversity and Universality:

> Transcultural nursing is a substantive area of study and practice focused on comparative cultural care (caring) values, beliefs, and practices of individuals or groups of similar or different cultures with the goal of providing culture-specific and universal nursing care practices in promoting health or well-being or to help people face unfavorable human conditions, illness, or death in culturally meaningful ways (p. 58).

The concept of culture in Leininger's theory borrows its meaning from anthropology. Culture is the "learned, shared, and transmitted knowledge of values, beliefs, norms, and life ways of a particular group that guides an individual or group in their thinking, decisions, and actions in patterned ways" (Leininger, 1995c, p. 60). Culture can be discovered in the actions of the people, in their words, in their norms or rules for behavior, and in the symbols that are important to the group. As the definition states, culture is learned and then passed down from generation to generation.

A key concept of Leininger's theory is that of cultural diversity. This refers to the differences or variations that can be found both between and among different cultures. By recognizing the variations, the nurse can avoid the problem of stereotyping and assuming that all people will respond to the same nursing care. A similar concept is that of cultural universality, the opposite of diversity, which refers to the commonalities or similarities that exist in different cultures. These ideas lead to an important goal of the theory—that is, "to discover similarities and differences about care and its impact on the health and well-being of groups" (Leininger, 1995c, p. 70).

Although nurses are familiar with the concept of professional care as the care provided by nurses after formal education, the concept of *generic care* may not be as well recognized. Generic, or folk, care is the use of remedies that have been passed down from generation to generation within a particular culture. As both Bailey (1991) and Snow (1993) point out, most people use generic care practices long before they seek professional care. Many healthcare professionals look upon the alternative or generic care practices and beliefs as merely based on ignorance or superstition. As Snow (1993) writes, many people learn that healthcare professionals ignore or make light of generic care activities, treating them as superstitions or "old wives' tales," and thus patients are afraid to report these beliefs or practices to them (p. 34). Leininger (1995c) states, "Interfacing generic and professional care into creative and meaningful nursing may well unlock the essential ingredients for quality healthcare" (p. 81).

This leads to two other important concepts that are implicit in the Theory of Culture Care Diversity and Universality. The first of these is *culture-specific care*. Culture-specific care refers to care that results from the identification and abstraction of care practices in a particular culture that will lead to the planning and application of nursing care that would "fit the specific care needs and life ways" of a client from that culture (Leininger, 1995c, p. 74). *Culturally congruent care* is the second important concept. This refers to the "cognitively based assistive, supportive, facilitative, or enabling acts or decisions" found in the cultural values, beliefs, and practices of an individual or group in order for the nurse "to provide meaningful, beneficial, satisfying care that leads to health and well-being" (Leininger, 1995c, p. 75). Leininger (1995c) states that culturally congruent nursing care "is the central idea and goal of the Theory of Culture Care" (p. 75).

CRITICAL THINKING IN NURSING PRACTICE WITH LEININGER'S THEORY

The nurse using Leininger's Theory of Cultural Universality and Diversity (1995a) should begin by becoming culturally aware of and sensitive first to individual cultures, then to group and family, institutional, regional, and community, societal and national, and, finally, global human cultures. This is accomplished by doing cultural research or by reading and studying the reports of studies already done by nurses in transcultural nursing. In doing research, the transcultural nurse is interested in obtaining information about a culture *from the people within that culture.* Therefore an open, naturalistic research approach is used in order to discover the subjective and objective aspects of the culture. Methods generally used are qualitative rather than quantitative and involve participation, observation, and interviews of informants.

The Sunrise Model (Figure 18-1) offers a visual image or map that will guide your exploration of culture. Leininger (1995d) has written, "This model should not be viewed as a theory per se, but rather as a depiction of the multiple components of the theory" (p. 107). In using the model, the nurse systematically moves through the major tenets of the theory with the goal of providing competent cultural care.

As can be seen from the model, culture care is the overriding component of the first part of the model. This is followed by the worldview and the cultural and social structure dimensions. *Worldview* refers to the way in which people of a culture look at their particular surroundings or universe to form certain values about their lives. As an example, in a study of Arab Muslims and culture care, Luna (1995) found that the "single most important feature of the world view of Islam is the concept of *Tawhid*" (p. 321). Luna explains that *Tawhid* refers to the "unity of the Supreme Being (Allah) and the subsequent unity of nature" (p. 321). She further points out that the Muslim belief that "the existence of God is not in isolation: rather all the world is united in God" (p. 321) must be taken

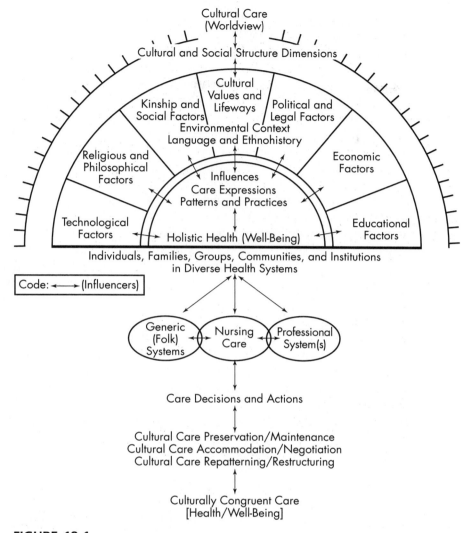

FIGURE 18-1

Sunrise Model to depict dimensions of the Theory of Culture Care Diversity and Universality. (From Leininger, M. M. *Journal of Transcultural Nursing 8*[2], p. 37, copyright © 1997 by Transcultural Nursing Society. Reprinted by permission of Sage Publications.)

into consideration in planning nursing care intervention for the Arab Muslims.

The social structure includes the components of technological, religious and philosophical, kinship, political and legal, economic, and educational factors. Again, these are studied through participation, observation, and interview research techniques. Some specific examples can be found in earlier transcultural research.

In many cultures, the family is an important element. Wenger and Wenger (1988) studied the Amish and found that the family is the basic unit in that culture. They discovered that in the community, although "individuals are valued as members of families, families themselves are the sociocultural units that make up the church district" (p. 43). Because of the extended family networks, Wenger and Wenger (1988) report that kinship thus "functions to tie the family and (religious) settlements together" (p. 44). Thus one can see how various elements of the social structure will influence other elements found in this section of the Sunrise Model.

Gelazis (1995), in her study of Lithuanian-Americans, discovered that "religious values and beliefs permeate the daily lives of Lithuanian Americans and are the basis for care expressions" (p. 435). She found that religion is "closely tied to cultural preservation, language, and education as well as other aspects . . . such as politics and welfare organizations" (Gelazis, 1995, p. 434). The nurse or student using the Sunrise Model for critical thinking can understand why the elements of the social structure have broken lines between each one to indicate an impact or movement from one element to another.

After the worldview, social structure dimensions, ethnohistory, and language of a culture are discovered, the findings are examined to reach a conclusion as to how they influence the care expressions, patterns, and practices in the culture being studied. The influence will be reflected in the diverse health systems of both generic or folk and professional systems. Nursing care is shown in the Sunrise Model as encompassing both of the above systems.

From the care expressions, patterns, and practices, the transcultural nurse determines nursing care decisions and actions. These decisions and actions can be seen as the following: (1) culture care preservation or maintenance, (2) culture care accommodation or negotiation, and (3) culture care repatterning or restructuring. As Leininger (1995d) defines them, nursing care preservation or maintenance is used to enable people of a particular culture to "retain or preserve relevant care values so that they can maintain their well-being, recover from illness, or face handicaps and/or death" (p. 106). Accommodation or negotiation involves actions and decisions that help the people in a culture "adapt to or negotiate with others for a beneficial or satisfying health outcome with professional care providers" (Leininger, 1995d, p. 106). "Repatterning or restructuring is used to help clients change or modify their health care patterns to provide a life way more beneficial or healthier while still respecting their cultural patterns and beliefs" (Leininger, 1995d, p. 106). Study can be of the individual, a family, groups, communities, and institutions. Table 18-1 will lead you through the steps of critical thinking guided by Leininger's Sunrise Model in Figure 18-1. Column one lists the actions of the nurse, and column two lists the components or tenets of the theory at each step of Leininger's Theory of Culture Care Diversity and Universality.

TABLE 18-1 Critical Thinking in Leininger's Theory	
Nursing Actions	**Components of the Theory**
1. The nurse uses participation, observation, and interviews within the culture.	To discover the worldview of the member or members of the culture; the cultural and social dimensions considering the cultural values and the life ways such as technological, religious and philosophical, kinship and social, political and legal, economic, and educational factors; and the influence of language, the ethnohistory, and the environmental context
2. The nurse analyzes the information gathered.	To discover patterns and themes related to health and well-being based on the factors from the model listed above
3. The nurse considers the care indicated according to the data.	To discover the generic (folk) care, nursing care, and professional systems of care indicated according to the data
4. The nurse develops a plan of care based on the data and presents it to the patient.	To plan for culture care preservation or maintenance, accommodation or negotiation, repatterning or restructuring
5. The nurse observes the outcome of culturally congruent care.	To promote health and well-being

CASE HISTORY OF DEBBIE

Debbie is a 29-year-old woman who was recently admitted to the oncology nursing unit for evaluation after sensing pelvic "fullness" and noticing a watery, foul-smelling vaginal discharge. A Papanicolaou smear revealed class V cervical cancer. She was found to have a stage II squamous cell carcinoma of the cervix and underwent a radical hysterectomy with bilateral salpingooophorectomy.

Her past health history revealed that physical examinations had been infrequent. She also reported that she had not performed breast self-examination. She is 5 feet, 4 inches tall and weights 89 pounds. Her usual weight is about 110 pounds. She has smoked approximately two packs of cigarettes a day for the past 16 years. She is gravida 2, para 2. Her first pregnancy was at age 16, and her second was at age 18. Since that time, she has taken oral contraceptives on a regular basis.

Debbie completed the eighth grade. She is married and lives with her husband and her two children in her mother's home, which she describes as less than sanitary. Her husband is unemployed. She describes him as emotionally distant and abusive at times.

She has done well following surgery except for being unable to completely empty her urinary bladder. She is having continued postoperative pain and nausea. It will be necessary for her to perform intermittent self-catheterization at home. Her medications are (1) an antibiotic, (2) an analgesic as needed for pain, and (3) an antiemetic as needed for nausea. In addition, she will be receiving radiation therapy on an outpatient basis.

Debbie is extremely tearful. She expresses great concern over her future and the future of her two children. She believes that this illness is a punishment for her past life.

NURSING CARE OF DEBBIE WITH LEININGER'S THEORY

The following is a capsule account of how a transcultural nurse would approach the care of Debbie in conjunction with other members of the healthcare team. The situation "in real life" would require much more research and analysis than can be presented here. However, a representative sample of the steps to take and the cultural care planning is given. Some of the material is taken from studies previously conducted by Morgan (1995, 1996).

Observation, Participation, and Interviews

Mary is the transcultural nurse who has been assigned by her home health agency to provide culture-specific care for Debbie. She will cooperate as a consultant on an ongoing basis with the other home health nurses who are giving Debbie physical care.

On her first visit, Mary finds that Debbie is an African-American who has lived in the small rural area of her southern state all her life. Debbie's mother's house, where Debbie and her family live, is wooden; the door and window frames are painted blue. Mary, who is knowledgeable about African-American beliefs, recognizes that the blue paint may be to prevent haunts, or "haints," from entering the house and frightening or harming the occupants. The use of the paint also indicates to Mary that the family probably is knowledgeable about voodoo and may use voodoo from the West Coast African Vondun religion. She will explore this after she has established a relationship with Debbie.

Although Mary has done research in African-American culture and knows a good bit about it, she realizes that she will have to explore Debbie and her family's beliefs, practices, and values that will be both similar and diverse from the group in general. Only after this exploration can culturally competent nursing care be planned.

When Mary approaches the house, she finds Debbie, her two children (ages 13 and 11), her mother, her grandmother, and an aunt sitting in front of the house. Several other small children are playing in the yard. Mary introduces herself as a nurse from the health department. She carefully calls Debbie by her last name. She asks for the names of the other people present and makes a note of those for future use. In the African-American community, great respect is given to the adults, particularly the elders in the family or community. Last names are a sign of that respect and should be used by outsiders.

Mary is asked to sit down with the family, and she engages them in conversation. Both the mother and the grandmother express concern over how Debbie is doing and mention that she "just looks too small and won't eat." Debbie's grandmother also worries that Debbie has "low blood." Mary knows that in the African-American community, the expression of "low" or "high" blood can be taken in many ways. It can mean anemia, too little blood in the body, low blood pressure, or blood that has "fallen" to the lower parts of the body. Conversely, it can mean too much blood, high blood pressure, or blood that has "risen" and affected the brain in some manner (Snow, 1993). Mary will get a nutritionist from the home health agency to work with Debbie on her anemia and weight loss because she knows from records that Debbie does indeed have anemia. She reassures the mother, grandmother, and Debbie herself that anemia is indeed something to work on and that she will arrange some help with it.

Mary notices the crosses around the necks of some of the family members and asks about their church. All regularly attend the African Methodist Episcopal Church just "down the road" from the house. All of the grown women tell Mary that they sing in the gospel choir, although Debbie adds that she has not had the energy to participate in the choir work since her operation. Debbie comments that her children and husband go there also. She volunteers that their pastor is a good man and that he "takes care of his flock."

As is the custom in the southern states (Westmacott, 1992), the front yard is the gathering place for families. There are flowers and bushes here and there, but the yard itself is dirt and is swept daily. The yard faces the street in front of the house, and Mary sees that everyone who passes by waves or "hails" the family in the front yard. The family responds with waves and smiles. Some neighbors stop and ask Debbie how she is doing and tell her that she can call them if they can help in any way.

Mary tells the family goodbye and makes arrangements to come back and talk to them again in a day or so. She explains that she would like to ask Debbie some more questions but does not want to tire her out during this first visit. She assures the family that the home health nurse that is Debbie's primary caregiver will be there every day for a while.

The next time Mary comes to the house, she finds Debbie lying on the sofa in the living room. A television is on in the room; a bathroom and kitchen can be seen from the living room; and a small fan blows on Debbie.

Mary, wanting to determine more about the technical aspects of Debbie's life, asks if the family has adequate refrigeration to preserve food and whether the bathrooms are working adequately. Debbie assures her that they are but says the main problem they have with water is that the neighborhood does not have sewer lines and that the grease trap in the back yard to handle sewerage often overflows.

Debbie also tells Mary that her husband has been better since she got sick but that he verbally mistreats her sometimes, calling her "dumb" because she did not finish high school like he did. She adds that her mother is a "good, strong woman" who protects her from her husband at times. She says she hopes her children can get a better education than she had. Debbie continues that she tries to learn about new things that she might have missed in school, and she particularly wants to learn more about her own body and her illness and operation.

Mary asks Debbie about her economic situation and Debbie answers that they "get by"—but barely. Her mother and grandmother work as housekeepers in motels in the nearby tourist area, and she worked in a textile mill before she got sick. However, she worked part-time and does not receive sick pack or unemployment benefits. Her husband picks up odd jobs now and then, but it is sporadic. She hastens to add that although she has not had an appetite since her surgery, the rest of the family have enough to eat. They grow some vegetables and often share food between neighbors, particularly when extra vegetables or fruit are grown and when the men go hunting or fishing and bring back their game and fish.

Mary notices that there are certain symbols in the house indicating a belief in both the Christian religion and possibly voodoo. There are pictures of Jesus in the house, and she also sees John the Conqueror oil, incense for luck and money, and two 7-day candles on the table. She asks Debbie about these, and Debbie states that although she and her family are Christians, "it is important to cover all bases" and that she and her mother do believe in the supernatural. In fact, she says she thinks that her illness and operation may have been because she was "fixed" or "rooted" (i.e., hexed) by someone. She also volunteers that she has relied on some generic medicines such as aspirin, ExLax, and cod liver oil as well as some herbs in addition to the medicines prescribed by her doctor.

Mary makes several other visits to Debbie while she, at the same time, consults with the other nurses caring for her. Her final report includes the care patterns and themes she has found, along with the cultural care suggestions to follow.

Themes Formulated from Mary's Research

The first patterns are that *protection, presence, and sharing* are viewed as important values to Debbie and her family. The theme growing from this pattern is that health and well-being are dependent on protection, presence, and sharing. Another theme is based on the patterns found in social structural factors. This theme is that spirituality, kinship, and economics have great influence on the health and well-being of Debbie and her family. A third theme that evolves from the observation, participation, and interview findings is that folk health beliefs and practices are used by the family to promote health and well-being.

Culture-Specific Care

From these themes, Mary forms the nursing care decisions and actions that she will share with the other home health nurses. To meet the goal of *culture care preservation or maintenance,* Mary realizes that religion can be used as a strengthening mechanism in Debbie's care. She suggests that arranging for visits and consultations with the pastor of Debbie's church is important. He may be able to help with Debbie's belief that her sins in the past affected her illness. At the same time, she tells both Debbie and her nurses that Debbie may benefit from consulting a "root doctor" to remove any hex that she may have suffered. Maintenance of strong caring by Debbie's relatives, fictive kin, and friends will also contribute to Debbie's well-being. Based on the pattern of presence being important, of the importance of language, and the desire for education, the nurses should plan their visits when they have time to sit with Debbie to talk and teach her about her body and situation.

Similarly, the findings from Mary's visits and the resulting patterns and themes she has discerned will lead to the second form of culture care—that is, *cultural care accommodation or negotiation.* Mary plans to negotiate with the city to try to take care of the unhealthy sewage situation and the grease traps overflowing in the yards of Debbie's neighborhood. City services and the local public health department will be contacted. With the finding of the importance of presence as caring and with Debbie's desire for further education about her body, the nurses will try to find a support group for women who have undergone hysterectomies for Debbie to attend. This offers a chance for Debbie to meet new friends and to learn about how others have coped with the operation. Mary (or the other nurses caring for Debbie) will investigate her prescribed medicines to determine whether they are compatible with the generic or folk methods Debbie uses. Mary will also teach the other nurses about voodoo and its importance so that they will not degrade it or view its practices as superstitions.

Finally, *cultural care repatterning or restructuring* is considered. A dietician will be sent to help Debbie with a menu that will be both agreeable to her and will contribute to weight gain and relief of her anemia. Meals on Wheels or a similar organization will be contacted to begin delivery of a hot lunch every day. The nurses will also attempt to help Debbie stop smoking. Other people in the household who smoke will be instructed about the health hazards to second-hand smoke around nonsmokers and the children. If smoking continues, the smoker is encouraged to do it outside.

Conclusion

Through the use of observation, participation, and interviews, Mary was able to discover the diverse and similar beliefs, practices, and values of Debbie and her family. Prior research and articles related to the African-American group were also used for the same purpose. Based on these beliefs, practices, and values, a nursing culturally congruent care plan could be devised for the client during her postoperative period.

CASE HISTORY OF AMERICAN HARE KRISHNA DEVOTEES

In a large American city, a temple devoted to the worship of Krishna can be found. Living at this temple are 17 Hare Krishna devotees. There are six married couples, two single men, and three single women. All are under 35 years of age except for one man and one woman, both of whom are in their forties. The majority of the devotees have 6 to 10 years in Krishna Consciousness. The majority of the members have some college education. Eight have university degrees, and all finished high school.

This case arose from a research study conducted by a graduate student working on a master's degree to become a certified nurse midwife. While Jane, the student, was in the temple conducting her transcultural study using the qualitative methods of observation, participation, and interviews, the devotees often asked her about health matters and particularly about having babies and the care of pregnant women.

Now that Jane is a certified nurse midwife, the devotees have asked her if she will be the primary caregiver for pregnant women of the temple. She agrees to see the women and their husbands both in the doctor's office with which she is affiliated as well as in regular visits to the temple and to deliver their babies in the hospital if the pregnancies are uncomplicated.

NURSING CARE OF AMERICAN HARE KRISHNA DEVOTEES WITH LEININGER'S THEORY

The following is an illustration of the use of the Leininger Theory of Culture Care Diversity and Universality with a group of people rather than an individual and a family. Again, it is only a representative sample of the use of the theory and Sunrise Model. The findings from the research are based on an earlier qualitative study done by Morgan (1992).

Ethnohistory, Worldview, and Social Structure Features

American Krishna Consciousness began in 1965, when His Divine Grace A. C. Bhaktivandanta Swami Prabhupada came to America from Delhi, India. Krishna Consciousness is a branch of the Hindu religion. The Krishna followers in this study belong to the *Bhakti* form of Hinduism, based on love and devotion to a personal God. The rules of life for the devotees is based on the *Bhagavad-Gita*, which was translated by Prabhubada from the original Sanskrit.

The goal of Krishna Consciousness is to achieve oneness with God (Krishna) through meditation and the chanting of the *mahamantra*, or supreme mantra. The chant, which is intoned by the devotees through-out the day, is "Hare Krishna, Hare Krishna, Krishna, Krishna, Hare, Hare, Hare Rama, Hare Rama, Rama, Rama, Hare, Hare." The translation is "O all-attractive, all-pleasing Lord, O energy of the Lord, please engage me in your devotional service" (Morgan, 1992, p. 7).

Discipline in Krishna Consciousness is strict. The four major rules of conduct are no eating of meat, fish, or game; no illicit sex; no intoxicants, which include drugs, alcohol, coffee, or tea; and no gambling. The devotees live communally in a large house that also serves as the temple. Jane often spends time in the house with the devotees. The couples may share a room, but the single men and women have separate quarters for each. The devotees usually wear traditional Indian clothing, particularly in the temple building. The men wear long flowing saffron-colored clothes called *dhotis*, whereas the women wear *saris*, colorful material that is wrapped around the whole lower body. The men shave their heads except for a tuft of hair on the back of the head called a *sikha*. The tuft is used by Krishna at the time of death to pull the devotee into his spiritual world. *Tilaki*, or clay, is placed on various parts of the body for both sanctification and protection.

In the temple the women do sewing, washing, ironing, and gardening activities. Jane participates in these activities. The men do all of the cooking because the food must be offered to Krishna to become sanctified before the devotees eat; only the Krishna men of upper status in the caste system can handle the food. In Krishna Consciousness, the male is considered to be of higher status than the female, and he is seen as the authority figure in the family and in the Temple.

Because the devotees live in a communal setting, they practice little private finance. The group is supported by private donations, by selling incense, soap, shampoos, and scented oil, and by the sale of the magazine of the movement, *Back to Godhead*. The men leave the temple to sell the magazine and flowers in public places such as airports and parks.

The devotees tell Jane that they view the world outside of the temple as being hostile and frightening. They realize that they are perceived by the public as being members of a cult, with all of the negative thoughts that surround such an image.

Cultural Beliefs and Values Related to Sexual Practices, Pregnancy, and Childbirth

The previously mentioned proscription against illicit sex requires some explanation. There is to be no sex among unmarried devotees. The married couples are not to have sexual intercourse for any reason other than the procreation of children to be raised in Krishna Consciousness. The couple hoping to conceive a baby may have sexual relations just once a month on what is termed the most auspicious day for conception. On that day, the couple is often excused from temple duties so they can devote the whole day to performing holy ceremonies to honor Krishna and to ask for his help. The couple says the Hare Krishna mantra 50 times. The husband then feeds his wife some sweet rice. During intercourse, the woman often tries to be less ardent and demonstrative than the man because it is believed that by doing this, the woman will conceive a boy. Jane found that the women often did not know at what point in their menstrual cycles ovulation occurs.

The Hare Krishnas have certain beliefs related to the child in the womb. In the Hindu religion, birth, life, and death are repeated many times in a cycle of resurrection until one reaches perfection and can ascend to live with Krishna. The person who has not lived a good life may come back to life in the form of an animal. Finally, the person will come back as a human.

The baby in the womb gets its nourishment from the mother and will suffer if she eats salty, bitter, or sour foods. The belief is that the baby lives in the womb in an environment of stools and urine, where worms are bred. The worms attack the baby and bite him or her until he or hse loses consciousness and remembers all of his or her past lives. Finally, he or she is born after regaining consciousness and praying in the uterus to Krishna and asking for relief from his or her former lives.

The devotees believe that prenatal care is important and that a first child should be delivered in a hospital since Prabhupada taught that the baby would be the first generation of American devotees to Krishna. When a Krishna woman goes into labor, she often prefers to have her "sisters" in Krishna with her in the hospital and for the birth. Women are very modest and don't want a man to see them undressed completely. They prefer to have a female attendant at the birth for the same reason. Another Krishna belief is that if the father sees the baby's delivery, he will shorten his life by 10 years.

Almost without exception, babies are breastfed. Prabubada taught that the mother should drink at least eight glasses of milk a day both during pregnancy and after the baby is born. Some of the mothers in Krishna Consciousness breastfeed their male children for 8 years. The belief is that by doing this, the boy will not lust after another woman's breast.

In terms of general healthcare, Jane discovered that the followers of Krishna observed what they termed holistic health practices. They depend on spiritual oneness with Krishna to keep them healthy and to heal them during sickness. If they get ill, they rely first on chanting and fasting. Herbs and nonprescription drugs are then used. Finally, if they are not helped by these measures, they seek professional medical care because they "couldn't serve Krishna" if they were too ill.

Themes Derived from the Study

The first theme from the study is that religion was the primary moving force in Krishna Consciousness and influences the worldview of the devotees. The next theme is that Krishna Consciousness affords the devotees a unity of purpose and strength in the face of hostility from the outside world. Another theme related to the findings is that the discipline of Krishna Consciousness is strictly obeyed and contributes to the health and well-being of the devotees. Specific to pregnancy and childbirth is the fourth theme, which states that bearing a child in Krishna Consciousness is highly valued and the process must be seen as a form of worship (Morgan, 1992).

Culturally Congruent Care

Culture care preservation or maintenance can be used to ensure that a devotee outside of the temple or in the hospital is furnished the lactovegetarian diet. If the patient desires it, food can be brought in from the temple because such food is considered blessed when it is first presented to Krishna. *Cultural care maintenance* should also be used to protect the modesty of the female devotee. This can be done by providing female doctors or advanced practice nurses and labor and delivery nurses who have been instructed in the need for such modesty. If a pregnant woman wants to have her husband at her side during the delivery of a baby, this can be arranged. However, because the modesty of the woman must be addressed and because of the belief that the husband can shorten his life by observing the birth, undue pressure on either the man or woman in this regard is unacceptable.

With *cultural care accommodation or negotiation*, Krishna devotees must be given a place in the hospital where they can chant and pray. It should be a place that will not distract the couple and will not bother other patients. The transcultural nurse may have to negotiate with the administrator of the hospital to get the couple a private room or, at the least, ample space for this activity to facilitate the birthing process. Often, chanting and praying along with meditation are the only forms of pain control acceptable to devotees.

When checking patients into the hospital or a healthcare provider's office or when permission permits must be signed, the nurse must remember that in Krishna belief the man has almost all of the authority for making decisions. However, the man and the woman should both be asked to sign.

Although breastfeeding and bonding with a baby right after birth are important to many mothers and healthcare providers, accommodation again must be made to individual cultural beliefs. Remembering that the baby in the uterus is thought to live in an environment of filth, feces, urine, and worms, the new mother may well wish to have her baby bathed before she begins these activities. Cultural care accommodation to this belief dictates a discussion with the mother about her desires as to when she wants to hold and feed the baby.

Because of the finding that, except during pregnancy and childhood, Krishna devotees seldom seek healthcare until it is a last resort, *cultural care repatterning or restructuring* is considered at these times. Brief reviews of immunization status, the nutritional information in light of the lactovegetarian diet, and questions related to the health of other devotees and family members who are not being followed by healthcare providers would be advantageous during the prenatal and pediatric periods.

Jane used a form of restructuring when she discovered that there was some confusion as to the timing of the fertile period in the woman's menstrual cycle. She presented the women devotees a book on natural family planning and a pregnancy wheel so that the time of ovulation could be more clearly identified.

Conclusion

The American Krishna devotees have a unique style of life in comparison to some other American groups and cultures. The use of the Leininger Theory of Culture Care Diversity and Universality with its focus on the worldview, ethnohistorical factors, social structural elements, and professional and generic healthcare beliefs and practices, enables the transcultural nurse to gain insight and new ways to understand the devotees and their care. The findings were an important means to plan and carry out culturally specific care during pregnancy and childbirth for the Krishna devotees.

CRITICAL THINKING EXERCISES

1. Consider your own cultural group. Describe the social structure factors, and analyze how they might have an impact on health.
2. Use your findings from critical thinking exercise #1 to plan some culturally congruent care for your culture.
3. Look around your living quarters. What symbols can you find that would give a clue to your cultural beliefs and practices? Hint: Your choice of music, videos, and artwork would be strong starting places. List and discuss other symbols you discover.
4. Think about the use of the words "you" and "they" in conversation. Can you give examples of how the use of these words could be divisive in discussing other cultures?
5. Leininger (1995c) states that "cultural imposition refers to the tendency of an individual or group to impose their beliefs, values, and patterns of behavior upon another culture for varied reasons" (p. 66). From your own experience or from observations in a healthcare setting, give some examples of cultural imposition.
6. Choose a cultural group and devise some interview questions that you might use in doing research with Leininger's Theory of Culture Care Diversity and Universality.

References

Bailey, E. J. (1991). *Urban African American health care.* Lanham, MD: University Press of America.

Gelazis, R. (1995). Lithuanian Americans and culture care. In M. M. Leininger (Ed.), *Transcultural nursing: Concepts, theories, research, and practices* (2nd ed., pp. 427-444). New York: McGraw-Hill.

Leininger, M. M. (1970). *Nursing and anthropology: Two worlds to blend.* New York: John Wiley & Sons.

Leininger, M. M. (1984). Care: The essence of nursing and health. In M. M. Leininger (Ed.), *Care: The essence of nursing and health* (pp. 3-15). Thorofare, NJ: Charles B. Slack. Reprinted (1990): Wayne State University Press.

Leininger, M. M. (1995a). Transcultural nursing: Development, focus, importance, and historical development. In M. M. Leininger (Ed.), *Transcultural nursing: Concepts, theories, research, and practices* (2nd ed., pp. 3-54). New York: McGraw-Hill.

Leininger, M. M. (1995b). *Transcultural nursing: Concepts, theories, research, and practices* (2nd ed.). New York: McGraw-Hill.

Leininger, M. M. (1995c). Transcultural nursing perspectives: Basic concepts, principles, and culture care incidents. In M. M. Leininger (Ed.), *Transcultural nursing: Concepts, theories, research, and practices* (2nd ed., pp. 57-92). New York: McGraw-Hill.

Leininger, M. M. (1995d). Overview of Leininger's theory of culture care. In M. M. Leininger (Ed.), *Transcultural nursing: Concepts, theories, research, and practices* (2nd ed., pp. 93-114). New York: McGraw-Hill.

Luna, L. J. (1995). Arab Muslims and culture care. In M. M. Leininger (Ed.), *Transcultural nursing: Concepts, theories, research, and practices* (2nd ed., pp. 317-333). New York: McGraw-Hill.

Morgan, M. G. (1992). Pregnancy and childbirth beliefs and practices of American Hare Krishna devotees within transcultural nursing. *Journal of Transcultural Nursing* 4(1), 5-10.

Morgan, M. G. (1995). African Americans and culture care. In M. M. Leininger (Ed.), *Transcultural nursing: Concepts, theories, research, and practices* (2nd ed., pp. 383-400). New York: McGraw-Hill.

Morgan, M. G. (1996). Prenatal care of African American women in selected USA urban and rural cultural contexts. *Journal of Transcultural Nursing,* 7(2), 3-9.

Snow, L. F. (1993). *Walkin' over medicine.* Boulder, CO: Westview Press.

Wenger, A. F. Z. & Wenger, M. (1988). Community and family care practices of Old Order Amish. In M. M. Leininger (Ed.), *Care: Discovery and uses in clinical and community nursing* (pp. 39-54). Detroit: Wayne State University Press.

Westmacott, R. (1992). *African-American gardens and yards in the rural South.* Knoxville: University of Tennessee Press.

Parse's Theory of Human Becoming in Nursing Practice

Gail J. Mitchell

"The goal of practice with the human becoming theory is quality of life from the person's perspective. Quality of life cannot be determined by those not living the life; thus the person is the only one who can describe his or her quality of life. With the human becoming practice methodology there is no set of standards a person must meet in order to have a "good" quality of life. The person constructs his or her own meaning of it. . . . The [human becoming] practice methodology, which focuses on the quality of life from the person's perspective, flows from the principles of the theory, bringing to life the belief system through the art of practice." (From R. R. Parse, Nursing Science Quarterly 9, *pp. 55-60, copyright © 1996 by Sage Publications, Inc. Reprinted by permission of Sage Publications, Inc.)*

HISTORY AND BACKGROUND

In the video series *Portraits of Excellence* (1990b), Parse establishes that her Theory of Human Becoming evolved over many years as she grew and matured with others and as she considered the values and ideas she engaged while living and learning. Her values led her to question the medical model as a suitable knowledge base for nursing. Parse found the medical model limiting, and she also found it inconsistent with her experience of how people make health decisions. Accordingly, she began searching, early in her nursing career, for a different way to know and practice nursing. From the beginning, Parse chose to focus on the lived experience of persons and their unique views of health. She believes that people coauthor their health, and she asserts that nurses do not have control of people nor of their health choices. Some 30 years ago, Parse had a vision of nursing that was based on dialogue, presence, and participation. Before the Theory of Human Becoming was fully formed in her thinking, Parse knew she wanted to contribute to the development of nursing as a unique science. The unique science she envisioned is consistent with basic tenets of the human science tradition (Mitchell & Cody, 1992), and it supports practices that truly honor the freedom and dignity of human beings (Parse, 1990b).

Parse's theory, originally called man-living-health, first appeared in print in 1981. The name of the theory was officially changed to human becoming in 1992 (Parse, 1992a). Parse (1981, 1987) explicitly presents the human becoming theory as a perspective grounded in human science—a perspective distinct from medicine and its related natural science methodologies. Parse (1981, 1987) referenced Dilthey, regarded by some as the architect of human science, as one person who influenced her thinking about science and about the possibility of systematically exploring the connectedness of life and the unity of lived experience. The Theory of Human Becoming focuses on lived experiences of unitary humans and the meanings and patterns of relating that create persons' unique processes of human becoming. This focus on lived experiences of unitary persons, their meanings, and their participation in health stands in stark contrast to the predominant focus in nursing—bio-psycho-social problem identification and the search for prescriptive interventions.

Parse (1981, 1998) named several thinkers who influenced her development of the assumptions underpinning the human becoming theory. Martha Rogers (1970, 1986, 1994), who originally conceptualized the Science of Unitary Human Beings, had a major influence on Parse's thinking. Additionally, the philosophers Sartre (1966), Merleau-Ponty (1963, 1973, 1974), and Heidegger (1962) anchored Parse's thinking in existential-phenomenological tenets. Parse developed a novel theory that is different from Rogers' work and more expansive than existential-phenomenological thought, yet the insights inspired by these authors are visible in the human becoming theory. The theory itself, which consists of three principles and nine concepts, was developed in deductive-inductive ways during the 1970s as Parse pondered the possibilities of a different kind of nursing (Parse, 1990b).

Since the original publication of her theory of nursing, Parse has published many articles and has authored, coauthored, and edited several texts that have contributed significantly to the discipline of nursing. A book on qualitative research (Parse, Coyne, & Smith, 1985) presents various research studies guided by the human becoming theory. This text was published before Parse had developed a research methodology consistent with her theory. Further development of practice and research methodologies appeared in print 2 years later in a general text on nursing science. The book *Nursing Science: Major Paradigms, Theories, and Critiques* describes various nursing theories and their alignment with two nursing paradigms named by Parse: the totality and the simultaneity paradigms (Parse, 1987). In 1995, Parse edited *Illuminations: The Human Becoming Theory in Practice and Research*. This text contains contributed works by various authors about the human becoming theory in practice and research. The book *Illuminations* also provides several evaluation studies that focus on explicating differences for nurses and clients when the human becoming theory guides practice. This same text presents a second research method, consistent with the human becoming theory that was first proposed and developed by Cody (1995b) in his hermeneutic analysis of Walt Whitman's *Leaves of Grass*.

In 1998, a revision of Parse's theory was published in her book *The Human Becoming School of Thought: A Perspective for Nurses and Other Health Professionals*. This marked an important development in the Theory of Human Becoming. In this second edition, Parse (1998) formally defined the human becoming school of thought as a

> human science system of interrelated concepts describing the unitary human's mutual process with the universe in cocreating becoming. Essential ideas are the human-universe mutual process, the coconstitution of health, the multi-dimensional meanings the unitary human gives to being and becoming, and the human's freedom in each situation to choose alternative ways of becoming (p. 10).

Currently, there are assumptions, principles, and practice and research methodologies within the human becoming school of thought. The phrase *school of thought* is more comprehensive than the human becoming theory itself. The human science system of interrelated concepts facilitates the development of other theories and research and practice methodologies that are consistent with the basic tenets of the system. The suggestion that the school of thought may also provide guidance for other healthcare professionals means that the essential ideas of the human becoming school of thought may provide a foundation for theory development in other disciplines. The human becoming school of thought presents another horizon for additional development in the human science tradition.

Numerous published articles describe the difference the human becoming theory makes in practice and how research enhances the understanding of lived experience while expanding the knowledge base of the human becoming theory. It is not possible to note all the contributions of authors in this brief history and background of the human becoming theory. Readers can access additional references on the world wide web at http://www.utoronto.ca/icps. To represent the scope of work related to the human becoming theory, selected examples of works that represent the breadth of practice and research activities with individuals and groups in various settings around the world are presented in this text.

The human becoming theory has guided practice in community settings (Banonis, 1995; Bunkers, Michaels, & Ethridge, 1997; Kelley, 1995), parishes (Bunkers, 1998b, 1999b), homeless shelters (Rasmusson, 1995; Rasmusson, Jonas, & Mitchell, 1991), and hospitals (Markovic, 1997; Mitchell, 1992; Mitchell & Copplestone, 1990). The theory has been shown to be a useful guide for practice with children (Cody, Hudepohl, & Brinkman, 1995), adolescents (Arndt, 1995), adults (Jonas-Simpson, 1997a; Mattice & Mitchell, 1990; Mitchell, 1988, 1993b; Wang, 1997), families (Butler, 1988; Cody, 1995c), and communities (Kelley, 1995). Nurses have used music (Jonas, 1995b; Jonas-Simpson, 1997a) and art (Baumann, 1999) in their work with Parse's theory. Most recently, nonnursing healthcare professionals have published papers depicting practice inspired by the human becoming school of thought (Elwood & Lewson, 1999).

The value of the human becoming theory has been considered from the perspectives of staff nurses (Quiquero, Knights, & Meo, 1991), managers (Mattice, 1991), advanced practice nurses (Bournes & DasGupta, 1997; Spenceley, 1995), administrators (Mitchell, 1997, 1998), and clients (Mitchell, Bernardo, & Bournes, 1997). Nurses have offered comparisons between human becoming and other nursing theories (Baumann, 1997a; Mitchell & Pilkington, 1990; Walker, 1996). Other authors have discussed how Parse's theory complements medical science (Mitchell & Cody, 1999). Baumann (1995) considered children's artistic expressions from the diverging perspectives of psychoanalytic and human becoming theory. Other scholars have explored how the theory changes the teaching-learning process (Bunkers, 1999a; Saltmarche, Kolodny, & Mitchell, 1998), curriculum development (Jacono & Jacono, 1996; Parse, 1981, 1987), and state board standards for decision making (Damgaard & Bunkers, 1998; Vander Woude, 1998).

The Theory of Human Becoming has been critiqued (Cowling, 1989; Phillips, 1987; Smith & Hudepohl, 1988) and evaluated in practice (Jonas, 1995a; Legault & Ferguson-Paré, 1999; Northrup & Cody, 1998; Santopinto & Smith, 1995). Human becoming theory has inspired many philosophical papers that clarify linkages with human science traditions (Mitchell & Cody, 1992), views of freedom (Mitchell, 1995), and ethical practices (Bournes, 2000; Milton, 1999; Mitchell, 1991b; Pilkington, 1999). Nurses have been inspired by the theory to explore paradox (Mitchell, 1993a; Wimpenny, 1993), metaphor (Banonis, 1995), true presence (Bernardo, 1998; Liehr, 1989), quality of life (Daly, Mitchell, & Jonas-Simpson, 1996; Fisher & Mitchell, 1998; Kelley, 1999; Parse,

1996c), persistence-change (Pilkington, 2000), and advanced nursing practice (Bunkers, Michaels, & Ethridge, 1997; Smith, 1995).

Research studies have enhanced understanding about lived experiences of aging (Futrell, Wondolowski, & Mitchell, 1994; Rendon, Sales, Leal, & Pique, 1995; Wondolowski & Davis, 1988), grieving (Cody, 1991, 1995a; Pilkington, 1993), suffering (Daly, 1995), persevering/struggling (Allchin-Petardi, 1998; Carson & Mitchell, 1998; Smith, 1990), recovering (Banonis, 1989), laughing (Parse, 1994a), and joy-sorrow (Parse, 1997b). The human becoming lens has helped nurses know more about how persons experience serenity (Kruse, 1999), health (Parse, Coyne, & Smith, 1985; Wondolowski & Davis, 1991), hope (Parse, 1999), and quality of life (Mitchell, 1998; Parse, 1996c; Pilkington, 1999, Wang, 1997). Research has been conducted with children (Bauman, 1994, 1996a, 1997b), older adults (Mitchell, 1990), families (Cody, 1995a), and with persons living with the diagnosis of cognitive impairment (Fisher & Mitchell, 1998; Parse, 1996c). The theory has global appeal and has provided meaningful direction outside the United States to nurses in Australia (Daly & Jackson, 1999), Japan (Takahashi, 1999), Finland (Toikkanen & Muurinen, 1999), Sweden (Willman, 1999), Taiwan (Liu, 1994; Wang, 1999), Korea (Kim, Shin, & Shin, 1998), Italy, (Zanotti & Bournes, 1999), the United Kingdom (Pilkington & Millar, 1999), and Spain (Rendon, Sales, Leal, & Pique, 1995).

Parse (1990b) suggests that the value of her work will be decided by future generations of nurses who live the theory, by the clients who experience practice with these nurses, and by the new knowledge that accompanies research guided by the theory. By viewing her work as an invitation to think and act differently, Parse provides new horizons for nursing as a human science focused on the lived experience of unitary human beings. Since the birth of human becoming theory, Parse has published many papers that continue to stretch nurses' thinking. Her commitment to scholarship and knowledge development is evident in her own work, especially as founder and editor of the journal *Nursing Science Quarterly,* and in the works of nurses who accept her invitation to think and act differently in practice and research.

OVERVIEW OF PARSE'S THEORY OF HUMAN BECOMING

The Theory of Human Becoming presents an alternative knowledge base for nurses to guide their practice and research activities. When first engaged, the human becoming theory can be experienced as familiar-yet-unfamiliar, simplistic-yet-complex, and clear-yet-obscure (Mitchell & Pilkington, 2000). It requires as much willingness on the part of the interested professional nurse and others to unlearn as it does to learn a new way of thinking. The Theory of Human Becoming appeals to nurses who, like Parse, find the biomedical model restrictive and dehumanizing. The principles and concepts are abstract, and the language Parse uses is nonlinear and can be both unsettling and uplifting in its fluidity and process orientation. The theory is a foundation of knowledge that is very deep. When informed by the lived experiences of persons, the theory becomes a dynamic and self-renewing source for understanding the human-universe-health process.

It is interesting and quite important to appreciate the meaning of the human-universe-health construct, especially in light of the idea that nursing's metaparadigm concepts have traditionally been thought of as separate entities—human, environment, health. In the Theory of Human Becoming, there is no separateness, nor is there a way to reduce the human and his or her mutual process with the universe. It is the unity of person with universe in mutual process that accounts for the major differences between the totality and simultaneity paradigms of nursing science (Parse, 1987). The essential ideas of unitary person, mutual process, situated freedom, multidimensional meanings, and coconstituted health provide the major conceptual ideas of the human becoming school of thought (Parse, 1998).

Parse (1990a) has described health in light of human becoming. She proposes that health is a synthesis of values and a personal commitment to be the person one wants to be. Persons are free to choose the meaning and significance of events. People are free to choose their attitudes, their concerns, and their hopes and dreams. Health, from Parse's perspective, relates to ways in which persons live their value priorities during the ups and downs that shape lived experience. Human dignity links with choice and with having one's value priorities respected by others. In any given moment from birth to death, people can and do choose their values and thus their health.

From the human becoming perspective, health cannot be given or taken, controlled or manipulated, judged, or diagnosed. Health is the way persons live their values in ways consistent with their desires, hopes, and dreams. Patterns of health are paradoxical and include times of disappointment as well as times of success, and times of joy as well as times of sorrow. From Parse's perspective, persons are the coauthors of their health, and no outsider can define the values that another person will cherish and live by. This view of health, along with the assumptions and principles of the human becoming theory, lays the foundation for the kind of practice directed by the theory.

The human becoming theory consists of three principles and nine concepts that flow from Parse's assumptions about humans and becoming. The nine assumptions are as follows (Parse, 1998):

1. The human is coexisting while coconstituting rhythmical patterns with the universe.

2. The human is open, freely choosing meaning in situation, bearing responsibility for decisions.
3. The human is unitary, continuously coconstituting patterns of relating.
4. The human is transcending multidimensionally with the possibles.
5. Becoming is unitary human-living-health.
6. Becoming is a rhythmically coconstituting human-universe process.
7. Becoming is the human's patterns of relating value priorities.
8. Becoming is an intersubjective process of transcending with the possibles.
9. Becoming is unitary human's emerging.

Three principles constitute the Theory of Human Becoming. These principles form the knowledge base that shapes the nurse's view of the human-universe-health process. The human becoming theory is unique in its identification of paradox as an inherent process of lived experience. Each principle has a central theme as well as paradoxical rhythms that help define human becoming. Taken together, these principles are like a landscape in that they form the background or fabric of knowledge that prepares the nurse's thinking and acting with clients in practice and research. These principles are values-based, and they are not to be "tested," at least not in the traditional sense of testing a theory. For example, a nurse would not set out to test the hypothesis that people choose meaning in situations or that people reveal and conceal who they are. A person either believes or does not believe in the assumptions and beliefs of unitary humans, mutual process, and situated freedom. It is a choice to practice with human becoming, a choice made most often because of the fit between one's personal values and the view of human becoming nursing. The principles of human becoming are to be integrated by professionals and then lived with others. Readers are encouraged to go to the original sources of Parse's work for a full discussion of the theoretical assumptions, principles, and concepts because each nurse interprets and lives the theory in consistent and yet unique ways.

Principle One

The first principle of the human becoming theory is "Structuring meaning multidimensionally is cocreating reality through the languaging of valuing and imaging" (Parse, 1998, p. 35). Meaning is the central theme of this principle. The first principle provides one of the three essential frames that shape what nurses think about human beings before they approach persons in practice. Structuring meaning multidimensionally is what humans do; every person constructs a unique view of the world that evolves at both explicit and tacit levels in the process of living and relating with others. The meaning of life situations is linked to the choices a person makes at many different realms of the universe regarding hopes, dreams, fears, doubts, and cherished beliefs. Nurses who integrate beliefs contained in the first principle approach persons as mysteries who assign unique meanings to their life situations. The first principle contains three concepts—imaging, valuing, and languaging.

Imaging is persons' explicit-tacit knowing of their personal realities. Explicit-tacit is a paradoxical process in which explicit awareness coexists with the secreted knowing of our realities. For instance, the reasons behind certain feelings or actions may be known, or the reasons may remain a mystery. Sometimes it is not possible to know "why?" Imaging is a process of knowing and of coming to know as persons accept and reject ideas, values, beliefs, and practices consistent with their worldview. The ways persons change the meaning of their personal realities occurs through processes such as questioning, speaking about what things mean, exploring personal views, picturing cherished possibilities, and comparing options and alternative views. Imaging is the creating of reality and one's reality reflects who one is as a unitary person.

Valuing is the second concept of the first principle about structuring meaning multidimensionally. *Valuing* is a process of choosing and embracing what is important. Values reflect choices and help to shape patterns of uniqueness. Persons act on values that are already integrated into their realities, and they appropriate new values into daily routines and decisions. Parse has suggested that people can know more about their own process of valuing by reflecting on those with whom they spend time, by thinking about what is important, and by considering what calls forth action in day-to-day living. She states that "values reflect choosing, prizing, and acting to beliefs [sic]" (Parse, 1998, p. 39). Confirming-nonconfirming is an important paradoxical process in light of the concept of valuing. Confirming is about embracing, accepting, and cherishing people, ideas, and projects that are most important. Nonconfirming is the opposite of confirming in that people, ideas, and projects may be denied, rejected, and ignored.

Languaging is the third concept of the first principle. *Languaging* is about the ways persons are with the world and in relationships with others and self. Speaking-being-silent and moving-being-still are para-doxical processes of languaging. This process suggests that people tell and do not tell things in their patterns of speaking and moving and during times when they keep quiet and remain still. Humans language their unique realities in their spoken words and in the choices about how to be with others. Languaging is a way of expressing meaning to and with others in the many situations that constitute daily living. According to Parse, we language our understandings of reality as our health. An outsider can describe observations about another's languaging, but only the person himself or herself is in a position to interpret or tell of its meaning.

Principle Two

The second principle of the human becoming theory states that "co-creating rhythmical patterns of relating is living the paradoxical unity of revealing-concealing and enabling-limiting while connecting-separating" (Parse, 1998, p. 42). The theme of this second principle is rhythmicity, and it focuses on the paradoxical rhythms that constitute patterns of becoming. The paradoxical concepts embedded in this principle appear to be opposites, but Parse (1998) presents them as two dimensions of the same rhythm. For instance, people often express opposing viewpoints about a situation. One of the most memorable descriptions of a paradox was reported by Pilkington (1993) in her study of grieving in women who experienced a miscarriage. These women described patterns of engaging and disengaging with the anguish of their loss. The women knew and needed to talk about their loss but also did not want to believe the reality. Thus they created ways to avoid speaking of it or being with others who reminded them of their loss. Three specific paradoxical unities embedded in the second principle are revealing-concealing, enabling-limiting, and connecting-separating.

Revealing-concealing concerns the ways persons disclose and do not disclose meanings, thoughts, feelings, values, concerns, and hopes. Human beings reveal and conceal all-at-once through their choices, actions, and words. Patterns of revealing-concealing are cocreated in that they vary in relation to who is present and what is happening. People reveal and conceal different things about themselves to different people and in different circumstances. Parse also links revealing-concealing to the mystery of humans and to the reality that persons are never fully revealed; there is always more to know about others and more to discover about self.

Enabling-limiting is the second paradoxical concept of the second principle. This concept concerns the choices persons make moment to moment and the inherent opportunities and limitations that accompany those personal choices. The concept is linked to the notion of doors opening and closing as people make choices and move on in life. People often comment about the unanticipated opportunities that come from hardships or the unwelcome hardships that accompany opportunity. Enabling-limiting is about choice, consequence, and discovery.

Connecting-separating is the third paradoxical concept of the second principle. This paradoxical concept concerns the ways persons can be with others while at the same time being separate from them or how persons can be together without being in the same location. Connecting-separating is also about the ways persons are with projects and ideas. As persons choose to participate in one project or as they choose to embrace a particular idea, there is at the same time a separating from that idea and other possible projects. People connect and separate with people, ideas, and situations. In this way, they show their unique patterns of human becoming.

Principle Three

The third principle of the human becoming theory states that "cotranscending with the possibles is powering unique ways of originating in the process of transforming" (Parse, 1998, p. 46). This principle brings forth ideas about change, struggle, and transcendence. It focuses on how human beings create themselves while moving with their hopes and dreams. The theme of this principle is transcendence and has three related concepts—powering, originating, and transforming.

Powering is the pushing-resisting process that propels people in life. It involves the way persons consider the possibilities that lie ahead and how they choose to go on and find a way to be with situations. To power is to risk losing something of value or even one's life. The pushing-resisting paradox inherent in powering emerges with conflict and tension at times. Conflict can happen with others or can occur within the private thinking of one person as conflicting ideas and options perpetuate the pushing-resisting of change and growth. People clarify value priorities and move on through powering.

Originating is about human uniqueness and the ways persons create their own becoming as they choose from all the possibles that could be. The paradox of conformity-noncomformity surrounds the concept of originating. People strive to be like others while simultaneously striving to be unique and different from others. In choosing how to become, persons face both certainty and uncertainty as they change and move beyond the "now" moment. It is never possible to know all the consequences of choices, yet people can move on with great certainty of direction. Originating is the unique choices people make when facing alternatives, and the consequences of those choices.

The third concept of the third principle is *transforming*. This concept represents a process of deliberately shifting one's patterns of health. The shift may be a choice to change one's attitude about a certain situation, or the shift may be a change in how one lives day-to-day routines or habits. The paradoxical process familiar-unfamiliar is embedded in the process of transforming. When new ideas or situations are encountered, persons logically look for connections to what they already know—to what is familiar. In this process of considering the unfamiliar in light of the familiar, people may discover something new about themselves and make change, or they may decide they do not like the new, in which case they may reject the idea or proposed change. People who decide to stop smoking or to leave a difficult relationship are transforming their patterns of becoming. The shifting of patterns may also happen as persons discover insights about themselves that were not apparent to them before. Transforming is about integrating unfamiliar ideas or activities into one's life. The unfamiliar gets woven with the familiar and becomes integrated within the unity and coherence of lived experience.

• • •

In summary, the three principles with their essential concepts form the knowledge base of the human becoming theory. This knowledge base is essential for nurses practicing the human becoming theory. Parse (1998) states, "The art of living human becoming is guided by the theoretical principles that espouse the human as free agent and meaning-giver, choosing rhythmical patterns of relating while reaching for personal hopes and dreams" (pp. 68-69). Parse maintains that nursing is a service to others. To help nurses to live the art of human becoming, Parse developed a practice methodology that sheds light on the nurse-person process.

THE HUMAN BECOMING PRACTICE METHODOLOGY

The essence of living human becoming is making a commitment to be truly present with others to bear witness and to participate with another's unique process of becoming. Parse (1998) distinguishes between the goal of the discipline of nursing and the goal of the nurse living the human becoming theory. She states that the goal of the discipline is quality of life from the person's perspective, whereas the goal of the nurse living the human becoming theory is to be truly present with others as they experience their quality of life. Quality of life, from Parse's view, is the *whatness* that makes life what it is. It encompasses the meanings, feelings, and thoughts of life experiences (Parse, 1994b). Parse (1998) says that "quality or whatness is the essence of something—in this case, the essence of life, the core substance that makes a life different and uniquely irreplaceable" (p. 69). From this understanding of quality of life, the nurse expresses a profound respect for each person's reality as it is expressed in the nurse-person process. Judgment about the person's reality, in any form, diminishes respect for that individual's quality of life and living.

Dimensions and Processes

Nurses live true presence with others with an awareness of and focus on the dimensions and processes of the human becoming theory. These dimensions and processes are as follows (Parse, 1998, pp. 69-70):

1. Illuminating meaning is explicating what was, is, and will be. Explicating is making clear what is appearing now through languaging.
2. Synchronizing rhythms is dwelling with the pitch, yaw, and roll of the human-universe process. Dwelling with is immersing with the flow of connecting-separating.
3. Mobilizing transcendence is moving beyond the meaning moment with what is not-yet. Moving beyond is propelling with envisioned possibles of transforming.

The dimensions and processes happen all-at-once in the nurse-person process. Nurses guided by the human becoming theory prepare to be present with others through focused attentiveness on the moment at hand and through immersion (Parse, 1998). The knowledge base—meaning the beliefs specified in the principles of the human becoming theory—prepare the nurse to be truly present with the person, family, or group. Nurses have opportunities to be with others and participate with them during times of change, struggle, upset, uncertainty, recovery, and hope. During these times, nurses invite persons to speak about their situations. In the telling, there are moments when insights are clarified, discoveries are made, and change is proposed as people see themselves and their situations in a new light.

Of critical importance for nurses is the understanding that another's universe-health process cannot be assessed, controlled, or manipulated by outsiders. The nurse has the privilege of being present to serve others; this service respects that every person is already living a process of complex unfolding, as he or she structures meaning multidimensionally while cocreating rhythmical patterns of relating and cotranscending with the possibles (Parse, 1981, 1998). The nurse's participation with others as lived through true presence makes a difference to persons, and this qualitative difference is the outcome of practice guided by human becoming.

CRITICAL THINKING IN NURSING PRACTICE WITH PARSE'S THEORY

A theory "is a structure for critical thinking, reasoning, and decision making in practice that provides a perspective of the person for whom the nurse cares and specifies the approach to be taken in the delivery of care" (Alligood, 1997, p. 32). The ability to reflect on and define coherence between knowledge and action is thus an indicator of critical thinking.

Parse (1996a) states that "critical thinking . . . is carefully choosing a direction in light of personal tacit and explicit knowing . . . and choosing a direction is moving beyond the moment with deliberateness" (p. 139).

In this text, the history of a woman named Debbie is provided for consideration from different theoretical perspectives. As previously noted, the practice of nursing and the focus of discussions with the human becoming theory do not follow the problem-solving process (assess, plan, and implement). Rather, nurses live true presence with persons to participate in the process of illuminating meaning, synchronizing rhythms, and moving beyond. Documentation with human becoming theory varies across settings. In general, however, the person's description of his or her health as well as the person's plans, hopes, and concerns are recorded. Typically, a nurse guided by human becoming documents paradoxical patterns that a person expresses and the specific decisions/actions that flow with the person's patterns. The recognition of change that is toward the desired goal is by the person, not by the nurse (see Box 19-1 later in this chapter). The nurse's responsibility is to record the person's evaluation, ongoing concerns, preferred choices, and meanings as they surface in the nurse-person process. The two situations described in the following represent the human becoming theory as a structure for thinking, reasoning, and choosing direction with deliberateness. Readers are encouraged to note the human becoming view of Debbie's situation, as presented in Box 19-1, and to compare it with the following assessment.

CASE HISTORY OF DEBBIE

Debbie is a 29-year-old woman who was recently admitted to the oncology nursing unit for evaluation after sensing pelvic "fullness" and noticing a watery, foul-smelling vaginal discharge. A Papanicolaou smear revealed class V cervical cancer. She was found to have a stage II squamous cell carcinoma of the cervix and underwent a radical hysterectomy with bilateral salpingooophorectomy.

Her past health history revealed that physical examinations had been infrequent. She also reported that she had not performed breast self-examination. She is 5 feet, 4 inches tall and weights 89 pounds. Her usual weight is about 110 pounds. She has smoked approximately two packs of cigarettes a day for the past 16 years. She is gravida 2, para 2. Her first pregnancy was at age 16, and her second was at age 18. Since that time, she has taken oral contraceptives on a regular basis.

Debbie completed the eighth grade. She is married and lives with her husband and her two children in her mother's home, which she describes as less than sanitary. Her husband is unemployed. She describes him as emotionally distant and abusive at times.

She has done well following surgery except for being unable to completely empty her urinary bladder. She is having continued postoperative pain and nausea. It will be necessary for her to perform intermittent self-catheterization at home. Her medications are (1) an antibiotic, (2) an analgesic as needed for pain, and (3) an antiemetic as needed for nausea. In addition, she will be receiving radiation therapy on an outpatient basis.

Debbie is extremely tearful. She expresses great concern over her future and the future of her two children. She believes that this illness is a punishment for her past life.

NURSING CARE OF DEBBIE WITH PARSE'S THEORY OF HUMAN BECOMING

The nurse guided by the human becoming theory approaches Debbie with the intent to be truly present with her as she struggles with this critical life situation. The Theory of Human Becoming guides the nurse to approach Debbie with openness, as an unknowing stranger who has opportunities to bear witness to Debbie's unfolding experience and to provide service as directed by Debbie as she lives her value priorities.

Practice with human becoming is a participatory experience in that the nurse's choices in relation to speaking and acting are guided by Debbie as she expresses her concerns, issues, wishes, hopes, and desires. The three principles of human becoming underpin the beliefs that the nurse holds about Debbie and her situation. The nurse caring for Debbie holds the following beliefs:

1. The nurse believes that Debbie structures the meaning of her experience at multidimensional realms. The meaning of Debbie's situation will be linked to her personal values, life experience, hopes, and fears. The nurse cannot know Debbie's meaning until she has the chance to bear witness to its unfolding in the nurse-person process. The meaning of the situation will be languaged by Debbie in her patterns of speaking-being-silent and moving-being-still. As she speaks about her situation, the meaning of the moment will be explicated for both Debbie and the nurse. The nurse believes that as Debbie speaks about the meaning that she is giving to her situation, there will be opportunities for Debbie to discover something new, something not explicitly known before. The discovery might be an insight that changes how Debbie looks at her situation, or it may lead her to a decision to choose a plan or to learn something new. Such opportunities for explicating meaning and discovering something new are created in the nurse-person process as nurses live true presence with others.

2. The nurse believes that Debbie lives her becoming in paradoxical patterns that involve others in her life. Debbie reveals and conceals her values as she connects and separates with others and with ideas in the enabling-limiting process of moving beyond. This means that the nurse is open to hear about how Debbie relates with others, how she views the value of her relationships and activities, whether and how she would like to change them, and the opportunities and restrictions she sees for herself. The nurse believes that if she goes with the flow of Debbie's exploration of paradoxical patterns, there will be opportunities for insight and plans for change—if that is what Debbie wants. The nurse believes that change and learning are chosen by persons themselves and that the nurse's unconditional regard and respect for this choosing enhances clarity and the discovery of new possibles.

3. The nurse believes that in the process of cotranscending with the possibles, Debbie finds ways to move beyond with the reality of her life situation. Debbie's way of being with the situation is a unique expression of her human becoming. Unique ways of moving beyond cannot be dictated by others. The nurse believes that Debbie's expressed concern for the future of her children is a place to invite additional discussion about her concerns and the possibilities she sees as she looks to the not-yet.

The practice dimensions and processes—illuminating meaning through explicating, synchronizing rhythms through dwelling with, and mobilizing transcendence through moving beyond—guide the nurse to be present as Debbie speaks about her meanings, concerns, and issues, as she sees them. The nurse will be with Debbie as she explores her situation and as she considers her options. The nurse will not judge or label Debbie based on the information provided. For instance, when Debbie states that she believes her illness is a punishment for her past life, the nurse goes with this belief and asks Debbie to say more about it. Regardless of what the nurse might think of this belief, the human becoming theory guides the nurse to respect that Debbie has expressed it and to view it as an opportunity to further explicate the meaning she has chosen. The nurse does not judge Debbie for her smoking or for any other decisions she has made in life. The opportunity with human becoming practice is to invite disclosure, exploration, and clarification in whatever way Debbie chooses. It is Debbie's life, and any attempt by the nurse to control or manipulate Debbie would violate the principles of the human becoming theory.

For the nurse guided by the human becoming theory, the information provided about Debbie with respect to her education, her home situation, her care, and her progress following surgery would all be explored from Debbie's perspective. From the perspective of Parse's theory, the statements made about Debbie and her choices in life have no usefulness on their own. In the course of day-to-day care, the nurse would explore

Debbie's experience of pain, her thoughts about going home, her priorities for learning, and her plans for change in light of her situation as she sees it. From these discussions, specific nursing activities that flow from and address the issues that Debbie identifies as important for her would be developed.

It is important to note the subtle but important difference between a nurse who makes recommendations and suggestions based on his or her values and a nurse who invites the client to lead this process of discussing issues, needs, and possibilities. The reality is that when nurses invite others to clarify their concerns and possibilities, a different nurse-person process unfolds. Until this is experienced or witnessed in practice, it is difficult to appreciate. For instance, some nurses might ask Debbie whether she has thought about quitting smoking. A nurse guided by the human becoming theory would learn about Debbie's views of her smoking and whether they are an area of importance in her description of her life situation. However, the human becoming nurse would not target smoking unless Debbie identified it as an area of concern. The human becoming nurse might ask Debbie questions such as the following:

- What is this situation like for you?
- What is most important for you?
- How would you like to change your situation?
- What would you like to know more about?
- What concerns you most?
- What are your hopes and dreams?

The nurse guided by human becoming theory trusts that persons will ask the questions and seek the information they need to move on and will seek answers from the nurse when they are ready to engage that information. Based on Debbie's descriptions, a plan of care based on her priorities and wishes would be constructed. The nurse's documentation would reflect Debbie's personal health description as it was stated in discussion with the nurse. Nursing actions would flow from Debbie's areas of interest or concern, and the effectiveness of nursing practice would be evaluated by asking Debbie to comment on her satisfaction with care.

For the purpose of enhancing understanding of the human becoming theory, a personal health description and patterns of becoming are presented in Box 19-1 as they might have happened with Debbie.

Human becoming nursing practice complements the medically driven, hospital-based care for which many nurses hold responsibility (Mitchell & Cody, 1999). Completing tasks or assessing vital signs do not detract from the opportunities to also practice nursing in relationships with others. From the human becoming perspective, nursing is a basic science that complements the practices of other healthcare professionals.

> **BOX 19-1**   **DEBBIE'S PERSONAL HEALTH DESCRIPTION,**
> **PARADOXICAL PATTERNS OF BECOMING,**
> **AND THEIR RELATED NURSING ACTIONS**

Debbie says her life is falling apart. She cannot think about anything except her children and what is going to happen to them. Debbie says she is having a lot of pain and she wants to be able to smoke a cigarette. She says that smoking is the only thing keeping her sane. Debbie wants to go home but she also wants to stay in the hospital because it will give her a bit more time to sort things out. She cries as she thinks about her situation and says her greatest worry is whether her husband and mother will take care of her children. Debbie wants her children to stay with their father, yet she does not want them with him because she is afraid he will not be there for them as they get older. Debbie wonders if her mother should keep the children. She says that on some days she just wishes she could walk away from all of them, yet she does not want to live without them; they are all she has. "Now," says Debbie, "I have to deal with everything happening here—cancer, pain, and the push to get me out of the hospital. They want me walking and taking care of this tube when I do not know how much I can handle right now."

AREAS FOR FURTHER DISCUSSION WITH DEBBIE

1. Ask Debbie to say more about how she is feeling. Explore her concerns about the catheter and how she wants to work with it. Explore what it will mean for Debbie to be expected to care for her own tube. Ask Debbie what she wants to know more about.
2. Explore Debbie's comment about having pain. Ask her to describe the pain, what helps it, what she would like to do about it, and how she would like to have assistance from the nurse/team.
3. Continue dialogue as directed by Debbie. Follow up on her concerns. Provide assistance and information as she directs.
4. Take any opportunity to be present with Debbie's family. Explore their concerns, issues, hopes, and how they are doing.

Paradoxical Patterns	Nursing Actions
1. Debbie wants to go home, yet she wants more time in the hospital	Explore Debbie's wish to go home: what she sees happening at home with her care, what she thinks she needs to get along at home. Explore her desire for more time in the hospital. Seek depth and clarity about all her issues, concerns, and needs. Explore what Debbie thinks will help her at this time. Follow up with her requests and/or issues.

DEBBIE'S EVALUATION

Two days later, Debbie says she is glad she is still in the hospital, especially because they discovered that she has a bladder infection, and now she must take antibiotics. She says she is still sad and worried. Debbie also says she feels somewhat better because she spoke with her mother and they have agreed to talk about how best to care for the children while Debbie is ill. Debbie says she is ready to go forward day-by-day and has no desire to look beyond tomorrow.

This means that a nurse will follow best medical practices when completing physical assessments or complex treatments and procedures and will also practice according to a nursing theory that is radically different from medicine. The for-better or for-worse of nursing happens in the nurse-person process as nurses live their values and beliefs with clients and families.

Human becoming practice does not take more time, although some nurses find they spend their time differently after they see the difference this practice makes in the lives of clients. Surprisingly, nurses who choose to live true presence and to study human becoming do so in the same hospitals and with all the same pressures regarding performance and efficiency as do nurses who practice in traditional ways. The difference with the human becoming theory happens in the nurse-person process, in the messages given and taken, in the words spoken and not spoken, in the intent to be present with another without judgment or expectation. Living the art of nursing, as defined in the Theory of Human Becoming, is not easier than traditional nursing. Indeed, it calls for critical thinking, courage, and maturity. However, the theory offers a repeating pattern of meaningful nursing practice. Persons, families, and groups let nurses know in many different ways that their human becoming practice makes a difference. In the following section, Mr. Frank expresses what it meant for him to work with a nurse who was guided by the human becoming theory.

NURSING PROCESS WITH MR. FRANK

Mr. Frank was referred to an advanced practice nurse for education and follow-up regarding a diagnosis of diabetes and the initiation of medication to control his blood sugar. The nurse introduces herself and welcomes Mr. Frank before inviting him to tell her about the reason for his visit.

Mr. Frank's Personal Health Description
Mr. Frank says he has always had "high sugar," but this past year the doctor tells him it is staying too high, so medication will be necessary. He says that things are pretty good overall, but he sees himself slowing down and feels a bit tired since his wife died more than 3 years ago. He smiles as he comments that doing her work is too hard on him. Mr. Frank uses a cane to get around. He says that is a bit difficult for him because the cane is a nuisance, but he is glad to have it because it helps him to stay on his feet.

Mr. Frank says his main concern is that he sometimes cannot remember where he is going or what he is doing. His daughter called the police two times to find him because he did not return to his apartment at the expected time. Mr. Frank says he was very embarrassed and worried with the attention from police, and he knows that his daughter is upset with him and is talking about putting him in a nursing home. Mr. Frank shakes his head and says that he cannot believe he is being treated like some kind of criminal.

Mr. Frank says that he knows he must take pills for his blood sugar and that, other than a bit of food, he is not in need of anything. Because he does not bother anyone else, he does not see why anyone should bother him. He says he wants to live but also that he would rather be dead than go to a nursing home. He is thinking about locking himself in his apartment if anyone tries to make him leave. The nurse asks him what would happen if he locked himself in his apartment. He hesitates before saying that his daughter would probably call the police; they would break down the door; and then he might be in real trouble. Mr. Frank sighs and says that maybe it would not be too bright to lock himself in his apartment.

NURSING CARE OF MR. FRANK WITH PARSE'S THEORY OF HUMAN BECOMING

The nurse asks Mr. Frank what would be a good idea for him. He indicates that he wants to get his blood sugar levels in order and keep living in his apartment. The nurse then asks Mr. Frank how he might accomplish those things. He establishes the following plans for himself:

1. Keep a record of my blood sugar reading every morning.
2. Take one pill a day as ordered by the doctor.
3. Follow diet unless it is necessary to eat more.
4. Talk to my daughter about staying in my apartment.
5. Find out about eating the right food.
6. Try to keep track of time so that my daughter does not need to call the police.

Over time, the nurse continues to work with Mr. Frank about the things on his list and asks whether or not he is satisfied with how things are going. The nurse explores with Mr. Frank the issues he describes as most important—like wanting to live in his own apartment, getting his blood sugar levels in order, and remembering things. During the next visit, Mr. Frank says that he has not yet talked to his daughter but that he really wants to talk to her. The nurse goes with his struggle of deciding when to speak with his daughter. The nurse asks him what he wants to say to her and where and when he thinks it would be best to talk to her. Mr. Frank says he can picture himself talking to her, but he is worried that she will get upset. The nurse asks Mr. Frank what will happen when she gets upset and how he thinks he will be at that time.

During the next visit with the nurse, Mr. Frank reports his sugar is staying between 5 and 10 mmol/L, which he thinks is great. Mr. Frank also states that he spoke with his daughter, and he smiles as he tells the nurse that they had a talk, that she did not get upset, and that she is going to spend some more time with him. Then Mr. Frank says that if it had not been for the nurse helping him, he would not have talked to his daughter. He said the nurse helped him find the way to talk to her, and now he is not so worried about going to a nursing home.

CONCLUSION

These moments with Debbie and Mr. Frank represent a slice of a practice that is complex and challenging to capture with mere words on paper. The nurse guided by human becoming theory lives true presence and invites the person's participation in a different way, as he or she coauthors his or her health and quality of life. Even people who cannot speak or who live with mental illness or cognitive impairment experience true presence in ways they describe as helpful, wonderful, meaningful, different, uplifting, and special. The practice looks and sounds like common sense and expected, but it requires a very deep level of thought and a very passionate commitment to promote human dignity. A thoughtful critique of one's history in nursing can be a place to start the critical thinking necessary to practice the human becoming theory.

CRITICAL THINKING EXERCISES

1. Reflect on your personal values and beliefs about nursing. Consider the following questions: What is most important for you in your nursing work? How do you know you make a difference with clients? What do you want clients to remember about you as a nurse? What kind of nurse would you want for yourself, for your loved ones?

2. Reflect on the assumptions and principles of the human becoming school of thought. Consider the essential beliefs of unitary humans, situated freedom, mutual process, and the person as coauthor of health. Examine your own beliefs and the congruence or lack of congruence with the essential beliefs of human becoming.

3. Consider the health descriptions of Debbie and Mr. Frank and identify how you would have practiced with them. Clarify the rationale for making your decisions with these two clients.

4. Examine your current practices in light of the beliefs of the human becoming theory. Consider the following questions: What is your main purpose or primary focus during discussions with clients? What do you hear yourself saying to people? What do your statements and questions tell you about your beliefs as a nurse? What are the primary messages you believe you are giving to clients in your practice?

5. To begin to change how you relate with clients, select a person and make the intent to go and be with the person for the purpose of understanding his or her reality. Ask the person an open-ended question such as "How are things going?" or "What are your concerns about this situation?" As the person describes his or her reality, ask questions that seek depth and clarity without summarizing, making suggestions, interpreting, or leading the discussion. (This typically takes some practice.) What did you learn about the person? What did you learn about yourself?

6. To practice the human becoming theory, study Parse's original books and the articles published about the theory in practice and research. Continue to examine your beliefs in light of what the theory is asking of you. Make the intent to be truly present with clients without judging or labeling their meanings or choices. Try to be with people in ways consistent with Parse's practice methodology—illuminating meaning, synchronizing rhythms, and mobilizing transcendence. Reflect on your words and actions with clients and evaluate the consistency with the human becoming theory.

References

Allchin-Petardi, L. (1998). Weathering the storm: Persevering through a difficult time. *Nursing Science Quarterly, 11,* 172-177.

Alligood, M. R. (1997). Models and theories: Critical thinking structures. In M. R. Alligood & A. Marriner-Tomey. *Nursing theory: Utilization and application* (pp. 31-45). St. Louis: Mosby.

Arndt, M. J. (1995). Parse's Theory of Human Becoming in practice with hospitalized adolescents. *Nursing Science Quarterly, 8,* 86-90.

Banonis, B. C. (1989). The lived experience of recovering from addiction: A phenomenological study. *Nursing Science Quarterly, 2,* 37-43.

Banonis, B. C. (1995). Metaphors in the practice of the human becoming theory. In R. R. Parse (Ed.), *Illuminations: The human becoming theory in practice and research* (pp. 87-95). New York: National League for Nursing.

Baumann, S. L. (1994). No place of their own: An exploratory study. *Nursing Science Quarterly, 7,* 162-169.

Baumann, S. L. (1995). Two views of children's art: Psychoanalysis and Parse's human becoming theory. *Nursing Science Quarterly, 8,* 65-70.

Baumann, S. L. (1996a). Feeling uncomfortable: Children in families with no place of their own. *Nursing Science Quarterly 9,* 152-159.

Baumann, S. L. (1996b). Parse's research methodology and the nurse-researcher-child process. *Nursing Science Quarterly, 9,* 27-32.

Baumann, S. (1997a). Contrasting two approaches in a community-based nursing practice with older adults: The medical model and Parse's nursing theory. *Nursing Science Quarterly, 10,* 124-130.

Baumann, S. L. (1997b). Qualitative research with children as participants. *Nursing Science Quarterly, 10,* 68-69.

Baumann, S. L. (1999). Art as a path of inquiry. *Nursing Science Quarterly, 12,* 106-110.

Bernardo, A. (1998). Technology and true presence in nursing. *Holistic Nursing Practice, 12*(4), 40-49.

Bournes, D. (2000). A commitment to honoring people's choices. *Nursing Science Quarterly, 13,* 18-23.

Bournes, D. & DasGupta, T. (1997). Professional practice leader: A transformational role that addresses human diversity. *Nursing Administration Quarterly, 21*(4), 61-68.

Bunkers, S. S. (1998a). Considering tomorrow: Parse's theory-guided research. *Nursing Science Quarterly, 11,* 56-63.

Bunkers, S. S. (1998b). A nursing theory-guided model of health ministry: Human becoming in parish nursing. *Nursing Science Quarterly, 11,* 7-8.

Bunkers, S. S. (1999a). The teaching-learning process and the Theory of Human Becoming. *Nursing Science Quarterly, 12,* 227-232.

Bunkers, S. S. (1999b). Translating nursing conceptual frameworks and theory for nursing practice. In A. Solari-Twadell & M. A. McDermott (Eds.), *Parish nursing: Promoting whole person health within faith communities* (pp. 205-214). Thousand Oaks, CA: Sage.

Bunkers, S. S., Michaels, C., & Ethridge, P. (1997). Advanced practice nursing in community: Nursing's opportunity. *Advanced Practice Nursing Quarterly, 2*(4), 79-84.

Butler, M. J. (1988). Family transformation: Parse's theory in practice. *Nursing Science Quarterly, 1,* 68-74.

Carson, M. G. & Mitchell, G. J. (1998). The experience of living with persistent pain. *Journal of Advanced Nursing, 28*(6), 1242-1248.

Cody, W. K. (1991). Grieving a personal loss. *Nursing Science Quarterly, 4,* 61-68.

Cody, W. K. (1995a). The meaning of grieving for families living with AIDS. *Nursing Science Quarterly, 8,* 104-114.

Cody, W. K. (1995b). Of life immense in passion, pulse, and power: Dialoguing with Whitman and Parse, a hermeneutic study. In R. R. Parse (Ed.), *Illuminations: The human becoming theory in practice and research* (pp. 269-307). New York: National League for Nursing.

Cody, W. K. (1995c). True presence with families living with HIV disease. In R. R. Parse (Ed.), *Illuminations: The human becoming theory in practice and research* (pp. 115-133). New York: National League for Nursing.

Cody, W. K. (1995d). The view of the family within the human becoming theory. In R. R. Parse (Ed.), *Illuminations: The human becoming theory in practice and research* (pp. 9-26). New York: National League for Nursing.

Cody, W. K., Hudepohl, J. H., & Brinkman, K. S. (1995). True presence with a child and his family. In R. R. Parse (Ed.), *Illuminations: The human becoming theory in practice and research* (pp. 135-146). New York: National League for Nursing.

Cody, W. K. & Mitchell, G. J. (1992). Parse's theory as a model for practice: The cutting edge. *Advances in Nursing Science, 15*(2), 52-65.

Cowling, W. R. (1989). Parse's theory of nursing. In J. J. Fitzpatrick & A. L. Whall (Eds.), *Conceptual models of nursing: Analysis and application* (2nd ed., pp. 385-399). Norwalk, CT: Appleton & Lange.

Daly, J. (1995). The view of suffering within the human becoming theory. In R. R. Parse (Ed.), *Illuminations: The human becoming theory in practice and research* (pp. 45-59). New York: National League for Nursing.

Daly, J. & Jackson, D. (1999). On the use of nursing theory in nursing education, nursing practice, and nursing research in Australia. *Nursing Science Quarterly, 12,* 342-345.

Daly, J., Mitchell, G. J., & Jonas-Simpson, C. M. (1996). Quality of life and the human becoming theory: Exploring discipline-specific contributions. *Nursing Science Quarterly, 9,* 170-174.

Damgaard, G. & Bunkers, S. S. (1998). Nursing science-guided practice and education: A state board of nursing perspective. *Nursing Science Quarterly, 11,* 142-144.

Dilthey, W. (1961). *Pattern and meaning in history.* New York: Harper & Row.

Elwood, K. H. & Lewson, B. (1999). Art therapy and audiology: Joining hands to hear the story of a resident in long term care. *Perspectives, 23*(4), 18-23.

Fisher, M. A. & Mitchell, G. J. (1998). Patients' views of quality of life: Transforming the knowledge base of nursing. *Clinical Nurse Specialist, 12*(3), 99-105.

Futrell, M., Wondolowski, C., & Mitchell, G. J. (1994). Aging in the oldest old living in Scotland: A phenomenological study. *Nursing Science Quarterly, 6,* 189-194.

Heidegger, M. (1962). *Being and time.* New York: Harper & Row.

Jacono, B. J. & Jacono, J. J. (1996). The benefits of Newman and Parse in helping nurse teachers determine methods to enhance student creativity. *Nursing Education Today, 16,* 356-362.

Jonas, C. M. (1995a). Evaluation of the human becoming theory in family practice. In R. R. Parse (Ed.), *Illuminations: The human becoming theory in practice and research* (pp. 347-366). New York: National League for Nursing.

Jonas, C. M. (1995b). True presence through music for persons living their dying. In R. R. Parse (Ed.), *Illuminations: The human becoming theory in practice* (pp. 97-104). New York: National League for Nursing.

Jonas-Simpson, C. (1997a). Living the art of the human becoming theory. *Nursing Science Quarterly, 10,* 175-179.

Jonas-Simpson, C. M. (1997b). The Parse research method through music. *Nursing Science Quarterly, 10,* 112-114.

Kelley, L. S. (1995). Parse's theory in practice with a group in the community. *Nursing Science Quarterly, 8,* 127-132.

Kelley, L. S. (1999). Evaluating change in quality of life from the perspective of the person: Advanced practice nursing and Parse's goal of nursing. *Holistic Nursing Practice, 13*(4), 61-70.

Kim, M. S., Shin, K. R., & Shin, S. R. (1998). Korean adolescents' experiences of smoking cessation: A prelude to research with the human becoming perspective. *Nursing Science Quarterly, 11,* 105-109.

Kruse, B. G. (1999). The lived experience of serenity: Using Parse's research method. *Nursing Science Quarterly, 12,* 143-150.

Legault, F. & Ferguson-Paré, M. (1999). Advancing nursing practice: An evaluation study of Parse's Theory of Human Becoming. *Canadian Journal of Nursing Leadership, 12*(1), 30-35.

Liehr, P. R. (1989). The core of true presence: A loving center. *Nursing Science Quarterly, 2,* 7-8.

Liu, S. L. (1994). The lived experience of health for hospitalized older women in Taiwan. *Journal of National Taipei College of Nursing, 1,* 1-84.

Markovic, M. (1997). From theory to perioperative practice with Parse. *Canadian Operating Room Nursing Journal, 15*(1), 13-16.

Mattice, M. (1991). Parse's theory of nursing in practice: A manager's perspective. *Canadian Journal of Nursing Administration, 4*(1), 11-13.

Mattice, M. & Mitchell, G. J. (1990). Caring for confused elders. *The Canadian Nurse, 86*(11), 16-18.

Merleau-Ponty, M. (1963). *The structure of behavior.* Boston: Beacon.

Merleau-Ponty, M. (1973). *The prose of the world.* Evanston, IL: Northwestern University Press.

Merleau-Ponty, M. (1974). *Phenomenology of perception.* New York: Humanities Press.

Milton, C. L. (1999). Ethical codes and principles: The link to nursing theory. *Nursing Science Quarterly, 12,* 290-291.

Mitchell, G. J. (1988). Man-living-health: The theory in practice. *Nursing Science Quarterly, 1,* 120-127.

Mitchell, G. J. (1990). The lived experience of taking life day-by-day in later life: Research guided by Parse's emergent method. *Nursing Science Quarterly, 3,* 29-36.

Mitchell, G. J. (1991a). Human subjectivity: The cocreation of self. *Nursing Science Quarterly, 4,* 144-145.

Mitchell, G. J. (1991b). Nursing diagnosis: An ethical analysis. *Image, 23*(2), 99-103.

Mitchell, G. J. (1992). Parse's theory and the multidisciplinary team: Clarifying scientific values. *Nursing Science Quarterly, 5,* 104-106.

Mitchell, G. J. (1993a). Living paradox in Parse's theory. *Nursing Science Quarterly, 6,* 44-51.

Mitchell, G. J. (1993b). Parse's theory in practice. In M. E. Parker (Ed.), *Patterns of nursing theories in practice* (pp. 62-80). New York: National League for Nursing.

Mitchell, G. J. (1995). The view of freedom within the human becoming theory. In R. R. Parse (Ed.), *Illuminations: The human becoming theory in practice and research* (pp. 27-43). New York: National League for Nursing.

Mitchell, G. J. (1997). Reengineered healthcare: Why nurses matter. *Nursing Science Quarterly, 10,* 70-71.

Mitchell, G. J. (1998). Standards of nursing and the winds of change. *Nursing Science Quarterly, 11,* 97-98.

Mitchell, G. J. (1999). Evidence-based practice: Critique and alternative view. *Nursing Science Quarterly, 12,* 30-35.

Mitchell, G. J., Bernardo, A., & Bournes, D. (1997). Nursing guided by Parse's theory: Patient views at Sunnybrook. *Nursing Science Quarterly, 10,* 55-56.

Mitchell, G. J. & Cody, W. K. (1992). Nursing knowledge and human science: Ontological and epistemological considerations. *Nursing Science Quarterly, 5,* 54-61.

Mitchell, G. J. & Cody, W. K. (1999). Human becoming theory: A complement to medical science. *Nursing Science Quarterly, 12,* 304-310.

Mitchell, G. J. & Copplestone, C. (1990). Applying Parse's theory to perioperative nursing: A nontraditional approach. *AORN Journal, 51*(3), 787-798.

Mitchell, G. J. & Pilkington, B. (1990). Theoretical approaches in nursing practice: A comparison of Roy and Parse. *Nursing Science Quarterly, 3,* 81-87.

Mitchell, G. J. & Pilkington, F. B. (2000). Comfort-discomfort with ambiguity: Flight and freedom in nursing practice. *Nursing Science Quarterly, 13,* 31-36.

Northrup, D. T. & Cody, W. K. (1998). Evaluation of the human becoming theory in practice in an acute care psychiatric setting. *Nursing Science Quarterly, 11,* 23-30.

Parse, R. R. (1981). *Man-living-health: A theory of nursing.* New York: Wiley.

Parse, R. R. (1987). *Nursing science: Major paradigms, theories, and critiques.* Philadelphia: W. B. Saunders.

Parse, R. R. (1990a). Health: A personal commitment. *Nursing Science Quarterly, 3,* 136-140.

Parse, R. R. [video]. (1990b). *Portraits of excellence.* Helene Fuld Health Trust. Oakland, CA: Studio Three Production.

Parse, R. R. (1992a). Human becoming: Parse's theory of nursing. *Nursing Science Quarterly, 5,* 35-42.

Parse, R. R. (1992b). Nursing knowledge for the 21st century: An international commitment. *Nursing Science Quarterly, 5,* 8-12.

Parse, R. R. (1992c). The performing art of nursing. *Nursing Science Quarterly, 5,* 147.

Parse, R. R. (1993a). The experience of laughter: A phenomenological study. *Nursing Science Quarterly, 6,* 39-43.

Parse, R. R. (1993b). Nursing and medicine: Two different disciplines. *Nursing Science Quarterly, 6,* 109.

Parse, R. R. (1994a). Laughing and health: A study using Parse's research method. *Nursing Science Quarterly, 7,* 55-64.

Parse, R. R. (1994b). Quality of life: Sciencing and living the art of human becoming. *Nursing Science Quarterly, 7,* 16-21.

Parse, R. R. (Ed.). (1995). *Illuminations: The human becoming theory in practice and research.* New York: National League for Nursing.

Parse, R. R. (1996a). Critical thinking: What is it? *Nursing Science Quarterly, 9,* 139.

Parse, R. R. (1996b). The human becoming theory: Challenges in practice and research. *Nursing Science Quarterly, 9,* 55-60.

Parse, R. R. (1996c). Quality of life for persons living with Alzheimer's disease: A human becoming perspective. *Nursing Science Quarterly, 9,* 126-133.

Parse, R. R. (1996d). Reality: A seamless symphony of becoming. *Nursing Science Quarterly, 9,* 181-183.

Parse, R. R. (1997a). The human becoming theory: The was, is, and will be. *Nursing Science Quarterly, 10,* 32-38.

Parse, R. R. (1997b). Joy-sorrow: A study using the Parse research method. *Nursing Science Quarterly, 10,* 80-87.

Parse, R. R. (1998). *The human becoming school of thought: A perspective for nurses and other health professionals.* Thousand Oaks, CA: Sage.

Parse, R. R. (1999). *Hope: An international human becoming perspective.* Sudbury, MA: Jones and Bartlett Publishers.

Parse, R. R., Coyne, B., & Smith, M. J. (1985). *Nursing research: Qualitative methods.* Bowie, MD: Brady.

Phillips, J. (1987). A critique of Parse's man-living-health theory. In R. R. Parse, *Nursing science: Major paradigms, theories, and critiques* (pp. 181-204). Philadelphia: W. B. Saunders.

Pilkington, F. B. (1993). The lived experience of grieving the loss of an important other. *Nursing Science Quarterly, 6,* 130-139.

Pilkington, F. B. (1999). An ethical framework for nursing practice: Parse's human becoming theory. *Nursing Science Quarterly, 12,* 21-25.

Pilkington, F. B. (2000). A unitary view of persistence-change. *Nursing Science Quarterly, 13,* 5-11.

Pilkington, F. B. (1999). A qualitative study of life after stroke. *Journal of Neuroscience Nursing, 31,* 336-347.

Pilkington, F. B. & Millar, B. (1999). The lived experience of hope with persons from Wales, UK. In R. R. Parse, *Hope: An international human becoming perspective* (pp. 163-189). Sudbury, MA: Jones and Bartlett Publishers.

Quiquero, A., Knights, D., & Meo, C. O. (1991). Theory as a guide to practice: Staff nurses choose Parse's theory. *Canadian Journal of Nursing Administration, 4*(1), 14-16.

Rasmusson, D. L. (1995). True presence with homeless persons. In R. R. Parse (Ed.), *Illuminations: The human becoming theory in practice and research* (pp. 105-113). New York: National League for Nursing.

Rasmusson, D. L., Jonas, C. M., & Mitchell, G. J. (1991). The eye of the beholder: Applying Parse's theory with homeless individuals. *Clinical Nurse Specialist Journal, 5*(3), 139-143.

Rendon, D. C., Sales, R., Leal, I., & Pique, J. (1995). The lived experience of aging in community-dwelling elders in Valencia, Spain: A phenomenological study. *Nursing Science Quarterly, 8,* 152-157.

Rogers, M. E. (1970). *An introduction to the theoretical basis of nursing.* Philadelphia: F. A. Davis.

Rogers, M. E. (1986). Science of Unitary Human Beings. In V. Malinski (Ed.), *Explorations on Martha Rogers' Science of Unitary Human Beings* (pp. 3-8). Norwalk, CT: Appleton-Century-Crofts.

Rogers, M. E. (1994). The Science of Unitary Human Beings: Current perspectives. *Nursing Science Quarterly, 7,* 33-35.

Saltmarche, A., Kolodny, V., & Mitchell, G. J. (1998). An educational approach for patient-focused care: Shifting attitudes and practice. *Journal of Nursing Staff Development, 14*(2), 81-86.

Santopinto, M. D. A. & Smith, M. C. (1995). Evaluation of the human becoming theory in practice with adults and children. In R. R. Parse (Ed.), *Illuminations: The human becoming theory in practice and research* (pp. 309-346). New York: National League for Nursing.

Sartre, J-P. (1966). *Being and nothingness.* New York: Washington Square.

Smith, M. C. (1990). Struggling through a difficult time for unemployed persons. *Nursing Science Quarterly, 3*, 18-28.

Smith, M. C. (1995). The core of advanced practice nursing. *Nursing Science Quarterly, 8*, 2-3.

Smith, M. C. & Hudepohl, J. H. (1988). Analysis and evaluation of Parse's theory of man-living-health. *The Canadian Journal of Nursing Research: Nursing Papers, 20*(4), 43-58.

Spenceley, S. M. (1995). The CNS in multidisciplinary pulmonary rehabilitation: A nursing science perspective. *Clinical Nurse Specialist, 9*, 192-198.

Takahashi, T. (1999). Kibou: Hope for persons in Japan. In R. R. Parse, *Hope: An international human becoming perspective* (pp. 115-128). Sudbury, MA: Jones and Bartlett.

Toikkanen, T. & Muurinen, E. (1999). Toivo: Hope for persons in Finland. In R. R. Parse, *Hope: An international human becoming perspective* (pp. 79-96). Sudbury, MA: Jones and Bartlett.

Vander Woude, D. (1998). Nursing theory-based regulatory decisioning model in South Dakota. *Issues, 19*(3), 14.

Walker, C. A. (1996). Coalescing the theories of two nurse visionaries: Parse and Watson. *Journal of Advanced Nursing, 24*, 988-996.

Wang, C. H. (1997). Quality of life and health for persons living with leprosy. *Nursing Science Quarterly, 10*, 144-145.

Wang, C-E. H. (1999). He-Bung: Hope for persons living with leprosy in Taiwan. In R. R. Parse, *Hope: An international human becoming perspective* (pp. 45-61). Sudbury, MA: Jones and Bartlett.

Willman, A. (1999). Hope: The lived experience for Swedish elders. In R. R. Parse, *Hope: An international human becoming perspective* (pp. 129-142). Sudbury, MA: Jones and Bartlett.

Wimpenny, P. (1993). The paradox of Parse's theory. *Senior Nurse, 13*(5), 10-13.

Wondolowski, C. & Davis, D. K. (1988). The lived experience of aging in the oldest old: A phenomenological study. *The American Journal of Psychoanalysis, 48*, 261-270.

Wondolowski, C. & Davis, D. K. (1991). The lived experience of health in the oldest old: A phenomenological study. *Nursing Science Quarterly, 4*, 113-118.

Zanotti, R. & Bournes, D. A. (1999). Speranza: A study of the lived experience of hope with persons from Italy. In R. R. Parse, *Hope: An international human becoming perspective* (pp. 97-114). Sudbury, MA: Jones and Bartlett.

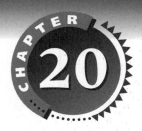

Newman's Theory of Health as Expanding Consciousness in Nursing Practice

Janet M. Witucki

"When we begin to think of ourselves as centers of consciousness ... within an overall pattern of expanding consciousness, we can begin to see that what we sense of our lives is part of a much larger whole. First the pattern of consciousness that is the person; then broadening the focus, the pattern of consciousness that is the family and physical surroundings; then the pattern that is the community, the person's larger environmental affiliations, such as work or school; and ultimately the pattern of the world. It is this pattern of the whole that is the phenomenon of nursing's practice." (From M. A. Newman, Health as expanding consciousness, *2nd ed., 1999: Jones and Bartlett Publishers, Sudbury, MA. WWW.jbpub.com. Reprinted with permission.)*

HISTORY AND BACKGROUND

The first published version of Newman's theory appeared in her book *Theory Development in Nursing* in 1979. In this early writing, Newman presented a viewpoint of health as a dialectic fusion of disease and nondisease, thus encompassing disease as a meaningful aspect of the totality of life experience. This viewpoint of health came about as a result of two influences: Newman's early experiences of her mother's 9-year struggle with amyotrophic lateral sclerosis, during which time Newman

Appreciation is expressed to Dr. Margaret A. Newman for critiquing and contributing to this chapter.

came to realize that an individual may be whole even though illness is present, and her exposure to Martha Rogers' work, which assisted her in conceptualizing health and illness as a single unitary process (Newman, 1986).

Evolution of the conceptualization of Health as Expanding Consciousness was influenced theoretically by several sources (Newman, 1986, 1990a, 1994a). Bentov's explanation (1977) of the evolution of consciousness, Moss' view (1981) of love as the highest level of consciousness, Bohm's theory of implicate order (1980), de Chardin's belief (1959) that consciousness continues to develop beyond physical life, and Young's stages (1976) of human development all contributed to Newman's ability to synthesize her thoughts and experiences into a cohesive and meaningful theory (Newman, 1986, 1994a). The Theory of Health as Expanding Consciousness evolved from a synthesis of these theoretical influences with Newman's own life experiences and thoughts.

Early application of this theory isolated and manipulated the basic theory concepts of space, time, and movement. Newman explored effects of changes in rates of walking on time perception in two studies (Newman, 1972, 1976) and the relationship between age, movement, and time perception of elders in another (Newman, 1982). Further work addressed the relationship between movement, time, and self-assessment of health (Engle, 1984). Schorr and Schroeder (1991) discovered decreased perceived duration of time with physical exertion. Depression was also related to decreased subjective time (Newman & Gaudiano, 1984), but Mentzer and Schorr (1986) found perceived duration of time not to be significantly related to age or perceived control. Finally, Schorr and Schroeder (1989) attempted to demonstrate a relationship between Type A behavior, temporal orientation, and death anxiety by using an extension of the Newman theory entitled Consciousness as a Dissipative Structure.

As work and research with the developing theory progressed, Newman made the discovery that research involving a person's pattern identification and the sharing of patterns with a person was actually nursing practice. She relates, "We discovered that our participation in the process made a difference in our own lives. We suspected that what we were doing in the name of research was nursing practice" (Newman, 1990a, p. 37). Within the theory, research is viewed as praxis. Theory, research, and practice are seen as one inseparable process (Newman, 1990a, 1990d). The professional nurse is viewed as a therapeutic partner who joins with the client in the search for pattern with its accompanying understanding and impetus for growth (Newman, 1987a).

A practice methodology of pattern identification and research/practice process was developed in 1990 (Newman, 1990a). This method reveals sequential patterns of persons' lives and facilitates recognition and insight into patterns as well as authentic involvement of the nurse-researcher in the movement toward higher consciousness. The theory and methodology have provided a basis for research/practice in a variety of clinical settings for diverse client populations and have been utilized extensively for exploring and understanding the experience of illness to individuals and families.

Some examples of theory application include conceptualization of breast cancer as a meaningful part of health (Kiser-Larsen, 1999; Moch, 1990; Roux, 1994), recognizing patterns in cancer patients (Endo, 1996; Newman, 1995b), expansion of consciousness in elderly women with chronic disease (Schorr, Farnham, & Ervin, 1991), life patterns of persons with coronary heart disease (Newman & Moch, 1991), patterns of persons with chronic obstructive pulmonary disease (Jonsdottir, 1998; Noveletsky-Rosenthal, 1996), and patterns of expanding consciousness in persons with HIV/AIDS (Lamendola & Newman, 1994). Additional application includes exploration of health patterning in persons with multiple sclerosis (Gulick & Bugg, 1992), help-seeking patterns in older wife caregivers of husbands with dementia (Witucki, 2000), pattern recognition in adolescent males incarcerated for murder (Dexheimer-Pharris, 1999), and giving and receiving of social support by spouse caregivers and their spouses (Schmitt, 1991). Newman's research as praxis also has described the lived experience of life-passing in middle adolescent females (Shanahan, 1993) and patterns of expanding consciousness in mid-life women (Picard, 2000). It has also been a basis for understanding the transformative experience of Japanese and Canadian primary family caregivers of relatives with schizophrenia (Yamashita, 1998, 1999), for exploring pain reduction with music therapy (Schorr, 1993), for facilitating pattern recognition of high-risk pregnant women (Kalb, 1990; Schroeder, 1993), and for exploring the nature of nursing practice with families of young children (Litchfield, 1997).

Marchione (1986) advocated application of the theory to individuals, families, and communities. Further, application of the theory to nursing management at Carondolet St. Mary's Hospital and Health Center in Tuscon, Arizona has been reported (Newman, Lamb, & Michaels, 1991; Ethridge, 1991; Michaels, 1992). Finally, Gustafson (1990) reported the application of Newman's theory and pattern recognition in parish nursing, and Magen, Gibbon, and Mrozek (1990) reported on implementation of the theory as one of several theories in care for the chronically mentally ill.

The theory has also been used to frame the description of a pinwheel model of bereavement and relevant nursing responses in a study by Solari-Twadell, Bunkers, Wang, and Snyder (1995). It has also been utilized in education to provide some content into the healing web model. This model was designed to integrate nursing education and nursing service together with private and public education programs for baccalaureate and associate degree nursing in South Dakota (Bunkers, Brendtro, Holmes, Howell, Johnson, Koerner, Larson, Nelson, & Weaver, 1992).

OVERVIEW OF NEWMAN'S THEORY OF HEALTH AS EXPANDING CONSCIOUSNESS

Newman's theory proposes a view of health as a unidirectional, unitary process of development (Newman, 1991). She acknowledges that Rogers' (1970) Science of Unitary Human Beings was a major influence in development of the Theory of Health as Expanding Consciousness. In Newman's theory, health is an expansion of consciousness that is defined as the informational capacity of the system and is seen as the ability of the person to interact with the environment (Newman, 1979, 1983, 1986, 1994a). Disease is a meaningful reflection of the whole and, as such, is viewed as a manifestation of health. Disease and nondisease are not separate entities but are dialectically fused into health as a pattern of the whole. Accordingly to Newman (1999), "Health is the pattern of the whole, and wholeness *is.* One cannot lose it or gain it" (p. 228). Disruptions in human beings, such as disease or catastrophic life events, often become catalysts that potentiate unfolding of life processes that persons naturally seek, thereby facilitating movement from one pattern of consciousness to another and transformation into order at a higher level—or expanded consciousness (Newman, 1997).

In the early development of the theory, Newman asserted that the phenomena of inquiry for nursing should be parameters of human wholeness and that there were characteristics of people that identified the whole (Newman, 1979). Major concepts identified by Newman at that time were time, space, movement, consciousness, and pattern.

Time

In the Theory of Health as Expanding Consciousness, time is not merely conceptualized as either subjective or objective but is also viewed in a holographic sense. According to Newman (1994a), "Each moment has an explicate order and also enfolds all others, meaning that each moment of our lives contains all others of all time" (p. 62). Further, time is considered an index of consciousness (Newman, 1983) because as consciousness expands, space-time transcends limitations of linear and physical boundaries to extend beyond what is the here-and-now. However, what is truly important is that one "be fully present in the moment and know that whatever the experience, it is a manifestation of the process of evolving to higher consciousness" (Newman, 1994a, p. 68).

The concept of time and timing is further described as a function of movement (Newman, 1983) and also as the "rhythm of living phenomena" (Newman, 1994a, p. 53). Time is important in revealing patterns because extending the time frame helps nurses and patients recognize patterns and reorganizing activities (Newman, 1994a). Temporal pattern synchronicity between persons and healthcare workers is also important to receptivity and health because these patterns are highly individualistic and influence how people respond to each other. Nurses who attempt to practice within this theoretical framework must be sensitive to synchronize their rhythms with those of persons with whom they are working. Newman refers to this as "the rhythm of relating" (1999, p. 227) and states that it is an indicator of the pattern of interacting consciousness. Through attuning themselves to the rhythms of others, nurses assist persons to identify patterns and move to higher levels of consciousness.

Space

Space is always linked with time and often is referred to as *space-time* or *time-space*. Newman posits that these two concepts are complimentary and inextricably linked to each other, with time being increased as one's life space decreases (Newman, 1979, 1983). Space has further been identified as life-space, personal space, and inner space (Newman, 1979), with personal space or territory very much involved in a person's struggles for self-determination and status (Newman, 1990a). As consciousness expands, the distinction between the self and the world becomes blurred. There is a "recognition that one's essence extends beyond the physical boundaries and is in effect boundarylessness, as one moves to higher levels of consciousness" (Newman, 1994a, p. 47).

Movement

Movement is defined as "the means whereby one perceives reality and therefore is a means of becoming aware of self" (Newman, 1983, p. 165). According to Newman (1994a), movement is a reflection of consciousness, indicates inner organization or disorganization of persons, and communicates the harmony of a person's pattern with the environment. It is integral to relationships and "is a means whereby time and space become a reality" (Newman, 1983, p. 165). Rate of movement is seen as a reflection of pattern (Newman, 1995b). Space, time, and movement are linked. In fact, "the intersection of movement-space-time represents the person as a center of consciousness and varies from person to person, place to place, and time to time" (Newman, 1986, p. 49). When natural movement is altered, space and time are also altered. When movement is restricted (physically or socially), it is necessary for one to move beyond oneself, thereby making movement an important choice point in the process of evolving human consciousness (Newman, 1994a).

Consciousness

Consciousness is defined in the theory as the informational capacity of the system (human beings) or the system's ability to interact with the environment (Newman, 1990a). Newman asserts that an understanding of her definition of consciousness is essential to understanding the theory. Consciousness includes not only cognitive and affective awareness but also the "interconnectedness of the entire living system, which includes physiochemical maintenance and growth processes as well as the immune system" (Newman, 1990a, p. 38). Consciousness is further conceptualized as coextensive in the universe and as the essence of all creation. Interaction, then, occurs openly, constantly, and instantaneously throughout the entire spectrum of consciousness (Newman, 1994a). The person does not just possess consciousness but *is* consciousness, as is all matter. The highest level of consciousness is absolute consciousness, which Newman equates with love that "embraces all experience equally and unconditionally" (Newman, 1994a, p. 48).

Movement through levels of consciousness occurs continuously and unidirectionally in stages and does not occur smoothly but rather in response to major disorganization and disharmony. Newman drew upon Prigogine's (1980) Theory of Dissipative Structures and Young's conceptualization (1976) of the evolution of human beings to describe the levels of consciousness in her theory and the dynamics of movement from one level to another. Figure 20-1 depicts the parallel between Newman's Theory of Expanding Consciousness and Young's stages of human evolution. According to Newman, "We come into being from a state of potential consciousness, are bound in time, find our identity in space, and through movement we learn the 'law' of the way things work and make choices that ultimately take us beyond space and time to a state of absolute consciousness" (Newman, 1994a, p. 26). Within the theory, physical self-development binds one in time and space as one develops and establishes personal territory (stages two and three). Movement provides a way of controlling the personal environment and also represents a choice point (stage four). When movement is restricted, as with illness or physical disability, "one becomes aware of personal limitations and the fact that the old rules don't work anymore" (Newman, 1990a, p. 39), and one experiences the disconnectedness, disorder, and disequilibrium that are precursors to moving to a higher level of consciousness. Transcendence (stage five)—or expansion of boundaries of self and awareness of broader life possibilities—occurs in response as new order is established at a higher level (Newman, 1994a). New ways of relating are discovered, and the freedom that comes with transcending old limitations is discovered (Newman, 1990d). The highest levels of consciousness occur at the sixth stage, in which timelessness occurs, and in the seventh stage, which is absolute consciousness.

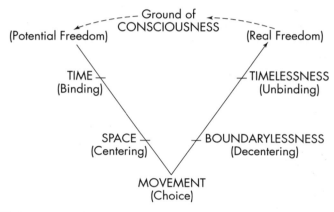

FIGURE 20-1

Parallel between Newman's Theory of Expanding Consciousness and Young's stages of human evolution. (From M. A. Newman, *Nursing Science Quarterly, 3*[1], 37-41; copyright © 1990 by Sage Publications, Inc. Reprinted with permission of Sage Publications, Inc.)

Pattern

Pattern is characterized by movement, diversity, and rhythm. It is constantly moving unidirectionally and evolving and may be enfolded in a larger pattern that is in the process of unfolding. Using Rogers' (1970) conceptualization of pattern, Newman (1986) states, "Pattern is information that depicts the whole, understanding of the meaning and relationships at once. It is a fundamental attribute of all there is and gives unity in diversity" (p. 13). Pattern is also a characteristic of wholeness and reveals the meaning of life (Newman, 1999). According to Newman (1987b), "*Whatever* manifests itself in a person's life is the explication of the underlying implicate pattern . . . the phenomenon we call health is the manifestation of that evolving pattern" (p. 37). This phenomenon also includes concepts of health and disease.

The evolution of consciousness is identified by patterns of increased quality and diversity of interaction with the environment (Newman, 1994a). Wholeness is identified in patterns of dynamic relatedness with one's environment (Newman, 1999). Expanding consciousness is seen in the evolving pattern, and episodes of pattern recognition are turning points in the process of an individual's evolving to higher levels of consciousness. Newman states that an individual's current pattern is a composite of "information enfolded from the past and information which will enfold in the future" (Newman, 1990a, p. 39). Viewing this pattern in relation to previous patterns represents an opportunity for new action and expansion of consciousness.

CRITICAL THINKING IN NURSING PRACTICE

From Newman's perspective, nursing is the study of "caring in the human health experience" (Newman, Sime, Corcoran-Perry, 1991, p. 3). The role of the nurse in this experience is to help clients recognize their own patterns (Newman, 1995b). Intervention is a form of "nonintervention," whereby the nurse's presence assists clients to recognize their own patterns of interacting with the environment (Newman, personal communication, May 17, 2000). Insight into these patterns provides clients with illumination of action possibilities, which then opens the way for transformation to occur (Newman, 1990a).

The nurse facilitates pattern recognition in clients by forming relationships with clients at critical points in their lives and by rhythmically connecting with them in an authentic way. The nurse-client relationship is characterized by "a rhythmic coming together and moving apart as clients encounter disruption of their organized, predictable state and moving through disorganization and unpredictability to a higher, organized state" (Newman, 1999, p. 228). The nurse comes together with clients at these critical choice points in their lives and participates with them in the process of expanding consciousness. The relationship is one of rhythmicity and timing. The nurse lets go of the need to direct the relationship or to "fix" things. As the nurse relinquishes the need to manipulate or control, there is a greater ability to enter into this fluctuating, rhythmic partnership with the client (Newman, 1999). Pattern identification is an element in the process, and personal transformation occurs (Newman, Sime, & Corcoran-Perry, 1991).

Newman utilizes a holographic pattern of intervention to describe the interaction process between nurse and client (Newman, 1986, 1989, 1994a). In this intervention, the nurse and client patterns interface in a way that is part of each person's pattern. Figure 20-2 depicts this model. The interference pattern expands to replace the original two patterns and becomes one pattern containing information about the whole of both. The nursing relationship involves the following: (1) a meeting of mutual concern of the nurse and client, (2) an interface or interpenetration of the two fields during which there is shared consciousness, and (3) a moving apart when the client is able to center without being connected to the nurse (Newman, 1994a).

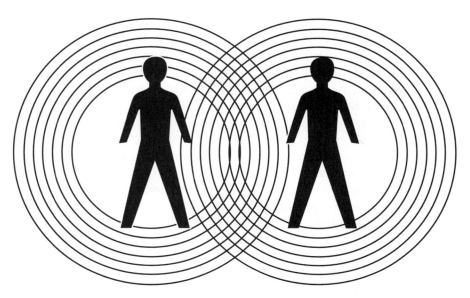

FIGURE 20-2

Interaction pattern of two persons. A holographic model of intervention. (From M. A. Newman, *Health as expanding consciousness,* 1994: National League for Nursing, New York, NY/Jones and Bartlett Publishers, Sudbury, MA. WWW.jbpub.com. New York: National League for Nursing. Reprinted with permission.)

A key aspect to assisting clients in pattern recognition is the nurse's sense into self or self-awareness (Newman, personal communication, May 17, 2000). There must be more to the relationship than mere observation. Sensing into the whole requires a sensing into oneself and a sense of stillness or centering is helpful to the process. Newman (1995b) elaborates, "The way to get in touch with the pattern of the other person is to sense into one's own pattern" (p. 88). The nurse resonates with the client and is fully present and in "synch" with the client to facilitate formation of shared consciousness in what has been described as a dance of empathic relating (Newman, 1999). As the nurse dialogues and shares impressions and feelings with the client, pattern recognition occurs. Verbalizing what the nurse senses in one's own pattern expresses the interpenetration of the two fields (Newman, personal communication, May 17, 2000) and facilitates the client getting in touch with self and becoming attuned to the larger pattern (Newman, 1989).

Newman's early suggestion was that the North American Nursing Diagnosis Association (NANDA) health assessment framework based on unitary person-environment patterns of interaction be utilized to facilitate clients' pattern recognition (Newman, 1995a). These nine patterns of interaction consist of the following: dimensions of choosing, communicating, exchanging, feeling, knowing, moving, perceiving, relating, and valuing (North American Nursing Diagnosis Association, 1989). At the time, the patterns were intended to guide nurses to make holistic observations of "person-environment behaviors that together depict a very specific pattern of the whole for each person" (Newman, 1995a, p. 261). Newman has since emphasized using terminology from individuals' own stories and patterns rather than utilizing the NANDA patterns (Newman, personal communication, May 17, 2000). Descriptions of the total pattern of the person are then presented as sequential patterns over time (Newman, 1990b).

Nurses can utilize the following method proposed by Newman (1990a) to elaborate the pattern of expanding consciousness: (1) establish the mutuality of the process of inquiry, (2) focus on the most meaningful persons and events in the client's life, (3) organize the data in narrative form and display it as sequential patterns over time, and (4) share the nurse's perception of the patterns with the client and seek revision or confirmation. Table 20-1 depicts critical thinking in nursing practice utilizing the elements of this method. Pattern recognition occurs with a burst of insight when everything fits together and the client can see clearly. Through this heightened understanding, the pathways for action unfold and open up, and one can take action (Newman, 1995b). The action indicated in response to pattern identification becomes apparent only as the pattern becomes apparent and the client discovers the new rules that apply to the situation (Newman, 1989). It is different for every situation. When pattern recognition occurs, clients sense that nurses know them and are able to assist in bringing about desired changes in their lives (Newman, Lamb, & Michaels, 1991). The client resonates with the nurse through the period of chaos and disequilibrium until a new rhythm emerges from the client's center of consciousness (Newman, 1999). The nurse and client then move apart.

Nurses practicing within the Newman framework are involved in a relationship process that coevolves as a function of the interpenetration of evolving fields of the nurse, client, and environment in a self-organizing and unpredictable way (Newman, 1994b). Nurses can be present at critical points for people and open up the possibility of freedom of choice, facilitating freedom by assisting clients in identification of patterns of their interaction with the environment. Insight regarding patterns opens up possibilities of different levels of interaction. By being open to whatever arises in the interaction with the client in an unconditional acceptance of the client's experience, the nurse in this process is fully present and is in "synch" with clients to facilitate forming of shared consciousness. Personal meaning becomes the main focus of nurse-client collaboration and mutuality (Newman 1990c). Nurses at-

TABLE 20-1	Critical Thinking and Newman's Theory (Elaboration of Application)	
Element	**Nursing Action/Interaction**
Meeting: Establish the mutuality of the process.	Recognizes disequilibrium in client as a choicepoint
	Prepares for interaction with client
	Shares perception of need for nurse-client interaction and relationship with client
Focus on the most meaningful persons and events in the client's life.	Opens self and grows with client
	Shows unconditional acceptance of client experience
	Becomes truly present with the client as the nurse and client fields interface and interpenetrate
Organize the data in narrative form and display it as sequential patterns over time.	Examines client's story in terms of patterns of relating at critical points in time and diagrams pattern to facilitate pattern identification
Share the nurse's perception of the pattern with the client.	Facilitates client recognition of pattern by sharing perceptions and patterns of relating in diagrammatic form
	Supports client unconditionally as insight into pattern occurs
Assist with client exploration of options.	Respects client choices in response to pattern recognition
	Provides assistance to client in implementing choices as client requests
Move apart.	Recognizes client gaining independence and gauges support accordingly

tend to the clients' agendas and are fully present with them, attending to what was important to them, what choices they are facing, and how the unfolding of those choices will take place. Clients become engaged in viewing and managing their health in creative ways (Newman, Lamb, & Michaels, 1991).

CASE HISTORY OF DEBBIE

Debbie is a 29-year-old woman who was recently admitted to the oncology nursing unit for evaluation after sensing pelvic "fullness" and noticing a watery, foul-smelling vaginal discharge. A Papanicolaou smear revealed class V cervical cancer. She was found to have a stage II squamous cell carcinoma of the cervix and underwent a radical hysterectomy with bilateral salpingooophorectomy.

Her past health history revealed that physical examinations had been infrequent. She also reported that she had not performed breast self-examination. She is 5 feet, 4 inches tall and weights 89 pounds. Her usual weight is about 110 pounds. She has smoked approximately two packs of cigarettes a day for the past 16 years. She is gravida 2, para 2. Her first pregnancy was at age 16, and her second was at age 18. Since that time, she has taken oral contraceptives on a regular basis.

Debbie completed the eighth grade. She is married and lives with her husband and her two children in her mother's home, which she describes as less than sanitary. Her husband is unemployed. She describes him as emotionally distant and abusive at times.

She has done well following surgery except for being unable to completely empty her urinary bladder. She is having continued postoperative pain and nausea. It will be necessary for her to perform intermittent self-catheterization at home. Her medications are (1) an antibiotic, (2) an analgesic as needed for pain, and (3) an antiemetic as needed for nausea. In addition, she will be receiving radiation therapy on an outpatient basis.

Debbie is extremely tearful. She expresses great concern over her future and the future of her two children. She believes that this illness is a punishment for her past life.

NURSING CARE OF DEBBIE WITH NEWMAN'S THEORY

The nurse working within the Newman theory focuses on assisting Debbie with pattern recognition. It is not clear from the data presented in this case study what Debbie's patterns of relating have been or currently are. Information of this type can be obtained only from the nurse-client interrelationship. However, insight that Debbie experiences as a result of the nurse-client relationship will open new opportunities for action and interaction. Nursing care will involve establishing a rhythm of relating (Newman, 1999), during which both the nurse and Debbie become transformed as pattern recognition occurs and as consciousness expands.

Meeting: Establish the Mutuality of the Process

The nurse working with Debbie recognizes Debbie's illness and surgery as a period of disruption and disorganization that represents a critical life choice point with a corresponding action potential for expanding consciousness. In preparation for beginning a relationship with Debbie, the nurse could utilize centering meditation as suggested by Picard, Sikul, and Natale (1998) to foster the capacity to be fully present. The nurse further uses self-reflection to examine personal values and beliefs that may affect the ability to unconditionally accept and share Debbie's experience. These personal values and beliefs are identified and set aside. Finally, the nurse approaches Debbie and shares his or her perception of the need to mutually examine Debbie's past life experiences to illuminate possible future options and actions.

Focus on the Most Meaningful Persons and Events in the Client's Life

The nurse opens self and grows with Debbie through nonjudgmental acceptance and empathically communicates in harmonic resonance and synchronization by "attending to the rhythm created by the silence between the signals" (Newman, 1999, p. 227). The focus is on the meaning of Debbie's evolving pattern. Through connecting and resonating with Debbie as they discuss meaningful life events and persons—such as health practices, pregnancies, the cancer and surgery, and relationships with her husband, mother, children, and others—patterns become apparent. Emphasis is placed on assisting Debbie to recognize her disease as a transformative opportunity to better know herself and to realize a fuller sense of self. The nurse's feelings are shared with Debbie during the interactions. Debbie determines the pace and frequency of interactions between herself and the nurse.

Organize the Data in Narrative Form and Display it as Sequential Patterns over Time

The nurse assists in the identification of Debbie's pattern of interaction with the environment. Dimensions such as choosing, communicating, exchanging, feeling, knowing, moving, perceiving, relating, valuing, and others are applied to Debbie's relationships with others and with herself. The importance of those relationships, choices, activities, and ways of relating are explored to identify past and present patterns of interacting. These patterns are then arranged sequentially over time to demonstrate the pattern of the whole. Past and present patterns are diagrammed and depict periods of disruption and key experiences.

Share the Nurse's Perception of the Pattern with the Client

The nurse shares pattern perceptions and feelings narratively and diagrammatically with Debbie in a nonjudgmental manner, concentrating on the present flow of interactions that reveal and suggest areas where attention may be needed to facilitate interaction between Debbie and her environment. Diagramming and sharing Debbie's patterns of relationships helps her to identify blocks to communicating and interacting.

Assist with Client Exploration of Options

As Debbie gains insight into her past and present patterns of interacting, new possibilities emerge, and she shares these with the nurse. The nurse assists her to explore options that have now become apparent, provides her with information, and arranges for referrals or other support that Debbie may need to implement her choices. Regardless of Debbie's choices, the nurse unconditionally supports her.

Move Apart

The shared rhythm and connectedness between the nurse and Debbie continues until a new pattern emerges from Debbie's own center of consciousness. When the chaos and disequilibrium of this major life event have been incorporated into the pattern of the whole and Debbie has moved to a higher level of consciousness, she determines that the nurse-client relationship is no longer necessary. There is a mutual agreement to terminate the relationship. Both Debbie and the nurse have been transformed.

CASE HISTORY OF CHARLOTTE

Charlotte is an 86-year-old woman caring for her 88-year-old husband, who was diagnosed with Alzheimer's disease 5 years ago. She has been diagnosed with macular degeneration and has had experimental surgery to attempt to correct this problem in her left eye. The vision in the operated eye has not yet improved, and there is uncertainty about whether it will improve at all. Charlotte states, "I may go completely blind. They had to try something." She has limited vision in her right eye and has not been able to drive since the surgery.

Charlotte and her husband have one daughter who lives about 10 minutes away and a son who lives out of state. They have not seen the son or his family for several years because Charlotte's husband refuses to travel and the son has a very demanding law practice that makes it difficult for him to visit. Their son has offered to pay their airfare to come visit, but the husband refuses to accept. Their daughter is in the midst of a divorce and "has troubles of her own."

Over the past year, Charlotte's husband has become increasingly difficult. His hearing has deteriorated, and his balance is also becoming a problem. He insists on trimming his own shrubs and cutting the lawn, even though he has difficulty starting and operating the equipment. He insists that Charlotte help him. Although she is fearful that they will both be injured, she does it anyway. She has regularly hired several young men to help, but her husband becomes verbally abusive to them. They usually quit after one visit. Home repairs need to be done, but Charlotte delays hiring anyone because of fear of her husband's reaction. She also states that "money is tight" and that she cannot afford to hire professional help.

Now that Charlotte cannot drive, she must depend on her daughter or her neighbors to get groceries and to transport her and her husband to doctor appointments. She does not go out otherwise. She stopped going to church because she did not feel safe going up the church steps and also because her husband became restless during church services. Most of her neighbors and friends have died or have stopped visiting. Church members and neighbors have offered to help, but Charlotte states that she is not comfortable asking people for help or "bothering" others. She cares for her home and her husband by herself but admits it is very difficult.

Charlotte is very concerned about the future for her husband and herself. She worries that they may not be able to live in their home much longer. She states that she has always been a very independent person. She was the oldest child of five and had to assume responsibility for her younger siblings when her father died and her mother was forced to return to work to support the family. Charlotte also describes a lengthy childhood disease that kept her out of school for many years. She states, "I learned how to take care of myself, but now what do I do?"

NURSING CARE OF CHARLOTTE WITH NEWMAN'S THEORY

Nursing care for Charlotte incorporates utilization of the elements of Newman's method to assist in pattern recognition for the purpose of illuminating new potentials for action. The nurse enters into a mutually transformative relationship with Charlotte by assisting her in this pattern recognition. Through relating to Charlotte in a synchronous manner, the nurse becomes dialectically involved with her to focus on the meaning of the evolving pattern.

Meeting: Establish the Mutuality of the Process

The nurse recognizes the current situation as a choice point that has attendant potential for increased interaction with environment and therefore expanded consciousness. As Charlotte's current options decrease and she becomes increasingly bound with restricted movement both outside and within her home, it becomes apparent that the old ways no longer work and that new ways of relating and doing things are necessary. The nurse prepares for entering into a relationship of unconditional acceptance with Charlotte. Initial contact with Charlotte is made, and the nurse shares the observation that an opportunity exists to examine her present circumstances and reflect on past life experiences for the purpose of illuminating possible future interactions that will assist both Charlotte and her husband. The nurse offers to engage in a mutual relationship with Charlotte that will assist in this process.

Focus on the Most Meaningful Persons and Events in the Client's Life

The nurse asks Charlotte to tell her story. Through dialoguing and interrelating with Charlotte, the nurse focuses on exploration of her past relationships with her husband, children, neighbors, friends, and church. They discuss past patterns of relating to her husband and of how some of these patterns are changed by present circumstances and how others are not changed are discussed. Charlotte's and her husband's relationships with their children and the changes in those relationships are also explored. Meaningful experiences in Charlotte's life—such as her childhood illness, her father's death, her husband's illness, and her own health problems—are mutually shared between Charlotte and the nurse. Emphasis is placed on understanding the meaning of these experiences. The nurse synchronizes her interaction with Charlotte in order to be fully present with her during the exploration of these life patterns. As the nurse resonates with Charlotte, feelings and impressions are shared. There are several such meetings arranged at Charlotte's request between the nurse and herself.

Organize the Data in Narrative Form and Display it as Sequential Patterns over Time

To identify patterns in Charlotte's story, the nurse configures her story to depict relationships at important moments in Charlotte's life. These patterns of relationships are arranged chronologically to illustrate particular significant events and people in Charlotte's life and to present a sequential view of the pattern of the whole. Charlotte's past and current relationships with her husband, children, and others together form this pattern.

It becomes apparent that Charlotte's predominant patterns have been those of valuing of independence and choosing to assume responsibility. Charlotte has always been the one to shoulder the burden and responsibility, first as a mother figure for her younger siblings, then as a self-reliant invalid during her childhood illness, next as the main disciplining and nurturing figure during the raising and rearing of her children, and finally as caregiver for her husband. During Charlotte's marriage, her husband has made the major decisions, but she had to assume the responsibility for implementation of those decisions. Although her husband is no longer capable, she continues to allow him to make decisions. This is demonstrated by her acceptance of his decision to refuse lawn or home maintenance help and by her attempts to repair their home or assist her husband with lawn care. Charlotte's vision problems have created sufficient disorganization and disequilibrium to become a choice point through which she can recognize that these past patterns of relating are no longer going to work.

Share the Nurse's Perception of the Pattern with the Client

The nurse shares pattern perception narratively and diagrammatically with Charlotte, who confirms and verifies the pattern identification. She states, "I never thought about it, but I have always been the one to handle things." Charlotte also shares that her brothers and sisters resented her "bossing them around" and that she really resented having the burden placed upon her. She states with a burst of insight, "You know, I really resent having to handle all this by myself, too."

Through continued dialogue between Charlotte and the nurse about past and present patterns, Charlotte comes to the realization that she does not need to shoulder the current situation by herself and in fact is not able to do so in a manner beneficial to either herself or her husband. Charlotte shares that she would really like to get help with the lawn and household but is afraid of her husband's reaction.

Assist with Client Exploration of Options

The nurse helps Charlotte explore how to introduce help that her husband would accept into the household. Charlotte feels that if the persons helping were older and more experienced, her husband might better accept them. The nurse assists Charlotte in contacting a senior citizens home assistance group that provides senior volunteers for just such situations. Through this group, Charlotte finds an elderly but physically fit "gentleman jack-of-all-trades" over whom her husband expresses reluctance at first, but he eventually looks forward to his visits. When the volunteer finishes the work, he often visits with Charlotte's husband while she goes shopping with a neighbor.

Charlotte still is unable to drive and has accepted that she needs assistance from neighbors, friends, and her daughter to shop and go to doctor appointments. She has also accepted the offer from some of the ladies of her church to bring a hot dish over once a week. She says she really enjoys not having to cook on Thursdays. The couple's son has been asking them to move into an assisted living facility not far from his residence. Although Charlotte admits that the idea appeals to her, she feels that her husband would not do well in that environment. She states, "He would just die if he couldn't be here in his own home." She is considering having a live-in couple for assistance in the future. The nurse is assisting Charlotte in exploring these options. Figure 20-3 diagrams Charlotte's pattern.

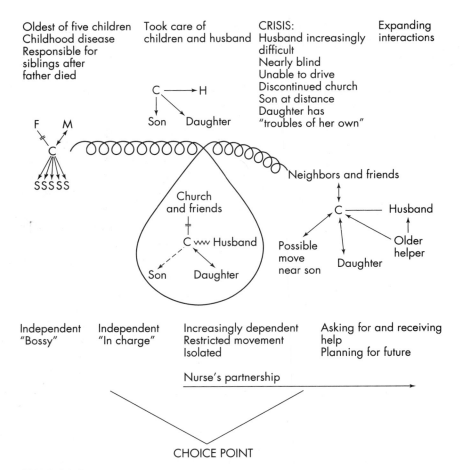

FIGURE 20-3

Diagram of Charlotte's pattern. (From Margaret Newman and Janet Witucki, 2000. Copyright Margaret Newman, St. Paul, MN, and Mosby/Harcourt Health Sciences, St. Louis, MO.)

Move Apart

The shared rhythm and connectedness between the nurse and Charlotte continues as the husband's condition deteriorates. During times of higher need, Charlotte and the nurse interact more often as the nurse assists Charlotte to determine what services she desires or needs and assists with access of services. However, Charlotte has been building her own support system and relies on the nurse less often. Charlotte stated recently, "I know I'm going to become more dependent and more aware of the outreach of people because many of my friends are reaching out." She has found that many people are willing to help her if she asks for and accepts their help.

CRITICAL THINKING EXERCISES

1. Select a friend or coworker and conduct an open-ended, tape-recorded, 60-minute interview focusing on past life events, persons, and interactions.
   (a) Practice being fully present with the person during the interview.
   (b) Identify patterns narratively and diagrammatically.
   (c) Share them with the person you interviewed.
2. Reflect on a time when you or someone close to you had a major catastrophic life event. How did this event change or transform you or him or her? How does this life experience support the Theory of Health as Expanding Consciousness?
3. Keep a journal for a week of events, your thoughts, feelings, and interactions as a method of self-reflection. Read and analyze the journal at the end of the week to facilitate self-knowledge.
4. Try a method of meditation for a week. Record the experience in your journal.

References

Bentov, I. (1977). *Stalking the wild pendulum.* New York: E. P. Dutton.

Bohm, D. (1980). *Wholeness and the implicate order.* London: Routledge and Kegan Paul.

Bunkers, S. S., Brendtro, M., Holmes, P. K., Howell, J., Johnson, S., Koerner, J., Larson, J., Nelson, J., & Weaver, R. (1992). The healing web: A transformative model for nursing. *Nursing & Health Care, 13,* 68-73.

de Chardin, T. (1959). *The phenomenon of man.* New York: Harper and Brothers.

Dexheimer-Pharris, M. D. (1999). The process of pattern recognition as a nursing intervention with adolescent males incarcerated for murder. Unpublished doctoral dissertation, University of Minnesota—Minneapolis; Minneapolis, Minnesota.

Endo, E. (1996). Pattern recognition as a nursing intervention with adults with cancer. Doctoral dissertation, University of Minnesota—Minneapolis; Minneapolis, Minnesota. *Dissertation Abstracts International,* 57-06B, 3653.

Engle, V. F. (1984). Newman's conceptual framework and the measurement of older adults' health. *Advances in Nursing Science, 7,* 24-36.

Ethridge, P. (1991). A nursing HMO: Carondolet St. Mary's experience. *Nursing Management, 22*(7), 22-27.

Gulick, E. E. & Bugg, A. (1992). Holistic health patterning in multiple sclerosis. *Research in Nursing & Health, 15,* 175-185.

Gustafson, W. (1990). Application of Newman's theory of health: Pattern recognition as nursing practice. In M. E. Parker (Ed.), *Nursing theories in practice* (pp. 141-161). New York: National League for Nursing.

Jonsdottir, H. (1998). Life patterns of people with chronic obstructive pulmonary disease: Isolation and being closed in. *Nursing Science Quarterly, 11,* 160-166.

Kalb, K. A. (1990). The gift: Applying Newman's theory of health in nursing practice. In M. E. Parker (Ed.), *Nursing theories in practice* (pp. 163-186). New York: National League for Nursing.

Kiser-Larsen, N. K. (1999). Life patterns of Native-American women experiencing breast cancer. Doctoral dissertation, University of Minnesota—Minneapolis; Minneapolis, Minnesota. *Dissertation Abstracts International,* 60-05B, 2062.

Lamendola, F. P. & Newman, M. A. (1994). The paradox of HIV/AIDS as expanding consciousness. *Advances in Nursing Science, 16*(3), 13-21.

Litchfield, M. C. (1997). The process of nursing partnership in family health. Doctoral dissertation, University of Minnesota—Minneapolis; Minneapolis, Minnesota. *Dissertation Abstracts International, 58-04B* 1802.

Magen, S. J., Gibbon, E. J., & Mrozek, R. (1990). Nursing theory application: A practice model. *Issues in Mental Health Nursing, 11,* 297-312.

Marchione, J. (1986). Application of the new paradigm of health to individuals, families, and communities. In M. A. Newman (Ed.), *Health as expanding consciousness* (pp. 107-134). St Louis: Mosby.

Mentzer, C. A. & Schorr, J. A. (1986). Perceived situational control and perceived duration of time: Expressions of life patterns. *Advances in Nursing Science, 9*(1), 12-19.

Michaels, C. (1992). Carondolet St. Mary's nursing enterprise. *Nursing Clinics of North America, 27,* 77-85.

Moch, S. D. (1990). Health within the experience of breast cancer. *Journal of Advanced Nursing, 15,* 1426-1435.

Moss, R. (1981). *The I that is we.* Millbrae, CA: Celestial Arts.

Newman, M. A. (1972). Time estimation in relation to gait tempo. *Perceptual and Motor Skills, 34,* 359-366.

Newman, M. A. (1976). Movement, tempo, and the experience of time. *Nursing Research, 25,* 273-279.

Newman, M. A. (1979). *Theory development in nursing.* Philadelphia: F. A. Davis.

Newman, M. A. (1982). Time an index of expanding consciousness with age. *Nursing Research, 31,* 290-293.

Newman, M. A. (1983). Newman's health theory. In I. Clements & F. Roberts (Eds.), *Family health: A theoretical approach to nursing care* (pp. 161-175). New York: John Wiley & Sons.

Newman, M. A. (1986). *Health as expanding consciousness.* St. Louis: Mosby.

Newman, M. A. (1987a). Nursing's emerging paradigm: The diagnosis of pattern. In M. McLane (Ed.), *Classification of nursing diagnoses* (pp. 53-60). St. Louis: Mosby.

Newman, M. A. (1987b). Patterning. In M. E. Duffy and N. J. Parker (Eds.), *Conceptual issues in health promotion: Report of proceedings of a wingspread conference* (pp. 36-50). Indianapolis: Sigma Theta Tau.

Newman, M. A. (1989). The spirit of nursing. *Holistic Nursing Practice, 3*(3), 1-6.

Newman, M. A. (1990a). Newman's theory of health as praxis. *Nursing Science Quarterly, 3*(1), 37-41.

Newman, M. A. (1990b). Nursing paradigms and realities. In N. L. Chaska (Ed.), *The nursing profession: Turning points* (pp. 230-235). St Louis: Mosby.

Newman, M. A. (1990c). Professionalism: Myth or reality. In N. L. Chaska (Ed.), *The nursing profession: Turning points* (pp. 49-52). St Louis: Mosby.

Newman, M. A. (1990d). Shifting to higher consciousness. In M. Parker (Ed.), *Nursing theories in practice* (pp. 129-138). New York: National League for Nursing.

Newman, M. A. (1991). Health conceptualizations. *Annual Review of Nursing Research* (Volume 9, pp. 221-243). New York: Springer.

Newman, M. A. (1994a). *Health as expanding consciousness* (2nd ed.). Sudbury, MA: James & Bartlett.

Newman, M. A. (1994b). Retrospective: Theory for nursing practice. *Nursing Science Quarterly, 7,* 153-157.

Newman, M. A. (1995a). Dialogue: Margaret Newman and the rhetoric of nursing theory. *Image, 27,* 261.

Newman, M. A. (1995b). Recognizing a pattern of expanding consciousness in persons with cancer. In M. A. Newman (Ed.), *A developing discipline: Selected works of Margaret Newman* (pp. 159-171). New York: National League for Nursing.

Newman, M. A. (1997). Evolution of Theory of Health as Expanding Consciousness. *Nursing Science Quarterly, 10,* 22-25.

Newman, M. A. (1999). The rhythm of relating in a paradigm of wholeness. *Image, 31,* 227-230.

Newman, M. A. Personal Communication. May 17, 2000.

Newman, M. A. & Gaudiano, J. K. (1984). Depression as an explanation for decreased subjective time in the elderly. *Nursing Research, 33,* 137-139.

Newman, M. A., Lamb, G., & Michaels, C. (1991). Nurse case management: The coming together of theory and practice. *Nursing & Health Care, 12,* 404-408.

Newman, M. A. & Moch, S. D. (1991). Life patterns of persons with coronary heart disease. *Nursing Science Quarterly, 4,* 161-167.

Newman, M. A., Sime, M., & Corcoran-Perry, S. (1991). The focus of the discipline of nursing. *Advances in Nursing Science, 14*(1), 1-6.

Noveletsky-Rosenthal, H. T. (1996). Pattern recognition in older adults living with chronic illness. Doctoral dissertation, Boston College; Chestnut Hill, Massachusetts. *Dissertation Abstracts International,* 57-10B, 6180.

North American Nursing Diagnosis Association. (1989). *Taxonomy I.* St. Louis: Author.

Picard, C. A. (2000). Uncovering pattern of expanding consciousness in mid-life women: Creative movement and the narrative as modes of expression. *Nursing Science Quarterly, 13*(2), 150-158.

Picard, C. A., Sikul, C., & Natale, S. (1998). Healing reflections: The transformative mirror. *International Journal for Human Caring, 2*(3), 40-47.

Prigogine, I. (1980). *From being to becoming.* San Francisco: W. H. Freeman.

Rogers, M. E. (1970). *An introduction to the theoretical basis of nursing.* Philadelphia: F. A. Davis.

Roux, G. M. (1994). Phenomenologic study: Inner strength in women with breast cancer. Doctoral dissertation, Texas Women's University—Denton. *UMI Dissertation Services,* No. 9417377.

Schmitt, N. (1991). Caregiving couples: The experience of giving and receiving social support. Doctoral dissertation, University of Minnesota—Minneapolis; Minneapolis, Minnesota. *UMI Dissertation Services.* No. 9212083.

Schorr, J. A. (1993). Music and pattern change in chronic pain. *Advances in Nursing Science, 15*(4), 27-36.

Schorr, J. A., Farnham, R. C., & Ervin, S. M. (1991). Health patterns in aging women as expanding consciousness. *Advances in Nursing Science, 13*(4), 52-63.

Schorr, J. A. & Schroeder, C. A. (1989). Consciousness as a dissipative structure: An extension of the Newman model. *Nursing Science Quarterly, 2,* 183-193.

Schorr, J. A. & Schroeder, C. A. (1991). Movement and time: Exertion and perceived duration. *Nursing Science Quarterly, 4,* 104-112.

Schroeder, C. A. (1993). Perceived duration of time and bedrest in high risk pregnancy: An exploration of the Newman model. *Dissertation Abstracts International, 54*(04B), p. 1894.

Shanahan, S. M. (1993). The lived experience of life-passing in middle adolescent females. *Masters Abstracts International, 32*(05), 1376.

Solari-Twadell, P., Bunkers, S., Wang, C., & Snyder, D. (1995). The pinwheel model of bereavement. *Image, 27,* 323-326.

Witucki, J. (2000). Help-seeking by older wife caregivers of demented husbands: A grounded theory approach. Unpublished doctoral dissertation, University of Tennessee—Knoxville; Knoxville, Tennessee.

Yamashita, M. (1998). Newman's Theory of Health as Expanding Consciousness: Research on family caregiving in mental illness in Japan. *Nursing Science Quarterly, 11,* 110-115.

Yamashita, M. (1999). Newman's theory of health applied in family caregiving in Canada. *Nursing Science Quarterly, 12,* 73-79.

Young, A. M. (1976). *The reflexive universe: Evolution of consciousness.* San Francisco: Robert Briggs.

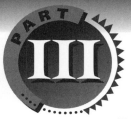

*E*xpansion

Continued development of the substantive body of nursing knowledge and utilization and application of that knowledge in the healthcare of society are essential to the future of the profession of nursing and professional nursing practice.

- Part II of this text has demonstrated utilization of philosophies, nursing models, and theories of nursing as structures to guide critical nursing thought.
- Areas of nursing practice for further theory utilization and application and the development of middle-range theories are plentiful.
- Nursing works—philosophies, models, and theories—are the values of the discipline of nursing and the promise of the future for professional nursing practice in the face of the healthcare challenges of this new century.

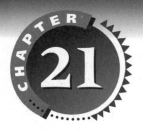

Areas for Further Development of Theory-Based Nursing Practice

Martha Raile Alligood

"Nursing's potential for meaningful human service rests on the union of theory and practice for its fulfillment." (Rogers, 1970)

"Systematic theory testing through application of nursing theories in practice with the participation of clinicians is essential for the enhancement of theory-based practice." (Silva & Sorrell, 1992)

Although practice based on nursing models and theories has been noted (see Chapter 2), there are many more areas of nursing practice that remain for theory development and expansion of theory-based practice. Bishop (1998) has noted the plea of both scholars and practitioners for "increased attention to the relationships between theory and practice" (p. 53) and identified these priorities (p. 53):

1. Continued development of nursing theories that are relevant to specialty practice engaged in by nurses,
2. Increased use of nursing theories in clinical decision making,
3. Increased collaboration between scientists and practitioners,
4. Efforts by nurse researchers to communicate findings from research to relevant practitioners, and
5. Increased emphasis on clinical research.

This text builds on Bishop's general concern: recognition of the importance of the relationship between theory and practice. The use of nursing models as critical thinking structures to guide clinical decision making (as presented in Chapters 1 and 3) addresses Bishop's second priority. This chapter focuses on her first priority and addresses it by doing the following: (1) suggesting examples of middle-range theories that might be derived from the grand theories of nursing models and (2) expanding the areas of nursing practice for their application.

New middle-range theories may be derived from models or grand theories that are relevant to specific areas of nursing practice. Middle-range theories are usually developed in relation to the specifics of actual clinical practice situations. However, ideas can be generated for new middle-range theory by using the grand theories to consider specific areas in which theory-guided practice has not been documented.

Middle-range theories are specific to practice (as discussed in Chapter 3). They indicate the situation or health condition, client population or age group, location or area of practice, and action of the nurse or the intervention. These specifics make middle-range theory applicable to nursing practice. They also multiply the possibilities for middle-range theories from one theory or grand theory because of the variety of the specifics already noted.

The areas of nursing practice in which theory-based practice has been reported were presented in Tables 2-1, 2-2, and 2-3 in Chapter 2. In this chapter, the tables are reversed, indicating areas in which theory-based practice has *not* been reported and *highlighting* opportunities for expansion. Table 21-1 presents possible areas for expansion in which practice with nursing models is described in terms of a situation or health condition with a medical focus. Table 21-2 presents areas for possible expansion in which practice with nursing models focuses on human development, type of practice, type of care, or health. Table 21-3 presents areas for expansion in which practice with nursing models focuses on a nursing intervention or nursing role.

These examples are presented to illustrate the nature of middle-range theory and to suggest ways for others to consider future directions of theory-based practice. This chapter may be useful to readers who are at various levels of nursing. Beginning students in nursing may find this chapter useful for learning what middle-range theory looks like and for identifying the specifics they contain for application in practice. Master's level students are often conducting their first research projects, and middle-range theories contain the specifics of practice for clinical theory-testing studies. Doctoral students who used the first edition as a text reported that this chapter was useful as a guide for development of middle-range theories to be tested in their dissertations.

TABLE 21-1   Areas of Practice for Expansion with Nursing Models Described in Terms of Medical Condition Focus

Practice Areas	Johnson	King	Levine	Neuman	Orem	Rogers	Roy
Acute care	•	•	•	•	•		•
Adolescent cancer	•	•	•	•	•	•	
Adult diabetes	•		•	•		•	•
AIDS management		•	•		•		
Alzheimer's disease	•	•	•	•	•	•	
Ambulatory care	•	•	•	•			•
Anxiety	•		•	•		•	•
Breast cancer	•	•	•		•	•	
Burns	•	•		•	•	•	•
Cancer	•	•		•			•
Cancer pain management		•	•	•	•	•	•
Cancer-related fatigue	•	•	•	•		•	•
Cardiac disease	•		•	•		•	
Cardiomyopathy	•	•	•	•	•	•	
Chronic pain	•	•		•	•		•
Cognitive impairment	•	•	•		•	•	•
Congestive heart failure	•	•		•	•	•	•
Critical care	•	•					
Guillain-Barré syndrome	•	•	•	•		•	•
Heart variations	•	•	•	•			•
Hemodialysis		•	•	•		•	•
Hypernatremia	•	•	•	•	•	•	
Intensive care	•	•	•				
Kawasaki disease	•	•	•	•	•	•	
Leukemia	•	•	•	•	•	•	
Long-term care	•	•		•		•	•
Medical illness			•		•		•
Menopause	•		•	•	•		•
Neurofibromatosis	•		•	•	•	•	•
Oncology		•	•	•			•
Orthopedics	•		•		•	•	•
Osteoporosis	•	•	•	•	•	•	
Ostomy care	•	•	•	•		•	•
Pediatric	•	•	•	•	•		•
Perioperative	•	•		•		•	
Polio survivors	•	•	•	•	•		•

Continued

TABLE 21-1	Areas of Practice for Expansion with Nursing Models Described in Terms of Medical Condition Focus—cont'd						
Practice Areas	**Johnson**	**King**	**Levine**	**Neuman**	**Orem**	**Rogers**	**Roy**
Postanesthesia	•	•	•	•	•	•	
Postpartum	•	•	•	•	•	•	
Posttrauma	•	•	•	•	•	•	
Preoperative adults	•	•		•	•	•	•
Preoperative anxiety	•		•	•		•	•
Pressure ulcers	•	•		•	•	•	•
Renal disease	•		•			•	•
Rheumatoid arthritis	•	•	•	•		•	•
Schizophrenia	•	•	•	•	•	•	
Substance abuse	•		•	•			•
Terminal illness	•	•	•	•	•		
Ventilator patient	•	•	•	•	•	•	
Ventricular tachycardia		•	•	•	•	•	•
Wound healing	•	•		•	•	•	•

CONCEPTUAL MODELS OF NURSING

Johnson

Middle-range theories may be derived from Johnson's Behavioral System Model and the grand Theory of the Person as a Behavioral System. Tables 2-1, 2-2, and 2-3 in Chapter 2 reflect areas to consider for expansion of Johnson's model in nursing practice. Since five applications of Johnson's model are included in the 50 situations or health conditions in Table 2-1, 45 potential areas for expansion of Johnson's theory (e.g., burns, leukemia, osteoporosis) are listed in Table 21-1. Likewise, since five applications are included in the 36 areas in Table 2-2, there are 31 possible areas for expansion in Table 21-2, such as nursing of women, risk reduction, and rehabilitation. Table 2-3 includes practice with specific nursing interventions, and because none was reported with Johnson's model, 19 areas for possible expansion are noted in Table 21-3. Based on the information in Tables 21-1, 21-2, and 21-3, an example of a middle-range theory from Johnson's grand theory might be: the risk for osteoporosis is reduced through behavioral counseling.

King

Middle-range theories may be derived from King's Theory of Goal Attainment. The details of the actual clinical situation specify the theory; however, use of Tables 21-1, 21-2, and 21-3 may help identify areas for

TABLE 21-2 Areas for Expansion with Nursing Models Based on Human Development, Type of Practice, Type of Care, or Type of Health

Practice Areas	Johnson	King	Levine	Neuman	Orem	Rogers	Roy
Battered women	•	•	•	•		•	•
Case management	•		•	•	•	•	•
Cesarean father	•	•	•	•	•	•	
Child health	•		•	•	•	•	•
Child psychiatric	•	•	•		•	•	•
Dying process	•	•	•	•	•		•
Emergency	•				•	•	
Gerontology	•		•				
High-risk infants	•		•	•	•	•	•
Holistic care	•	•		•	•	•	•
Homeless	•	•		•	•	•	•
Hospice	•	•		•		•	•
Managed care	•		•		•	•	•
Mental health		•	•				
Neonates	•	•	•	•	•	•	
Nursing administration	•		•				•
Nursing adolescents			•	•		•	•
Nursing adults	•						•
Nursing children		•		•			
Nursing community			•				
Nursing elderly	•						
Nursing families	•		•		•		•
Nursing home residents	•	•	•	•	•		
Nursing infants	•	•		•		•	
Nursing in space	•	•	•	•	•		•
Nursing service	•	•	•	•	•		•
Nursing women	•	•	•	•			•
Occupational health	•	•	•	•		•	•
Palliative care	•	•	•	•	•	•	•
Pregnancy	•	•	•	•		•	•
Psychiatric nursing	•	•	•	•	•		•
Public health	•	•	•		•	•	•
Quality assurance		•	•	•	•	•	•
Rehabilitation	•	•					
Risk reduction	•	•	•		•	•	•
Transcultural	•		•	•	•	•	•

TABLE 21-3	Areas for Expansion of Nursing Intervention or Role						
Practice Areas	Johnson	King	Levine	Neuman	Orem	Rogers	Roy
Breastfeeding	•	•	•		•	•	
Community presence	•	•	•	•	•		•
Counseling	•	•	•	•	•		•
Family therapy	•		•		•	•	•
Group therapy	•		•	•	•		
Health patterning	•	•	•	•	•		•
Humor	•	•	•	•	•		•
Imagery	•	•	•	•	•		•
Intentionality	•	•	•	•	•		•
Knowing participation	•	•	•	•	•		•
Laughter	•	•	•	•	•		•
Leadership and scholarship	•	•	•		•	•	•
Life-patterning difficulties	•	•	•	•	•		•
Life review	•	•	•	•	•		•
Movement	•	•	•	•	•		•
Nutrition	•	•	•		•	•	•
Parenting	•		•		•	•	•
Storytelling	•	•	•	•	•		•
Therapeutic touch	•	•	•	•	•		•

expansion of King's theory for nursing practice. Ten of the 50 areas listed in Table 2-1 reported the use of King's theory. Thus Table 21-1 offers 40 health conditions—such as breast cancer, cancer related fatigue, and oncology—for possible expansion. In Table 2-2, 13 of the 36 client groups or areas of practice were represented by publications based on King's theory. Twenty-three areas of practice for possible expansion remain in Table 21-2, such as hospice, occupational health, and nursing of women. Three of the 19 nursing interventions in Table 2-3 were King theory–based interventions, which suggests 16 areas for possible expansion (e.g., health patterning, life review, nutrition) (see Table 21-3). Therefore a middle-range theory from King's Theory of Goal Attainment might be: mutual goal setting in women with breast cancer and cancer-related fatigue leads to attainment of the goal to conserve energy.

Levine

Middle-range theories may be derived from Levine's Theory of Therapeutic Intention. The details of actual clinical situations specify the theory; however, Tables 21-1, 21-2, and 21-3 may be used to stimulate thinking and expand the use of Levine's model in practice. Ten of the 50 areas were applications of Levine's model in Table 2-1, leaving 40 areas (e.g., hemodialysis, posttrauma, ostomy care) for expansion in Table 21-1. Nine of the 36 client groups or areas of practice reported using Levine's model in Table 2-2, leaving 27 areas for expansion, such as nursing of adolescents, gerontology, and high-risk infants (see Table 21-2). Specific nursing interventions based on Levine's model were not found in Table 2-3, so Table 21-3 lists 19 possible areas for expansion. A middle-range theory derived from Levine's Theory of Therapeutic Intention might be: therapeutic regimens that facilitate holistic adaptation of adolescents in posttrauma foster their health.

Neuman

Middle-range theories may be derived from Neuman's Theory of Optimal Client Stability. The details of actual clinical situations specify the theory; however, Tables 21-1, 21-2, and 21-3 lead to ideas for possible expansion. Seven of the 50 conditions were reported in nursing practice guided by the Neuman model in Table 2-1. This identifies 43 areas of practice in Table 21-1 for possible expansion, such as Alzheimer's disease, rheumatoid arthritis, and hemodialysis. Thirteen of the 36 client groups or areas of practice in Table 2-2 were addressed in publications based on Neuman's model, leaving 23 areas for possible expansion (e.g., occupational health, psychiatric nursing, quality assurance), as noted in Table 21-2. Five of the 19 nursing interventions that use the Neuman model were reported in Table 2-3; therefore Table 21-3 lists 14 areas for possible expansion, such as group therapy, storytelling, and life-patterning difficulties. A middle-range theory derived from Neuman's Theory of Optimal Client Stability might be: occupational health of rheumatoid arthritis patients is stabilized by identifying stressors that lead to life-patterning difficulties.

Orem

Middle-range theories are derived from Orem's self-care deficit or dependent-care theory. The details of actual clinical situations provide the specifics of the theory; however, Tables 21-1, 21-2, and 21-3 may be used to stimulate thinking for theory expansion possibilities. Use of Orem's model in practice was reported in 19 of the 50 areas included in Table 2-1, and 31 areas for possible expansion are listed in Table 21-1, such as AIDS management, breast cancer, and leukemia. Although 15 of the 36 client groups or areas of practice were addressed in publications based on Orem's theory in Table 2-2, 21 areas for expansion (e.g., child health, nursing of families, the dying process) remain in Table 21-2. Specific interventions based on Orem's theories as reported in Table 2-3 were not found; therefore the 19 areas of possible expansion are noted in Table 21-3. A middle-range theory derived from Orem's Self-Care Deficit Theory might specify fostering self-care in AIDS patients in the dying process through nutrition.

Rogers

Middle-range theories may be derived from Rogers' Theory of Accelerating Change. The details from actual clinical situations specify the theory; however, ideas for theory expansion can be generated from Tables 21-1, 21-2, and 21-3. Fifteen of the 50 conditions included in Table 2-1 were addressed by nurses whose practice was guided by Rogerian science, leaving 35 areas for possible expansion (e.g., adolescent cancer, orthopedics, anxiety) listed in Table 21-1. Nurses reported practice in 15 of the 36 client groups or areas of practice in Table 2-2, which means 21 areas for possible expansion are listed in Table 21-2, such as nursing adolescents, nursing infants, and palliative care. Fourteen of the 19 interventions in Table 2-3 were based on nursing practice with Rogers; therefore five areas for expansion remain in Table 21-3, such as breastfeeding, parenting, and family therapy. A middle-range theory derived from Rogers' Theory of Accelerating Change might be: patients with anxiety identify family therapy as a measure that is palliative.

Roy

Middle-range theories may be derived from Roy's Theory of the Person as an Adaptive System. The details from actual clinical practice normally generate the specifics of the theory; however, ideas for theory expansion that reflect new areas for theory-based practice are developed in Tables 21-1, 21-2, and 21-3. In Table 2-1, 19 of the 50 health conditions were addressed by nurses practicing with Roy's model, leaving 31 areas for expansion listed in Table 21-1, such as anxiety, menopause, and oncology. Eleven of the 36 client groups or areas of practice in Table 2-2 were included in publications based on Roy's model, which means there are 25 areas for expansion in Table 21-2, such as nursing adolescents, holistic care, and nursing of women. Two of the 19 nursing interventions in Table 2-3 were based on Roy's model, which leaves 17 areas for possible expansion (e.g., imagery, nutrition, humor) listed in Table 21-3. A middle-range theory derived from Roy's Theory of the Person as an Adaptive System might be: adolescents experiencing anxiety adapt through the intervention of imagery for improved coping.

PHILOSOPHIES AND THEORIES OF NURSING

In addition to the opportunities for expansion of theory-guided practice noted thus far in the chapter, Part II (the application section in this second edition) has been expanded to include examples of philosophies and theories of nursing that are theoretical works that also guide research and practice. Philosophies include Nightingale's classic work (1946), which guides the nurse by identifying environmental factors that are pertinent to nursing from the patients' surroundings. Watson's work (1988) emphasizes transpersonal caring and proposes 10 carative factors to guide the process of the nurse with the patient. Benner's work (1984) also emphasizes the importance of caring and proposes that the events of each nurse-patient relationship are unique and are best understood through hermeneutic interpretation of the human process. These works have implicit theory and explicit propositions that contribute to our understanding of nursing and systematically guide nursing practice.

The theories of nursing are at various levels of abstraction, and their applications vary according to the specifics of each theory (as discussed in Chapter 3). Orlando's theory (1990) is specific to the process you use in interaction with the patient. Her work guides your practice as it specifies deliberate action based on your interaction with the patient. Therefore it is widely applicable in most nursing situations, but it is specific to the interaction process. Modeling and Role-Modeling Theory (Erickson, Tomlin, & Swain, 1983) guides the nurse to a comprehensive understanding of patients' situations and engages them in mutually developed interventions through a specific process of the nurse with the patient. Mercer's theory (1986) is very specific to the maternal role. Her work builds on Rubin's earlier work and provides you with the wisdom of years of study of the maternal role. It guides you to foster maternal role development in patients through attention to specified characteristics. Leininger's work (1991) is a theory specific to culture. Her Theory of Culture Care Diversity and Universality guides you to the cultural dimension of each patient and provides you with a view of the patient situation from that perspective. Care is designed while taking into account a full array of cultural dimensions, including the healthcare delivery system culture and folk practices. Parse's work (1992) is a Theory of Human Becoming. This work recognizes the nurse-patient relationship as the heart of nursing, emphasizes the importance of the presence of the nurse, and facilitates the patient's process rather than the nurse's. Newman's Theory of Health as Expanding Consciousness (1994) guides the nurse to view the patients and their health (wellness and illness) in a holistic manner. Her work focuses on recognizing manifestations of pattern as all of the events of a person's life are understood in a pattern of the whole. These theories are more specific to aspects of practice than the nursing models are, and, as has been illustrated, each contributes to theory-based nursing practice in its own unique way.

CONCLUSION

This chapter has addressed Bishop's first priority (1998) by suggesting areas for additional middle-range theories and possible new areas for theory-guided practice. The importance of the implementation of theory-based nursing practice to the future development of the discipline cannot be overemphasized. Smith (1993) has pointed out that "some knowledge base or perspective guides all nursing practice" (p. 8). Therefore it is extremely important for every nurse to be explicit as to how practice decisions are being made.

This text recognizes the vital nature of theory development but places particular emphasis on the importance of theory utilization in this theory era. Nursing philosophies, models, and theories that demonstrated their capacity to be decision-making structures that guide nursing practice have been set forth in Chapters 5 through 20. The challenge for nurses is to move beyond the focus on nursing process and nursing action to a patient focus with application of theories in theory-based practice. This has been identified as key to survival of the nursing discipline in this twenty-first century (Fawcett, 1999). With that goal in mind, the American Academy of Nursing's Expert Panel on Nursing Theory–Guided Practice (2000) has set forth the following definition:

> Nursing theory-guided practice is a human health service to society based on the discipline-specific knowledge articulated in the nursing frameworks and theories. The discipline-specific knowledge reflects the philosophical perspectives embedded in the ontological, epistemological, and methodological processes that frame nursing's ethical approach to the human-universe-health process (p. 177).

As nurses implement theory-guided practice using the various theoretical works identified in this text in the many areas of nursing practice, development of the nursing profession continues. The use of substantive knowledge in service to society benefits those whom we serve, the patients. Silva (1999) has suggested that "nursing will be best remembered . . . for what nurses did or failed to do" in this new century (p. 222).

References

American Academy of Nursing's Expert Panel on Nursing Theory–Guided Practice. (2000). *Nursing Science Quarterly, 13*(2), 177.

Benner, P. (1984). *From novice to expert: Excellence and power in clinical nursing practice.* Menlo Park, CA: Addison-Wesley.

Bishop, S. (1998). Theory development process. In A. Marriner-Tomey & M. R. Alligood (Eds.), *Nursing theorists and their work* (4th ed., pp. 43-54). St. Louis: Mosby.

Erickson, H., Tomlin, E., & Swain, M. (1983). *Modeling and role-modeling: A theory and paradigm for nursing.* Englewood Cliffs, NJ: Prentice-Hall.

Fawcett, J. (1999). The state of nursing science: Hallmarks of the 20th and 21st centuries. *Nursing Science Quarterly, 12*(4), 311-315.

Leininger, M. (1991). *Culture care diversity and universality: A theory of nursing.* New York: National League for Nursing.

Mercer, R. (1986). *First-time motherhood: Experiences from teens to forties.* New York: Springer.

Newman, M. (1994). *Health as expanding consciousness* (2nd ed.). New York: National League for Nursing.

Nightingale, F. (1946). *Notes on nursing: What it is and what it is not.* Philadelphia: J. B. Lippincott.

Orlando, I. (1990). *The dynamic nurse-patient relationship: Function, process and principles.* New York: National League for Nursing.

Parse, R. (1992). Human becoming: Parse's theory of nursing. *Nursing Science Quarterly, 5*(1), 35-42

Rogers, M. E. (1970). *Theoretical basis of nursing.* Philadelphia: F. A. Davis.

Silva, M. C. (1999). The state of nursing science: Reconceptualizing for the 21st century. *Nursing Science Quarterly, 12*(3), 221-224.

Silva, M. & Sorrell, J. (1992). Testing of nursing theory: Critique and philosophical expansion. *Advances in Nursing Science, 14*(4), 12-23. Aspen Publishers, Inc.

Smith, M. (1993). Case management and nursing theory-based practice. *Nursing Science Quarterly, 6*(1), 8-9.

Watson, J. (1988). *Nursing: Human science and human care.* New York: National League for Nursing.

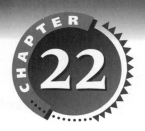

Conceptual Models of Nursing, Nursing Theories, and Nursing Practice: Future Directions

Jacqueline Fawcett

"If we want to ensure the survival of our discipline, all of us must fall in love with nursing [knowledge] now and develop a passion for the destiny of the discipline of nursing." (From J. Fawcett, Nursing Science Quarterly 12, *pp. 311-315, copyright © 1999 by Sage Publications, Inc.)*

Nursing knowledge, in the form of conceptual models of nursing and nursing theories, has been developed by several nurse scholars who have devoted a great deal of time to observing clinical situations, thinking about what is important to nursing in those situations, and then publishing their ideas in books and journals. Nursing knowledge continues to evolve as nursing students, clinicians, and researchers use those conceptual models and theories to guide their clinical practice and research and then report the results at conferences and in publications. Thus all nurses can contribute to the evolution of nursing knowledge and the subsequent advancement of nursing practice.

The purpose of this chapter is to discuss the use of conceptual models of nursing and nursing theories as guides for nursing practice. The chapter begins with a discussion of the dangers that come from *not* using nursing knowledge, followed by articulation of the philosophical value of using explicit nursing models and theories to guide nursing practice.

Next, strategies that can be adopted by the individual nurse to implement nursing model–based and nursing theory–based nursing practice are identified. Recommendations for the work needed to determine the scientific value of conceptual models of nursing and nursing theories are then offered. The chapter concludes with a futuristic proposal that links conceptual models of nursing with the five types of theories necessary for nursing practice.

THE DANGER OF *NOT* USING NURSING KNOWLEDGE

A significant danger to the advancement of the discipline of nursing has come from the rapid growth of nurse practitioner programs. In particular, the emphasis on practitioner skills in contemporary nursing education programs has diverted attention away from *nursing* models and theories and toward the medical model as the base for practice. As a result, both the human experiences of health and nursing have been medicalized (Chinn, 1999), and independent functioning has been equated with physician skills (McBride, 1999). Furthermore, nurses have increasingly imitated physicians and now are performing tasks "traditionally within the domain of medical practice" (Orem, 1995, p. 41). Therefore it should not be surprising that at least some nurses are said to resemble "quasi practitioners of medicine" (Orlando, 1987, p. 412), physician's assistants (Rogers, in Huch, 1995), physician substitutes (McBride, 1999), physician extenders (Sandelowski, 1999), junior doctors (Meleis, 1993), mini-doctors (Barnum, 1998), or pseudo doctors (Kendrick, 1997) engaged in nursing-qua-medicine (Watson, 1996) and primary care medicine rather than primary care nursing (Barrett, 1993). In effect, so-called advanced practice nursing has evolved into limited medical practice rather than full nursing practice. As Sandelowski (1999) has pointed out, nurses continue to perform work that relieves deliberately controlled shortages of physicians, which preserves their market value but has led to what is quickly becoming an oversupply of nurse practitioners (Anderson, 1999; Barnum, 1998).

Another danger comes from the use of nonnursing research as documentation for evidence-based nursing practice. This danger arises from two sources: (1) research done by members of other disciplines who have no understanding of the nursing conceptual models and theories that should be used to guide nursing research, and (2) research done by nurses who have abandoned nursing models and theories in favor of conceptual models and theories from other disciplines as guides for their research. The findings of research from either source should not be used as the evidence on which to base nursing practice because such research simply is not *nursing* research and therefore has nothing to do with *nursing* practice (Fawcett, 2000b).

THE PHILOSOPHICAL VALUE OF USING EXPLICIT NURSING KNOWLEDGE

Nursing, as Rogers (1985) maintains, has "no dependent functions" (p. 318). She explains that "like all other professions, nursing has many collaborative functions, which are indispensable to providing society with a higher order of service than any one profession can offer. Moreover, no profession has the knowledge, competence, or prerogative to delegate anything to another profession. Each profession is responsible for determining its own boundaries within the context of social need" (p. 381).

Clearly, the value of using *nursing* knowledge to guide nursing practice needs to be underscored, so that all nurses can become nursing practitioners (not "nurse practitioners") (Orem, 1995), senior nurses (Meleis, 1993), or maximally functioning nurses (Barnum, 1998). These nurses have the courage to follow the independent path of professional nursing (Orlando, 1987) and have the freedom and autonomy that comes from engaging in nursing-qua-nursing (Hawkins & Thibodeau, 1996; Watson, 1997). Recognition of the philosophical value of using explicit nursing models and theories to guide nursing research and nursing practice is documented in numerous publications, many of which are listed at the end of Chapter 2. In addition, the use of conceptual models of *nursing* and *nursing* theories in research and practice is the hallmark of professional nursing. As Rogers (1992) so eloquently puts it, "The practice of nurses . . . is the creative use of this knowledge in human service" (p. 29).

The use of nursing models and theories in nursing research and practice "distinguishes nursing as an autonomous health profession" and represents "nursing's unique contribution to the healthcare system" (Parse, 1995, p. 128). Furthermore, Anderson (1995) points out that the use of a "well-developed body of knowledge distinguishes a profession from a trade" (p. 247). She goes on to explain that as a professional discipline, nursing "must ensure that we have a solid scholarly and scientific foundation upon which to base our practice" (p. 247). It is therefore incumbent on all nurses to use *nursing* models and *nursing* theories and to evaluate that use in a systematic manner.

Research findings indicate that nurses feel vulnerable and experience a great deal of stress as they attempt to achieve professional aspirations within a continuously changing, medically dominated, and bureaucratic healthcare delivery system (Graham, 1994) that is focused more on economic issues than on humanistic issues. As structures for critical thinking within a distinctively nursing context, conceptual models of nursing and nursing theories provide the intellectual skills that nurses need to survive at a time when cost containment through the reduction of professional nursing staff is the *modus operandi* of healthcare delivery systems administrators.

Feeg (1989) and Fawcett (2000a) explain that the conceptual models of nursing and nursing theories collectively identify the distinctive nursing territory within the vast arena of healthcare. Each nursing model and theory provides a holistic orientation that reminds nurses of the focus of the discipline—concern for the "wholeness or health of humans, recognizing that humans are in continuous interaction with their environments" (Donaldson & Crowley, 1978, p. 119). Furthermore, each conceptual model of nursing and nursing theory provides a nursing discipline–specific lens for viewing clinical situations and facilitates the identification of details that are relevant to nursing from the plethora of available information. In addition, nursing models and theories help nurses to explicate what they know and why they do what they do. In other words, nursing models and theories facilitate the communication of nursing knowledge and how that knowledge governs the actions performed on behalf of or in conjunction with people who require healthcare. Ultimately, nursing research and nursing practice that is based on an explicit conceptual model of nursing or nursing theory is "for our patients' sake" (Dabbs, 1994, p. 220).

IMPLEMENTING NURSING KNOWLEDGE–BASED NURSING PRACTICE: PROCESS AND STRATEGIES

A discussion of the way that a conceptual model is used to guide nursing research is beyond the scope of this book. Readers can learn more about constructing conceptual-theoretical-empirical structures for nursing research by reading *The Relationship of Theory and Research* (Fawcett, 1999a) as well as by extrapolating the following substantive and process elements from nursing practice to nursing research.

The substantive and process elements of implementing conceptual model–based or theory-based nursing practice at the clinical agency level have been discussed in detail by Fawcett (2000a). In this chapter, the focus narrows to the process that occurs and the strategies that can be used by the individual nurse when implementing nursing practice based on nursing theories or conceptual models of nursing. Understanding and telling others about the process and using the strategies now should ensure that nursing knowledge is used to guide practice in the future.

In Chapters 1 and 3, Alligood points out that the first step toward implementing nursing practice based on conceptual models of nursing or nursing theories is "the decision to do so." The authors of Chapters 5 through 20 certainly made that decision.

The second step is to recognize that the adoption of an explicit conceptual model of nursing or nursing theory—or a change from one explicit model or theory to another—requires an adjustment in thinking about nursing and clinical situations. More specifically, the successful implementation of the conceptual model of nursing–based or nursing theory–based nursing practice requires recognition of the fact that the nurse needs time to evolve from the use of one frame of reference for practice to another frame of reference. Time is required regardless of whether the original frame of reference is an implicit one or a different explicit model or theory. The process that occurs during the period of evolution is referred to as perspective transformation.

Perspective Transformation

Drawing from Mezirow's early work (1975, 1978) in the development of adult learning theory, Rogers (1989), a Canadian nurse who is not related to the theorist who developed the Science of Unitary Human Beings, explained that perspective transformation is based on the assumption that each person has a particular meaning perspective that is used to interpret and understand the world. She defined and described perspective transformation as the process

> whereby the assumptions, values, and beliefs that constitute a given meaning perspective come to consciousness, are reflected upon, and are critically analyzed. The process involves gradually taking on a new perspective along with the corresponding assumptions, values, and beliefs. The new perspective gives rise to fundamental structural changes in the way individuals see themselves and their relationships with others, leading to a reinterpretation of their personal, social, or occupational worlds (Rogers, 1989, p. 112).

Thus the process of perspective transformation involves the shift from one meaning perspective or frame of reference about nursing and nursing practice to another, from one way "of viewing and being with human beings" to another (Nagle & Mitchell, 1991, p. 22).

Rogers (1989) points out that the cognitive and emotional aspects of perspective transformation represent a major change for each nurse. Moreover, she underscores the importance of recognizing, appreciating, and acknowledging that during the process of perspective transformation, each nurse evolves from feeling "a [profound] sense of loss followed by an ultimate sense of liberation and empowerment" (Rogers, 1992, p. 23). Clearly, perspective transformation requires considerable effort and a strong commitment to change (Nagle & Mitchell, 1991).

Perspective transformation encompasses nine phases: stability, dissonance, confusion, dwelling with uncertainty, saturation, synthesis, resolution, reconceptualization, and return to stability (Rogers, 1992). The prevailing period of stability is disrupted when the idea of implementing conceptual model of nursing–based or nursing theory–based nursing practice or changing the model or theory is introduced. Dissonance occurs as the nurse begins to examine his or her current frame of reference for practice in light of the challenge to adopt or change a conceptual model or theory. As the nurse begins to learn the content of the new conceptual model or theory, he or she begins to appreciate the discrepancy between the current way of practice and what nursing practice could be. A phase of confusion follows. As the nurse struggles to learn more about the model or theory and its implications for practice, a feeling of "lying in limbo" between frames of reference prevails (Rogers, 1992, p. 22). Throughout the phases of dissonance and confusion, the nurse often feels anxious, angry, and unable to think. Rogers (1992) explained that these distressing emotions "seem to arise out of the grieving of a loss of an intimate part of the self. The existing [frame of reference] no longer makes sense, yet the new [model or theory] is not sufficiently internalized to provide resolution" (p. 22).

The phase of confusion is followed by the phase of dwelling with uncertainty. At this point, the nurse acknowledges that confusion "is not a result of some personal inadequacy" (Rogers, 1992, p. 22). As a consequence, anxiety is replaced by a "feeling of freedom to critically examine old ways and explore the new [model or theory]" (Rogers, 1992, p. 22). The phase of dwelling with uncertainty is spent immersed in information that often seems obscure and irrelevant. It is a time of "wallowing in the obscure while waiting for moments of coherence that lead to unity of thought" (Smith, 1988, p. 3).

The phase of saturation occurs when the nurse feels that he or she "cannot think about or learn anything more about the nursing [model or theory]" (Rogers, 1992, p. 22). The phase does not represent resistance but rather "the need to separate from the difficult process of transformation, [which] is part of the natural ebb and flow of the learning experience" (Rogers, 1992, p. 22).

The phase of synthesis occurs as insights render the content of the new conceptual model or theory coherent and meaningful. The formerly obscure practice implications of the conceptual model or theory become clear and worthy of the implementation effort. Increasing tension is followed by exhilaration as insights illuminate the connections between the content of the conceptual model or theory and its use in nursing practice (Rogers, 1992; Smith, 1988). "These insights," Smith (1988) explains, "are moments of coherence, flashes of unity, as though suddenly the fog lifts and clarity prevails. These moments of coherence push one beyond to deepened levels of understanding" (p. 3).

The phase of resolution is characterized by "a feeling of comfort with the new nursing [model or theory]. The feelings of dissonance and discontent . . . are resolved and the anxiety is dissipated" (Rogers, 1992,

p. 23). During this phase, "nurses describe themselves as changed, as seeing the world differently and feeling a distinct sense of empowerment" (Rogers, 1992, p. 23).

The phase of reconceptualization occurs as the nurse consciously reconceptualizes nursing practice using the new conceptual model of nursing or nursing theory (Rogers, 1992). During this phase, the nurse compares the activities of practice—from patient assessment through shift reports—according to the old and new ways of thinking and changes those activities so that they are in keeping with the new model or theory. The final phase, return to stability, occurs when nursing practice is clearly based on the new conceptual model of nursing or nursing theory.

Strategies to Facilitate Perspective Transformation

Rogers (1989) identified several strategies that can be used to facilitate perspective transformation. These strategies are especially effective during the early phases of perspective transformation, when the nurse is moving from the original to the new frame of reference for practice.

One strategy is to use analogies to facilitate understanding of the terms, conceptual model, and theory. Analogies such as a chair or book can be used for concepts (conceptual), the analogy of a model home or model airplane can be used for models, and the analogy of a conjecture can be used for theory. Rogers (1989) notes that the acts of conceptualizing and theorizing can be demystified "by stating that it is not a process reserved for intellectuals but rather a cognitive process of all humans that begins in infancy as a baby puts together all the pieces to form the concept of mother" (p. 114).

Two other strategies are directed toward identification of the nurse's existing frame of reference for nursing practice. One of those strategies is to list words that reflect the nurse's view of nursing practice. Similarly, the nurse could depict his or her view of nursing practice in drawings or collages of photographs. Another strategy is to think about the details of, reasons for, and outcomes of a recent interaction with a patient.

Once the nurse has gained a clear understanding of the original frame of reference, he or she needs to explore the difference between the current state of nursing practice and what practice would be like if her or she were using the new conceptual model or theory. This can be accomplished through the use of provocative strategies. One provocative strategy is to think about how situations such as childbirth and death are currently managed and how they could be managed using the new model or theory. Another strategy is to describe what is unique about nursing practice or what would be done if physicians' orders did not need to be followed.

Rogers (1989) points out that as the nurse becomes aware of the differences between the present and the potential future practice of nursing, he or she experiences cognitive dissonance or discomfort that comes from "the awareness of the 'what is' versus 'what [c]ould be'" (p. 115). She concludes by noting that when cognitive dissonance "has been experienced by nurses both individually or collectively, then perspective transformation can occur, and a climate for the implementation of a nursing [model or theory] will have been created" (p. 116).

Subsequent stages of perspective transformation and the implementation of conceptual model–based or theory-based nursing practice are facilitated by constant reinforcement. Accordingly, all nursing activities should be tied to the conceptual model or theory in a systematic manner. The novice user of an explicit conceptual model or theory should not become discouraged if initial experiences seem forced or awkward. Adoption of an explicit conceptual model of nursing or nursing theory requires restructuring the nurse's way of thinking about clinical situations and use of a new vocabulary. However, repeated use of the model or theory should lead to more systematic and organized endeavors. Broncatello (1980) comments,

> The nurse's consistent use of any model [or theory] for the interpretation of observable client data is most definitely not an easy task. Much like the development of any habitual behavior, it initially requires thought, discipline, and the gradual evolvement of a mind set of what is important to observe within the guidelines of the model [or theory]. As is true of most habits, however, it makes decision making less complicated (p. 23).

THE SCIENTIFIC VALUE OF USING EXPLICIT NURSING KNOWLEDGE

The scientific value of using conceptual models of nursing and nursing theories as guides for nursing research and nursing practice has begun to be documented in the form of the credibility of each conceptual model and the empirical adequacy of each theory. Inasmuch as a review of the relevant literature is beyond the scope of this chapter, readers are referred to extensive evaluations in *Analysis and Evaluation of Contemporary Nursing Knowledge: Nursing Models and Theories* (Fawcett, 2000a). However, much more work in evaluating conceptual models of nursing and nursing theories remains.

Communicating the Scope and Substance of Nursing Practice

The decision to implement conceptual model–based or theory-based nursing practice typically is undertaken in response to the quest for a way to articulate the scope and substance of professional nursing practice to the public and to other healthcare professionals as well as to improve the conditions and outcomes of nursing practice. Consequently, one potential outcome of conceptual model of nursing–based or nursing theory–based nursing practice is enhanced understanding of the roles of nurses in healthcare by administrators, physicians, social workers, dietitians, physical therapists, occupational therapists, respiratory therapists, and other healthcare team members as well as by those individuals, families, and communities who participate in nursing. Research is needed to determine the extent to which the role of nursing within the healthcare delivery system is better understood when practice is based on an explicit conceptual model of nursing or on nursing theory.

Documentation of Nursing Practice

The methodology of conceptual model of nursing–based or nursing theory–based nursing practice is operationalized by the documents and technology used to guide and direct nursing practice, to record observations and results of interventions, and to describe and evaluate nursing job performance. In other words, the methodology encompasses the standards for nursing practice, department and unit objectives, nursing care plans, care maps, patient database and classification tools, flow sheets, Kardex forms, computer information systems, quality assurance tools, nursing job description and performance appraisal tools, and other relevant documents and technologies (Fawcett, 1992; Fitch, Rogers, Ross, Shea, Smith & Tucker, 1991; Laurie-Shaw & Ives, 1988; Weiss & Teplick, 1993). Each existing document and all current technology must be reviewed for congruence with the conceptual model of nursing or nursing theory and revised as necessary. Although revisions often are needed and the work may seem overwhelming at the outset, the importance of having documents and technologies that are congruent with the conceptual model or theory cannot be overemphasized. Indeed, this congruence may be regarded as the *sine qua non* of conceptual model of nursing–based or nursing theory–based nursing practice. Although at least one computer software program (Bliss-Holtz, Taylor, & McLaughlin, 1992) and many clinical documentation tools (Fawcett, 2000a; Weiss & Teplick, 1993) have been developed, systematic studies to determine the utility of the software and the validity and reliability of the tools are needed.

Nurse-Sensitive Patient Outcomes

The evidence needed for evidence-based nursing practice must be nurse-sensitive. That is, the evidence must connect *nursing* actions to patient outcomes. The documentation of conceptual model of nursing–based or nursing theory–based practice can provide the required empirical evidence of nurse-sensitive patient outcomes. For example, Poster and Beliz (1988, 1992) found that 90% of the 38 adolescent psychiatric inpatients studied had an adaptive change in at least one behavioral subsystem after 1 week of Johnson's Behavioral System Model–based nursing practice (1990). Furthermore, on average, the patients demonstrated significant improvement in all behavioral subsystems during the discharge phase of hospitalization. Dee, van Servellen, and Brecht (1998) added empirical research evidence of Johnson's Behavioral System Model–based nursing practice with their findings of improvement in all behavioral subsystems for inpatients under managed behavioral healthcare contracts. More specifically, the study results revealed statistically significant differences in the dependency, affiliative, aggressive, and achievement subsystems from admission to discharge.

Measuring Satisfaction

Another potential outcome of conceptual model of nursing–based or nursing theory–based nursing practice is the nurse's increased satisfaction with the conditions and outcomes of his or her nursing practice through an explicit focus on and identification of nursing problems and actions as well as through enhanced communication and documentation (Fitch, Rogers, Ross, Shea, Smith, & Tucker, 1991). Still another potential outcome is patients' and their families' increased satisfaction with the nursing that is received. The evidence regarding nurse, patient, and family satisfaction is primarily in the form of anecdotal evidence from just a few clinical agencies (e.g., Scherer, 1988; Studio Three, 1992). However, empirical evidence is beginning to emerge. For example, Moreau, Poster, and Niemela (1993) reports that nursing practice based on Johnson's Behavioral System Model (1990) was well received by the nurses and members of the multidisciplinary team. Moreover, the nurses reported an increase in job satisfaction and retention and a decrease in role conflict. Niemela, Poster and Moreau (1992) reported that the nurses experienced increased general satisfaction and role clarity and decreased role tension. In addition, the nurses reported that they increased communication with patients' family members.

Additional empirical evidence comes from Messmer's report (1995) of an increase in female patients' satisfaction with nursing on a general surgical inpatient pilot unit that implemented King's General Systems Framework–based nursing practice (1981) compared with the satisfaction of patients on two other units that were not yet using the framework. Still other empirical evidence comes from a study by Hanucharurnkul and Vinya-nguag (1991), who found that patients who received a nursing intervention based in part on King's Theory of Goal Attainment (1981) reported greater satisfaction with nursing than those who did not receive the intervention.

A plethora of instruments have been designed to measure nurse and patient satisfaction. However, only a few of these instruments (e.g., Marckx, 1995) measure satisfaction with nursing practice that is based on an explicit conceptual model of nursing or nursing theory. Thus valid and reliable instruments need to be developed before more systematic, multisite studies, which are necessary to fully document nurse, patient, and family satisfaction, are undertaken.

Utility of Nursing Models and Theories Across Populations

The literature associated with the conceptual models of nursing and nursing theories included in this text challenges nurses to consider each model and theory for possible expansion of application to a wide range of nursing specialties and for many different clinical populations (see Chapters 2 and 21). Aggleton and Chalmers (1985) noted that the literature "might encourage some nurses to feel that it does not really matter which model of nursing is chosen to inform nursing practice within a particular care setting" (p. 39). They also noted that that literature might "encourage the view that choosing between models is something one does intuitively, as an act of personal preference. Even worse, it might encourage some nurses to feel that all their everyday problems might be eliminated were they to make the 'right choice' in selecting a particular model for use across a care setting" (p. 39). However, critical appraisals of the literature have not yet revealed the extent to which the fit of the conceptual model or theory to particular clinical populations might have been forced. Indeed, the issue of forced fit has not yet been addressed in the literature. This is an area for future research.

Furthermore, little attention has been given to the extent to which a particular conceptual model or theory is modified to fit a given situation (Germain, Personal Communication, October 21, 1987). Although modifications certainly are acceptable, they should be acknowledged, and serious consideration should be given to renaming the conceptual model or theory to indicate that modifications have been made. Clearly, systematic exploration of the practice implications of various conceptual models, coupled with more practical experience with each model and theory in a variety of settings, is required.

A VISION FOR THE FUTURE

Throughout this chapter, discussion has focused on conceptual model of nursing–based *or* nursing theory–based nursing practice. A more comprehensive and futuristic focus links the various concepts of each conceptual model with many theories. Those theories more fully specify the content of the conceptual model. To date, discussion of such so-called conceptual-theoretical structures for nursing practice has emphasized scientific or empirical theories (Fawcett, 1999a, 2000a). However, Carper (1978) and White (1995) also identified other types of theories that are necessary for nursing practice, including ethical nursing theories, theories of personal knowing in nursing, esthetic nursing theories, and sociopolitical nursing theories (Table 22-1). Their work "not only highlighted the centrality of empirically derived theoretical knowledge, but [also] recognized with equal importance and weight, knowledge gained through clinical practice" (Stein, Corte, Colling, & Whall, 1998, p. 43).

Empirical nursing theories are objective in nature and are developed by means of empirical research (see Table 22-1). In contrast, ethical nursing theories, theories of personal knowing in nursing, and esthetic nursing theories are "subjective forms of knowledge acquired through experience and envisioned as fundamental to humane, personalized, and [moral] nursing [practice]" (Stein, Corte, Colling, & Whall, 1998, p. 44). These types of theories are developed by means of nonempirical modes of inquiry (see Table 22-1). Sociopolitical nursing theories, according to White (1995), help nurses to understand the context of nursing practice, and they facilitate acceptance of multiple perspectives of a situation. The knowledge embedded in sociopolitical nursing theories comes from hearing and acknowledging the many voices involved in nursing practice. Carper (1978) and Chinn and Kramer (1999) have pointed out that each type of nursing theory is an essential component of the integrated knowledge base for professional practice, and no single type of theory should be used in isolation from the others. When all five types of nursing theories are linked with the concepts of a conceptual model of nursing (Table 22-2), holistic and humanistic nursing practice becomes a reality. Table 22-2 is a worksheet that encourages each nurse to think about which concepts of a particular conceptual model of nursing should be more fully specified by which type or types of nursing theories. For example, the Roy Adaptation Model concept of adaptation might be linked with empirical nursing theories about stimuli that evoke adaptive responses and stimuli that evoke ineffective responses as well as with esthetic nursing theories that help the nurse to interpret a particular patient's behavior. Moreover, the Roy Adaptation Model concept of nursing management of stimuli might be linked with ethical nursing theories that stipulate whether certain stimuli should be managed, with personal theories that help the nurse to use herself or himself in a therapeutic manner, and with sociopolitical nursing theories that sensitize the nurse to the context of the clinical situation and the voices to be heard in making decisions about what stimuli to manage and how to manage them.

TABLE 22-1   Five Types of Nursing Theory and Modes of Inquiry

Type of Nursing Theory	Characteristics	Mode of Inquiry
Empirics	Factual descriptions, explanations, or predictions based on subjective or objective group data Publicly verifiable Discursively written as empirical theories	Empirical research with emphasis on replication of studies.
Ethics	Emphasizes the values of nurses and nursing Focuses on the value of changes and outcomes in terms of desired ends Addresses questions of moral obligation, moral value, and non-moral value Discursively written as standards, codes, and normative ethical theories	Dialogue and justification of values, with emphasis on clarification of values about rights and responsibilities in practice
Personal knowledge	Concerned with the knowing, encountering, and actualizing of the self Concerned with wholeness and integrity in the personal encounter between nurse and patient Addresses the quality and authenticity of the interpersonal process between each nurse and each patient Expressed as autobiographical stories about the authentic genuine self	Self-reflection and response from others, with emphasis on actualization of the authentic self through opening and centering the self
Esthetics	Focuses on particulars rather than universals Emphasizes the nurse's perception of what is significant in the individual patient's behavior Addresses manual and technical skills Expressed as criticism of the art-act of nursing and through works of art	Envisioning of possibilities and rehearsing the art and acts of nursing, with emphasis on developing appreciation of esthetic meanings in practice and inspiration for the development of the art of nursing
Sociopolitical knowledge	Provides the context or cultural location for nurse-patient interactions and the broader context in which nursing and healthcare take place Focuses on exposing and exploring alternate constructions of reality Expressed as transformation and critique	Critique and hearing all voices

Constructed from Carper, B. A. (1978). Fundamental patterns of knowing in nursing. *Advances in Nursing Science, 1*(1), 13-23; Chinn, P. L. & Kramer, M. K. (1999). *Theory and nursing: Integrated knowledge development* (5th ed.). St. Louis: Mosby; and White, J. (1995). Patterns of knowing: Review, critique, and update. *Advances in Nursing Science, 17*(4), 73-86.

TABLE 22-2   Linkage of Nursing Conceptual Model Concepts with Five Types of Nursing Theories

Type of Nursing Theory	Conceptual Model Concept$_1$	Conceptual Model Concept$_2$	Conceptual Model Concept$_3$	Conceptual Model Concept$_n$
Empirical				
Esthetic				
Ethical				
Personal				
Sociopolitical				

CONCLUSION

The belief that explicit nursing discipline–specific knowledge—rather than knowledge from medicine, psychology, sociology, social work, pharmacology, and other fields—is the proper guide for nursing practice has permeated the discussion in this chapter. The continued reliance on nonnursing perspectives, coupled with a rejection of nursing knowledge, reflects the thinking of an oppressed group (Bent, 1993). However, no one is forcing or even encouraging nurses to use nonnursing knowledge. Nurses must therefore break the intellectual chains associated with self-imposed oppression by rejecting nonnursing knowledge as the fundamental basis of practice and embracing nursing knowledge in the form of explicit conceptual models of nursing and nursing theories.

References

Aggleton, P. & Chalmers, H. (1985). Critical examination. *Nursing Times, 81*(14), 38-39.
Anderson, C. A. (1995). Scholarship: How important is it? *Nursing Outlook, 43,* 247-248.
Anderson, C. A. (1999). Hitting the wall. *Nursing Outlook, 47,* 153-154.

Barnum, B. S. (1998). The advanced nurse practitioner: Struggling toward a conceptual framework. *Nursing Leadership Forum, 3,* 14-17.

Barrett, E. A. M. (1993). Nursing centers without nursing frameworks: What's wrong with this picture? *Nursing Science Quarterly, 6,* 115-117.

Bent, K. N. (1993). Perspectives on critical and feminist theory in developing nursing praxis. *Journal of Professional Nursing, 9,* 296-303.

Bliss-Holtz, J., Taylor, S. G., & McLaughlin, K. (1992). Nursing theory as a base for computerized nursing information system. *Nursing Science Quarterly, 5,* 124-128.

Broncatello, K. F. (1980). Auger in action: Application of the model. *Advances in Nursing Science, 2*(2), 13-23.

Carper, B. A. (1978). Fundamental patterns of knowing in nursing. *Advances in Nursing Science, 1*(1), 13-23.

Chinn, P. L. (1999). From the editor. *Advances in Nursing Science, 21*(4), v.

Chinn, P. L. & Kramer, M. K. (1999). *Theory and nursing: Integrated knowledge development* (5th ed.). St. Louis: Mosby.

Dabbs, A. D. V. (1994). Theory-based nursing practice: For our patients' sake. *Clinical Nurse Specialist, 8,* 214, 220.

Dee, V., van Servellen, G., & Brecht, M. (1998). Managed behavioral healthcare patients and their nursing care problems, level of functioning, and impairment on discharge. *Journal of the American Psychiatric Nurses Association, 4,* 57-66.

Donaldson, S. K. & Crowley, D. M. (1978). The discipline of nursing. *Nursing Outlook, 26,* 113-120.

Fawcett, J. (1992). Conceptual models and nursing practice: The reciprocal relationship. *Journal of Advanced Nursing, 17,* 224-228.

Fawcett, J. (1999a). *Relationship of theory and research* (3rd ed.). Philadelphia: F. A. Davis.

Fawcett, J. (1999b). The state of nursing science: Hallmarks of the 20th and 21st centuries. *Nursing Science Quarterly, 12,* 311-315.

Fawcett, J. (2000a). *Analysis and evaluation of contemporary nursing knowledge: Nursing models and theories.* Philadelphia: F. A. Davis.

Fawcett, J. (2000b). But is it nursing research? *Western Journal of Nursing Research, 22,* 524-525.

Feeg, V. (1989). Is theory application merely an intellectual exercise? *Pediatric Nursing, 15,* 450.

Fitch, M., Rogers, M., Ross, E., Shea, H., Smith, I., & Tucker, D. (1991). Developing a plan to evaluate the use of nursing conceptual frameworks. *Canadian Journal of Nursing Administration, 4*(1), 22-28.

Germain, C. P. Personal Communication. October 21, 1987.

Graham, I. (1994). How do registered nurses think and experience nursing: A phenomenological investigation. *Journal of Clinical Nursing, 3,* 235-242.

Hanucharurnku[l], S. & Vinya-nguag, P. (1991). Effects of promoting patients' participation in self-care on postoperative recovery and satisfaction with care. *Nursing Science Quarterly, 4,* 14-20.

Hawkins, J. W. & Thibodeau, J. A. (1996). *The advanced practice nurse: Current issues* (4th ed.). New York: Tiresias Press.

Huch, M. H. (1995). Nursing and the next millennium. *Nursing Science Quarterly, 8,* 38-44.

Johnson, D. E. (1990). The behavioral system model for nursing. In M. E. Parker (Ed.), *Nursing theories in practice* (pp. 23-32). New York: National League for Nursing.

Kendrick, K. (1997). What is advanced nursing? *Professional Nurse, 12*(10), 689.

King, I. M. (1981). *A theory for nursing: Systems, concepts, process.* New York: John Wiley & Sons.

Laurie-Shaw, B. & Ives, S. M. (1988). Implementing Orem's self-care deficit theory: Part II—Adopting a conceptual framework of nursing. *Canadian Journal of Nursing Administration, 1*(2), 16-19.

McBride, A. B. (1999). Breakthroughs in nursing education: Looking back, looking forward. *Nursing Outlook, 47,* 114-119.

Marckx, B. B. (1995). Watson's theory of caring: A model for implementation in practice. *Journal of Nursing Care Quality, 9*(4), 43-54.

Meleis, A. I. (1993, April). Nursing research and the Neuman model: Directions for the future. Panel discussion with B. Neuman, A. I. Meleis, J. Fawcett, L. Lowry, M. C. Smith, & A. Edgil, conducted at the Fourth Biennial International Neuman Systems Model Symposium, Rochester, NY.

Messmer, P. R. (1995). Implementation of theory-based nursing practice. In M. A. Frey & C. L. Sieloff (Eds.), *Advancing King's systems framework and theory of nursing* (pp. 294-304). Thousand Oaks, CA: Sage.

Mezirow, J. (1975). *Education for perspective transformation: Women's re-entry programs in community colleges.* New York: Center for Adult Education, Teachers College, Columbia University.

Mezirow, J. (1978). Perspective transformation. *Adult Education, 28,* 100-110.

Moreau, D., Poster, E. C., & Niemela, K. (1993). Implementing and evaluating an attending nurse model. *Nursing Management, 24*(6), 56-58, 60, 64.

Nagle, L. M. & Mitchell, G. J. (1991). Theoretic diversity: Evolving paradigmatic issues in research and practice. *Advances in Nursing Science, 14*(1), 17-25.

Niemela, K., Poster, E. C., & Moreau, D. (1992). The attending nurse: A new role for the advanced clinician . . . adolescent inpatient unit. *Journal of Child and Adolescent Psychiatric and Mental Health Nursing, 5*(3), 5-12.

Orem, D. E. (1995). *Nursing: Concepts of practice* (5th ed.). St. Louis: Mosby.

Orlando, I. J. (1987). Nursing in the 21st century: Alternate paths. *Journal of Advanced Nursing, 12,* 405-412.

Parse, R. R. (1995). Commentary. Parse's Theory of Human Becoming: An alternative guide to nursing practice for pediatric oncology nurses. *Journal of Pediatric Oncology Nursing, 12,* 128.

Poster, E. C. & Beliz, L. (1988). Behavioral category ratings of adolescents in an inpatient psychiatric unit. *International Journal of Adolescence and Youth, 1,* 293-303.

Poster, E. C. & Beliz, L. (1992). The use of the Johnson Behavioral System Model to measure changes during adolescent hospitalization. *International Journal of Adolescence and Youth, 4,* 73-84.

Rogers, M. E. (1985). The nature and characteristics of professional education for nursing. *Journal of Professional Nursing, 1,* 381-383.

Rogers, M. E. (1989). Creating a climate for the implementation of a nursing conceptual framework. *Journal of Continuing Education in Nursing, 20,* 112-116.

Rogers, M. E. (1992). Nursing science and the space age. *Nursing Science Quarterly, 5,* 27-34. Quoted material copyright © 1992 by Sage Publications, Inc. Reprinted by permission of Sage Publications, Inc.

Rogers, M. E. (1992, February-April). *Transformative learning: Understanding and facilitating nurses' learning of nursing conceptual frameworks.* Paper presented at Sigma Theta Tau Conferences, "Improving Practice and Education Through Theory." Chicago, IL; Pittsburgh, PA; Wilkes-Barre, PA.

Sandelowski, M. (1999). Venous envy: The post–World War II debate over IV nursing. *Advances in Nursing Science, 22*(1), 52-62.

Scherer, P. (1988). Hospitals that attract (and keep) nurses. *American Journal of Nursing, 88,* 34-40.

Smith, M. J. (1988). Wallowing while waiting. *Nursing Science Quarterly, 1,* 3.

Stein, K. F., Corte, C., Colling, K. B., & Whall, A. (1998). A theoretical analysis of Carper's ways of knowing using a model of social cognition. *Scholarly Inquiry for Nursing Practice, 12,* 43-60.

Studio Three. (1992). *The nurse theorists: Excellence in action—Callista Roy.* Athens, OH: Fuld Institute of Technology in Nursing Education.

Watson, M. J. (1996). Watson's theory of transpersonal caring. In P. Hinton Walker & B. Neuman (Eds.), *Blueprint for use of nursing models: Education, research, practice, and administration* (pp. 141-184). New York: National League for Nursing.

Watson, J. (1997). The Theory of Human Caring: Retrospective and prospective. *Nursing Science Quarterly, 10,* 49-52.

Weiss, M. E. & Teplick, F. (1993). Linking perinatal standards, documentation, and quality monitoring. *Journal of Perinatal and Neonatal Nursing, 7*(2), 18-27.

White, J. (1995). Patterns of knowing: Review, critique, and update. *Advances in Nursing Science, 17*(4), 73-86.

GLOSSARY

accountability The assumption of responsibility for action taken as a professional. It implies the use of professional judgment in determining appropriate actions. Thus it requires the use of a discipline's knowledge base in anticipating consequences.

action process (1) The person perceives an object or objects with any one of his or her five senses; (2) the perceptions stimulate automatic thought; (3) each thought stimulates an automatic feeling; (4) the person acts.

adaptation The process of change whereby individuals retain their integrity, or wholeness, with the realities of their environment. It is an expression of the integration of the entire organism.

agency Ability, capability, or power to engage in action in Orem's theory.

attachment Formation of an emotional bond with another person that lasts for a lifetime, such as the bond between a parent and a child.

automatic personal response (1) A nurse responds by withholding from the patient his or her immediate reaction—perception, thought, or feeling; (2) the patient cannot verify or correct any part of the reaction; (3) the patient makes assumptions about the nurse's verbal and nonverbal behavior; (4) the nurse acts without knowledge of the patient's reaction, which causes a situational conflict.

basic conditioning factors (BCFs) Factors identified by Orem that influence individual health-related demands and ability to engage in self-care; for example, age, gender, health state, and family patterns.

behavioral system balance A system's ability to maintain a certain level of behavior within an acceptable range. Synonyms are *stability* and *steady state*.

behavioral system imbalance Disturbances in structure, function or functional requirements in one or more subsystem that may be described in terms of insufficiency, discrepancy, dominance, or incompatibility.

central (centrality) That which is focal, pivotal, principal, or essential.

change The essence of life or process of adaptation that is directed, purposeful, meaningful, and eminently understandable.

comportment Style and manner of action and interacting, which includes gestures, posture and stance (Benner, Hooper-Kyriakidis, & Stannard, 1999).

conceptual models A set of interrelated concepts that symbolically represent and convey a mental image of a phenomenon. Conceptual models of nursing identify concepts and describe their relationships to the phenomena of central concern to the discipline: person, environment, health, and nursing (Powers & Knapp, 1995).

conceptualization The process of creative thinking that involves imagination, invention, contemplation, consideration, reflection, judgment, and conclusion.

conservation The keeping-together function of the nurse, specified by Levine as a product of adaptation.

criteria for a profession A set of standards that a discipline or group uses as a gauge to recognize its level of development.

criterion A standard by which something is measured or evaluated.

critical thinking A disciplined process in which one actively and skillfully uses reason and logic as a guide to belief and action in decision making.

critical thinking structures Organized systems of thought—such as nursing philosophies, conceptual models, or theoretical frameworks—that guide the reasoning process leading to decisive action.

cultural diversity Differences or variations that can be found both between and among different cultures.

developmental self-care requisites Needs or goals that arise from maturational changes in the life cycle, such as pregnancy, or from situational events throughout human development, such as the death of a significant other.

deduction An approach to thinking and reasoning that proceeds from the general to the particular.

diagnostic statement A product of the assessment process in Neuman's model that reflects systematic consideration of actual or potential environmental stressors.

disequilibrium The absence of client system balance in Neuman's Systems Model.

external regulatory force Role of the nurse specified by Johnson to preserve the organization and integration of the client's behavior at an optimal level under conditions in which the client's behavior constitutes a threat to physical and psychosocial health.

folk care The use of remedies for illness or injury passed down from generation to generation within a particular culture. Also known as *generic care.*

functional requirements/sustenal imperatives Protection, nurturance, and stimulation that the behavioral system must receive from the environment to survive and develop.

'good' Something that, if achieved, will benefit a person or a group of persons; for example, healthcare is a 'good.'

grand theory Propositions derived from a conceptual model or framework that are at a sufficiently high level of abstraction to generate many middle-range applications specific to practice level details.

health deviation self-care requisites Self-care deficits that arise when persons are ill, injured, have defects or disabilities, or are undergoing diagnosis or treatment.

hermeneutics Derived from biblical exegesis, a term for interpretation or explication. As used in research, hermeneutics refers to describing and studying "meaningful human phenomena in a careful and detailed manner as free as possible from prior theoretical assumptions, based instead on practical understanding" (Packer, 1985, p. 1081-1082).

induction An approach to thinking and reasoning that proceeds from the particular to the general.

infant cues Infant sounds and behaviors that send signals to parents and others for needs to be met.

manifestation What is perceivable of field patterning (Rogers) or the aspect of the field that our perceptions can recognize.

metaparadigm The worldview of a discipline, the most global perspective that subsumes more specific views and approaches to the central concepts with which a discipline is concerned. Nursing's metaparadigm generally is thought to consist of the central concepts of person, environment, health, and nursing (Powers & Knapp, 1995).

middle-range theory The least abstract set of related concepts that propose a truth specific to the details of nursing practice.

moral Appraisal of actions according to whether these are praiseworthy or blameworthy. An action is normally praiseworthy to the degree that it is focused on achieving a 'good' of some sort for another person or group of persons.

moral imperative Action or practice that is absolutely required in order to promote a particular 'good.'

mutual patterning The process by which the human and environmental field process is evolving. Known patterns are identified in the human/environmental field process.

naturalistic research A qualitative research approach used to discover the subjective and objective aspects of a group or culture.

normal science "[R]esearch firmly based upon one or more past scientific achievements, achievements that some particular scientific community acknowledges for a time [as a paradigm] supplying the foundation for its further practice" (Kuhn, 1970, p. 10).

nurse-patient situation A dynamic whole. Each nurse and each patient affect one another's behavior and is unique for each situation. The patient's behavior stimulates the nurse's immediate reaction and becomes the starting point of the nurse's investigation.

nursing art Expressive and skillful activities of nurses tailored by the individual nurse according to the blending of knowledge and values in actions for a personal style of practice.

nursing science Knowledge of practice produced through the unique interrelationship of theory and research in approaches aimed at understanding the phenomena of interest to the discipline.

nursing system All the actions and interactions of the nurse and client and/or family in a nursing situation at a point in time.

patient's presenting behavior The patient's behavior, regardless of its form, may be a plea for help but may not be what it appears to be. Orlando emphasizes that it is not reliable for determining the meaning of the patient's behavior or for the help required without the nurse's further investigation.

perceived dissonance A perception of disharmony or discomfort in the human/environmental field process in Rogers' theory.

perspective transformation The process whereby the assumptions, values, and beliefs that constitute a given meaning perspective come to consciousness, are reflected upon, and are critically analyzed. The process involves gradually taking on a new perspective along with corresponding fundamental structural changes in the way individuals see themselves and their relationships with others. This leads to a reinterpretation of their personal, social, or occupational worlds. The nine phases of perspective transformation are stability, dissonance, confusion, dwelling with uncertainty, saturation, synthesis, resolution, reconceptualization, and return to stability.

provocative facts The presenting symptoms alerting one to a problem.

role identity Taking on a role. In Mercer's Theory of Maternal Role Attainment, it is seeing oneself in the role and having a sense of comfort about it.

scholarship Development and communication of knowledge.

self-care agency The individual's learned ability or power to perform self-care, including knowledge, skill, and motivation for self-care actions that promote life, health, and well-being.

self-care deficit An inadequacy of the individual's self-care ability to meet the therapeutic self-care demand.

spiritual distress A disruption of the human spirit. The human spirit gives meaning and purpose to life, serves to integrate the whole human being, and connects the individual to self, others, the universe, and the creator. In spiritual distress, the individual may lose sight of the meaning and purpose of life or connectedness.

stability Equilibrium or client system balance in Neuman's Systems Model.

stressor Intrapersonal, interpersonal, or extrapersonal conditions or situations identified by Neuman as threats to the stability or integrity of the client system.

substantive Substantial, essential, having a solid basis, or independent in existence.

subsystem A minisystem with its own unique goal and function that is maintained as long as its relationship to other subsystems is in a steady state, functional requirements are provided, and/or the environment is not disturbed.

theory A set of statements that tentatively describe, explain, or predict relationships among concepts that have been systematically selected and organized as an abstract representation of some phenomenon (Powers & Knapp, 1995, p. 170-171). These systematic organized perspectives serve as guides for nursing action in administration, education, research, and practice.

theory application The operation of a system of ideas in action.

theory development A knowledge-building process in the context of syntax, structure, and growth.

theory utilization Orchestrating systematic ideas to accomplish a purpose.

therapeutic self-care demand The self-care actions that should be performed by the individual at a point in time to maintain health and promote well-being.

therapeutic self-care requisite The need or goal that will be met by satisfying the therapeutic self-care demand.

transcendence Going beyond what is customary or rising above the everyday physical world in some way.

transition Passing from one phase to another. It involves letting go of previous attitudes and behaviors and taking on new attitudes and behaviors.

trophicognosis A nursing care judgment achieved through the use of Levine's scientific process.

universal self-care requisites Human needs for self-care that promote structural and functional integrity of the person and well-being—including maintenance of air, food, water, and elimination; balance between activity and rest; solitude and social interaction; prevention of hazards; and the promotion of normalcy.

References

Benner, P., Hooper-Kyriakidis, P., & Stannard, D. (1999). *Clinical wisdom and interventions in critical care: A thinking in action approach.* Philadelphia: W. B. Saunders.

Kuhn, T. S. (1970). *The structure of scientific revolutions* (2nd ed.). Chicago: University of Chicago Press.

Packer, M. J. (1985). Hermeneutic inquiry in the study of human conduct. *American Psychologist,* *40*(10), 1081-1093.

Powers, B. A. & Knapp, T. R. (1995). *A dictionary of nursing theory and research* (2nd ed.). Thousand Oaks, CA: Sage.

Index

Page numbers followed by b indicate boxes;
page numbers followed by f indicate figures;
page numbers followed by t indicate tables.